MCQs in Reproductive Endocrinology and Infertility

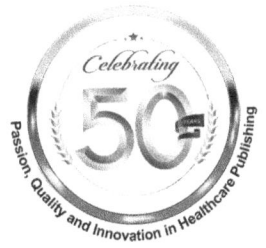

MCQs in Reproductive Endocrinology and Infertility

Rashmi Vohra
MBBS (GMC, Patiala), MS OBG (IGMC, Shimla)
Resident
MCh Reproductive Medicine and Surgery (SRIHER)
Chennai, Tamil Nadu, India

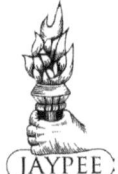

JAYPEE BROTHERS MEDICAL PUBLISHERS
The Health Sciences Publisher
New Delhi | London

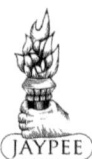 **Jaypee Brothers Medical Publishers (P) Ltd**

Headquarters
Jaypee Brothers Medical Publishers (P) Ltd
4838/24, Ansari Road, Daryaganj
New Delhi 110 002, India
Phone: +91-11-43574357
Fax: +91-11-43574314
Email: jaypee@jaypeebrothers.com

Overseas Office
J.P. Medical Ltd
83 Victoria Street, London
SW1H 0HW (UK)
Phone: +44 20 3170 8910
Fax: +44 (0)20 3008 6180
Email: info@jpmedpub.com

Website: www.jaypeebrothers.com
Website: www.jaypeedigital.com

© 2020, Jaypee Brothers Medical Publishers

The views and opinions expressed in this book are solely those of the original contributor(s)/author(s) and do not necessarily represent those of editor(s) of the book.

All rights reserved. No part of this publication may be reproduced, stored or transmitted in any form or by any means, electronic, mechanical, photocopying, recording or otherwise, without the prior permission in writing of the publishers.

All brand names and product names used in this book are trade names, service marks, trademarks or registered trademarks of their respective owners. The publisher is not associated with any product or vendor mentioned in this book.

Medical knowledge and practice change constantly. This book is designed to provide accurate, authoritative information about the subject matter in question. However, readers are advised to check the most current information available on procedures included and check information from the manufacturer of each product to be administered, to verify the recommended dose, formula, method and duration of administration, adverse effects and contraindications. It is the responsibility of the practitioner to take all appropriate safety precautions. Neither the publisher nor the author(s)/editor(s) assume any liability for any injury and/or damage to persons or property arising from or related to use of material in this book.

This book is sold on the understanding that the publisher is not engaged in providing professional medical services. If such advice or services are required, the services of a competent medical professional should be sought.

Every effort has been made where necessary to contact holders of copyright to obtain permission to reproduce copyright material. If any have been inadvertently overlooked, the publisher will be pleased to make the necessary arrangements at the first opportunity. The **CD/DVD-ROM** (if any) provided in the sealed envelope with this book is complimentary and free of cost. **Not meant for sale.**

Inquiries for bulk sales may be solicited at: jaypee@jaypeebrothers.com

MCQs in Reproductive Endocrinology and Infertility

First Edition: 2020

ISBN: 978-93-89776-75-1

Dedicated to

The Godliness in all of us.

Preface

Friends

The journey of a medical student starts with admission to MBBS course and as the time passes it progresses through multiple hardships as well as pleasures of learning. The acquisition of medical knowledge not only lets you practice the noble profession but also quenches the thirst for knowing the deep mysteries of human body and function. Many alphabets like MD, DNB are added to the original as per the requirement and the zeal in this journey. DM and MCh used to be another set of these alphabets in the past. *Now they have become essentials.* Ever increasing number of the aspirants appearing in entrance exams for these courses stands testimony for this.

When I decided to appear for NEET SS I found myself surrounded with vast vacuum of dearth of books guiding me through the competitive examinations. I did not know how to beat the competition for scantly available super specialization seats with scantier available guidance to pursue my dream of becoming Reproductive Endocrinologist. That is why I decided to write the book, immediately after starting my MCh in Reproductive Medicine and Surgery degree, for helping the students appearing in future. Believe me I had to work doubly hard to take out time, along with my regular academic and clinical curriculum, in order to accomplish this feat. That is why I find myself bereft of words to describe the satisfaction of seeing this work of passion in your hands.

The compilation of these MCQs has been done with meticulous care and understanding that these will stimulate the process of generating an examination-based approach to your studies. Although the compilation question might not appear to be exhaustive yet they fulfill the aim of stimulating the process of your thinking. In due course of time you will be devising your own MCQs while going through the texts of Reproductive Endocrinology if you are able to grasp the essence of the book. Although I do not claim that you will find these MCQs in the competitive examinations *'as such'* yet I am confident that this book is going to help you fulfill your aim of achieving success in any competitive examination for the purpose.

Friends, **'To error, is human'** is an old idiom, to which I add that **'to *rectify, is a good friend***'! I hope that you will help me rectify the mistakes in this edition by communicating them to me.

With the best wishes

Rashmi Vohra

Acknowledgements

This book I owe to

"My husband, **Dr Ankush Goyal** without whose support and continuous motivation, I could not have done this. Despite being so busy in his own work, he tried giving me as much as possible. This book I owe to him."

My sister, Dr Shweta Vohra and brother-in-law Dr Jacky Garg. They both were the continuous motivation behind this laborious work. Sincere thanks to my parents, my brother, my son and my dog.

My sincere thanks to my mam Dr Rita Mittal, Professor IGMC, Shimla. She has always been my support from the very beginning of my career.

A special thanks to my teachers, Prof N Sanjeeva Reddy who is eminent teacher and my mentor for the field of Reproductive Medicine, thank you sir for teaching me basics of the subject and always being there for clarifying my doubts.

I want to thank Dr Mona Pandurangi, Dr Radha V, Dr Siddhartha Nagireddy, and Dr Ashish Soni for teaching me new concepts.

Thanks to my colleagues and friends Dr Hiya Agrawal, Dr Chandana Bhat, Dr Ashu Pilania, Dr Tejas Gundewar, Dr Vivek Kakkad, Dr Niket Shah and Dr Harsh Nihlani.

My sincere thanks to Jaypee Brothers Medical Publishers (P) Ltd, for accepting and publishing my book.

Contents

1. Basics of Molecular Biology 1
2. Hormone Biosynthesis, Metabolism and Mechanism of Action 6
3. Neuroendocrinology 15
4. Endocrinology of Menstrual Cycle 22
5. Endocrinology of Pregnancy 32
6. Normal and Abnormal Sexual Development 42
7. Endocrinology of Pubertal Development 62
8. Endocrinology of Amenorrhea 74
9. Chronic Anovulation and Polycystic Ovary Syndrome 88
10. Endocrinology of Hyperprolactinemia 101
11. Endocrinology of Hirsutism 110
12. Endocrinology of Obesity 120
13. Endocrinology of Reproduction and Thyroid 127
14. Endocrinology of Endometriosis 135
15. Fibroids and Reproduction 144
16. Infertility 151
17. Embryology 162
18. Drugs in Reproductive Endocrinology 177
19. Miscellaneous 184

CHAPTER 1

Basics of Molecular Biology

Multiple Choice Questions

1. Apart from nucleus, which organelle contains DNA?
   a. Mitochondria   b. Golgi Apparatus
   c. Ribosomes   d. Microtubules

2. All of the following are true regarding mitochondria, *except:*
   a. Diseases due to mitochondrial genes are inherited from mother
   b. Mitochondria contain dsDNA
   c. Diseases due to mitochondrial genes are inherited from both parents
   d. The mitochondria in sperm are eliminated during fertilization

3. Chromosomes with lowest and highest number of genes, respectively:
   a. x, 1   b. y, 21
   c. x, 22   d. y, 1

4. A unit of DNA within a chromosome that can be activated to transcribe a specific RNA:
   a. Gene   b. Exon
   c. Intron   d. Toroid

5. The location of a gene on a particular chromosome is designated as:
   a. Band   b. Arm
   c. Locus   d. Region

6. What percentage of genes in human genome is actually involved in encoding protein synthesis?
   a. 2%   b. 4%
   c. 6%   d. 10%

7. 7q31.1 is the location for the cystic fibrosis gene. What does the number 1 signifies in this?
   a. Chromosome number
   b. Arm symbol
   c. Region number
   d. Band number

8. Correct order of arrangement in mitosis:
   a. Interphase > Prophase > Metaphase > Anaphase > Telophase
   b. Interphase > Metaphase > Prophase > Anaphase > Telophase
   c. Interphase > Anaphase > Prophase > Metaphase > Telophase
   d. Anaphase > Interphase > Metaphase > Prophase > Telophase

9. Barr body or the sex chromatin can be seen in female cells in which phase of cell cycle?
   a. Prophase   b. Interphase
   c. Metaphase   d. Anaphase

10. Maximal chromosomal condensation is seen in which phase of cell cycle?
    a. Interphase   b. Prophase
    c. Anaphase   d. Metaphase

11. Oocyte is arrested in which phase of prophase?
    a. Diplotene   b. Leptotene
    c. Pachytene   d. Zygotene

12. Crossing over or recombination (DNA exchange of homologous segments between two of the four strands) occur in which phase of prophase?
    a. Pachytene   b. Leptotene
    c. Diplotene   d. Zygotene

13. Nucleotide is the basic building block of DNA. It consists of all *except:*
    a. Deoxyribose sugar   b. Ribose sugar
    c. Phosphate group   d. Nucleic acid base

14. RNA differs from DNA in that it is single stranded, its sugar moiety is ribose, and it substitutes uracil for:
    a. Thymine   b. Cytosine
    c. Adenine   d. Guanine

15. Not a stop codon:
    a. UGG   b. UAG
    c. UAA   d. UGA

16. Process of messenger RNA production of peptide chain is known as:
    a. Transcription   b. Translation
    c. Gene expression d. Transformation

17. **True about MicroRNAs all *except*:**
    a. 18 to 25 nucleotides
    b. Regulate target gene expression at both the transcriptional and translational level
    c. Over 1,500 mRNAs have been identified
    d. Protein-coding small RNAs

18. **Concept of cellular context, similar agents having different actions in different tissues is explained by:**
    a. Adapter proteins
    b. Homeoproteins
    c. Epiproteins
    d. Proteomics

19. **Sequence of gene expression**
    a. Transcription > epigenetic modifications > translation
    b. Translation > transcription > epigenetic modifications
    c. Transcription > translation > epigenetic modifications
    d. Epigenetic modifications > Transcription > translation

20. **Numerical abnormalities due to nondisjunction, is seen in which phase of mitosis or meiosis?**
    a. Anaphase
    b. Prophase
    c. Telophase
    d. Metaphase

21. **With autosomal dominant inheritance, what is the risk of inheritance for child with two heterozygous parents and with one heterozygous parent, respectively?**
    a. 75%, 50%
    b. 50%, 50%
    c. 100%, 50%
    d. 75%, 0%

22. **Which of the following is not included in epigenetic change?**
    a. Glycosylation
    b. Methylation
    c. Translation
    d. Proteolytic cleavage

23. **Enzyme involved in production of complementary DNA:**
    a. Reverse transcriptase
    b. Deoxyribonuclease
    c. DNA Polymerase
    d. Restriction endonuclease

24. **Electrophoresis to separate and quantitate proteins?**
    a. Southern blotting
    b. Northern blotting
    c. Western blotting
    d. Slot blotting

25. **Sequence of PCR in correct order:**
    a. Denaturation > annealing > amplification
    b. Denaturation > amplification > annealing
    c. Annealing > amplification > denaturation
    d. Amplification > denaturation > annealing

Basics of Molecular Biology

Answer with Explanations

1. **a. Mitochondria**

   (Ref: Speroff 8th/ed p4; U Satyanarayana biochemistry 4th/ed p6)

   Mitochondria are double membrane bound organelle.

   ## Mitochondria

   - Mitochondrial DNA is the small circular chromosome.
   - Mitochondria and mitochondrial DNA are passed almost exclusively from mother to offspring.
   - The Mitochondrial matrix contains a circular double stranded DNA (**mtDNA**), RNA and ribosomes.

2. **b. Mitochondria contain dsDNA**

   Ref: Speroff 8th/ed p4; Robbins Basic Pathology 10th/ed p14

   - Mitochondrial diseases are transmitted from the mother.
   - With the exception of DNA within mitochondria, all of our DNA is packaged in a nucleus surrounded by a nuclear membrane.
   - Mitochondria are believed to be descendants of primitive bacteria engulfed by our ancestors, and they still contain some important genes.
   - Because ova are rich in mitochondria, diseases due to mitochondrial genes (for example, Leber's optic neuropathy) are transmitted by the mother.
   - The mitochondria in sperm are eliminated during fertilization.
   - Because the ovum contributes to vast majority of cytoplasmic organelles to fertilized zygote, mitochondrial DNA is virtually entirely **maternally inherited**.

3. **d. y, 1**

   Ref: Speroff 8th/ed p4

   The chromosomes vary in size, ranging from 50 million to 250 million base pairs.

   Chromosome **1** contains the most genes (2,968), and the **Y** chromosome has the smallest number (231).

4. **a. Gene**

   Ref: Speroff 8th/ed p4; U Satyanarayana biochemistry 4th/ed p543

   A single **gene** is a unit of DNA within a chromosome that can be activated to transcribe a specific RNA.

   The word **gene** refers to the **functional unit of DNA** that can be transcribed.

5. **c. Locus**

   Ref: Speroff 8th/ed p4

   The location of a gene on a particular chromosome is designated its **locus**.

6. **a. 2%**

   Ref: Speroff 8th/ed p5; Harper's illustrated biochemistry 31st/ed p872

   - Because there are 22 pairs of autosomes, most genes exist in pairs. The pairs are homozygous when similar and heterozygous when dissimilar.
   - Only **2%** of the human genome consists of genes that encode protein synthesis.

7. **d. Band Number**

   Ref: Speroff 8th/ed p5

   The usual human karyotype is an arrangement of the chromosomes into pairs, usually after proteolytic treatment and Giemsa staining to produce characteristic banding patterns, allowing a blueprint useful for location. The staining characteristics divide each arm into regions, and each region into bands that are numbered from the centromere outward.

   A given point on a chromosome is designated by the following order: chromosome number, arm symbol (p for short arm, q for long arm), region number, and band number.

8. **a. Interphase > Prophase > Metaphase > Anaphase > Telophase**

   Ref: Speroff 8th/ed p6

9. **b. Interphase**

   Ref: Speroff 8th/ed p5

   During Interphase, all normal cell activity occurs *except:* active division. It is during this stage that the inactive X chromosome (the **Barr body** or the sex chromatin) can be seen in female cells.

10. **d. Metaphase**

    Ref: Speroff 8th/ed p5

    During **metaphase**, the chromosomes migrate to the center of the cell, forming a line designated the equatorial plate. The chromosomes are now maximally condensed. The spindle, microtubules of protein that radiate from the centrioles and attach to the centromeres, is formed.

11. a. Diplotene

Ref: Yen & Jaffe's 8th/ed p 134

Oocytes are arrested in **diplotene** stage of prophase of **first** meiotic division.

- During embryonic development, oocytes within the ovary are found as clusters, or germ cell cysts. These clusters form by both aggregation as well as clonal division.
- Meiotic progression in oocytes ceases at the diplotene stage of prophase I when germ cells are enclosed by somatic cells into individual follicles called primordial follicles.
- Oocytes in primordial follicles remain arrested until released to complete meiosis I during ovulation and form the "ovarian reserve", which is thought to ultimately determine reproductive lifespan.
- Massive germ cell loss also occurs in humans, with an estimated 1 million oocytes surviving at birth from approximately 6 million in the fetal human ovary.

12. a. Pachytene

Ref: Speroff 8th/ed p6

- **Pachytene** is the stage in which crossing over or recombination can occur (DNA exchange of homologous segments between two of the four strands).
- Chiasmata are the places of contact where crossovers occur (and can be visualized). This movement of blocks of DNA is a method for creating genetic diversity.

13. b. Ribose Sugar

Ref: Speroff 8th/ed p8; U Satyanarayana Biochemistry 4th/ed p71

- **RNA contains D-ribose** while **DNA contains D-deoxyribose**.

Each molecule of DNA has a deoxyribose backbone, identical repeating groups of deoxyribose sugar linked through phosphodiester bonds. Each deoxyribose is attached in order (giving individuality and specificity) to one of four nucleic acids, the nuclear bases:
A purine—adenine or guanine.
A pyrimidine—thymine or cytosine.

14. a. Thymine

Ref: Speroff 8th/ed p9; U Satyanarayana Biochemistry 4th/ed p70

RNA differs from DNA in that it is single stranded, its sugar moiety is ribose, and it substitutes uracil for **thymine**. The nucleic acids differ with respect to second pyrimidine base **DNA contains thymine (T) whereas RNA contains uracil (U)**.

15. a. UGG

Ref: Speroff 8th/ed p13; Harper's Illustrated Biochemistry 31st/ed p958

- Three codons (UAG, UAA, UGA) are called **stop codons**, because they specify a stop to translation of RNA into protein (like a period at the end of a sentence).
- By contrast, an **open reading frame** is a long series of base pairs between two stop codons; therefore, an open reading frame encodes the amino acid sequence of the protein product.

16. b. Translation

Ref: Speroff 8th/ed p15; Harper's Illustrated Biochemistry 31st/ed p956,957

Gene expression is composed of the following steps: transcription of DNA to RNA, RNA processing to produce functional messenger RNA by splicing out introns, **translation** of messenger RNA on a ribosome to a peptide chain, and protein structural processing to the functional form.

17. d. Protein-coding small RNAs

Ref: Speroff 8th/ed p15; Harper's illustrated biochemistry 31st/ed p912

- MicroRNAs are **non-protein-coding** small RNAs of 18 to 25 nucleotides
- Over 1,500 mRNAs have been identified.
- MicroRNAs are transcribed from genes and regulate target gene expression at both the transcriptional and translational levels.
- All eukaryotic cells have two major classes of RNA, the **protein coding RNAs**, or **mRNAs**, and two forms of abundant **nonprotein coding RNAs** delineated on the basis of size: the large ribosomal RNAs (**rRNAs**) and long noncoding RNAs (**lncRNAs**) and small noncoding transfer RNAs (**tRNAs**), the small nuclear RNAs (**snRNAs**) and the micro and silencing RNAs (**miRNAs** and **siRNAs**)

18. a. Adapter proteins

Ref: Speroff 8th/ed p15

Final result of hormonal activity and gene expression is a reflection of cellular context, the nature and activity of transcription factors as influenced by specific intracellular **adapter proteins**. This explains how similar agents (and similar transcription factors, e.g., the estrogen receptor) can have different actions in different tissues.

19. c. Transcription > Translation > Epigenetic modifications

Ref: Speroff 8th/ed p16

The final expression of a gene may not end with the translation process.

Further (posttranslational) processing of proteins occurs, such as glycosylation (the gonadotropins) or proteolytic cleavage (conversion of pro-opiomelanocortin to ACTH). These are referred to as "epigenetic" modifications.

20. a. Anaphase

Ref: Speroff 8th/ed p17; Robbins Basic Pathology 10th/ed p262

Numerical abnormalities usually are due to nondisjunction, a failure of separation at **anaphase**, either during mitotic division or during meiosis.

In humans, the normal chromosome count is 46 (i.e., 2n = 46).

- Any exact multiple of the haploid number (n) is called **euploid**.
- Chromosome numbers such as 3n and 4n are called **polyploid**. Polyploidy generally results in a spontaneous abortion.
- Any number that is not an exact multiple of n is called **aneuploid**.

The chief cause of aneuploidy is nondisjunction of a homologous pair of chromosomes at the first meiotic division or a failure of sister chromatids to separate during the second meiotic division.

Failure of pairing of homologous chromosomes followed by random assortment (anaphase lag) also can lead to aneuploidy.

21. a. 75%, 50%

Ref: Speroff 8th/ed p17; U Satyanarayana biochemistry 4th/ed p739

With two heterozygous parents, each child has a 75% risk of being affected. With one heterozygous parent, each child has 50% risk of being affected.

22. c. Translation

Ref: Speroff 8th/ed p18; Harper's illustrated biochemistry 31st/ed p1020

- **Epigenetics** is the study of changes in gene expression not directly caused by DNA sequence changes.

Mechanisms include modifications of DNA without changing the DNA sequence, such as
- Methylation of DNA to turn off gene expression
- Altering the histone proteins that are responsible for the overall structure of chromatin
- The production of new forms of RNA
- Alterations in cellular proteins that influence gene expression.

Each of these mechanisms can be transmitted to offspring and be responsible for imprinting.

23. a. Reverse Transcriptase

Ref: Speroff 8th/ed p19; U Satyanarayana biochemistry 4th/ed p688

Reverse transcriptase is DNA polymerase that is RNA dependent.

It is called reverse transcriptase because the flow of information is from RNA to DNA, the reverse of the usual direction of flow.

This enzyme permits the copying of essentially any RNA molecule into single-stranded DNA; such DNA is called **complementary DNA** because it is a mirror image of the messenger RNA.

When certain retroviruses (genetic material RNA) infect cells, a complementary DNA (**cDNA**) is made from their RNA by the enzyme **reverse transcriptase**.

24. c. Western blotting

Ref: Speroff 8th/ed p19; U Satyanarayana biochemistry 4th/ed p587

Electrophoresis to separate and quantitate proteins is called **Western blotting**, and antibodies are used for the hybridization identification process.

Like Northern blotting, Western blotting tests gene expression, not just the presence of a gene. The terms Northern and Western represent intentional witticisms in response to Southern blotting.

Hybridization without electrophoresis by placing a drop of the cell extract directly on filter paper is called dot or slot blotting.

25. a. Denaturation > annealing > amplification

Ref: Speroff 8th/ed p21; U Satyanarayana biochemistry 4th/ed p594

The first step involves separating DNA into its single strands by denaturation with heat (92°C); then the temperature is lowered (40°C), causing the primers to stick (anneal) their complementary regions on the DNA. The temperature is raised to 62°C, and DNA polymerase then synthesizes a new strand beginning and ending at the primers, forming a new double-stranded DNA.

The double-stranded DNA of interest is denatured to separate into two individual strands. Each strand is then allowed to hybridize with a primer (renaturation). The primer-template duplex is used for DNA synthesis (the enzyme-DNA polymerase). These three steps—**denaturation, renaturation** and **synthesis** are repeated again and again to generate multiple forms of target DNA.

CHAPTER 2

Hormone Biosynthesis, Metabolism and Mechanism of Action

Multiple Choice Questions

1. Intercellular communication involving the local diffusion of regulating substances from a cell to nearby (contiguous) cells is known as:
   a. Paracrine communication
   b. Autocrine
   c. Endocrine
   d. Intracrine

2. The corticoids as well as the progestins have pregnane nucleus as the basic structure consists of:
   a. 27 carbon series
   b. 19 carbon series
   c. 18 carbon series
   d. 21 carbon series

3. Which steroid is not produced by Normal human ovary?
   a. Estrogens
   b. Cortisol
   c. Progestins
   d. Androgens

4. Incorrect for cytochrome p450 enzymes:
   a. Dehydrogenase enzymes
   b. Termed 450 because of a pigment (450) absorbance shift when reduced
   c. P450 enzymes can metabolize many substrates
   d. The human genome contains genes for 57 cytochrome P450 enzymes

5. The rate-limiting step in steroidogenesis is the transfer of cholesterol from the outer mitochondrial membrane to the inner mitochondrial membrane mediated by following enzyme:
   a. P450 c17
   b. P450 11
   c. P450 arom
   d. P450 scc

6. Most important protein proposed as regulators of acute intracellular cholesterol transfer:
   a. Steroidogenic acute regulator (StAR) protein
   b. Sterol carrier protein 2 (SCP2)
   c. Steroidogenesis activator polypeptide (SAP)
   d. Peripheral benzodiazepine receptor (PBR)

7. False about aromatization:
   a. Mediated by P450arom
   b. Found in mitochondria
   c. Aromatase cytochrome P450 derived from chromosome 15
   d. Inactivating mutation of *CYP19A1* present at birth with virilization

8. In which case 17β-hydroxysteroid dehydrogenase enzymes are involved?
   a. Preganenolone to 17-hydroxypregnenolone
   b. Estradiol to estrone
   c. Cholesterol to pregnenolone
   d. Androstenedione to estrone

9. False about two cell system involved in ovarian follicular steroidogenesis:
   a. FSH receptors are induced by LH
   b. FSH receptors are present on granulosa cells
   c. FSH induces LH receptors on granulosa cells
   d. FSH induces aromatase enzyme activity in granulosa cells

10. What is not true about insulin like growth factor?
    a. Enhances LH stimulation of androgen production in theca cells
    b. Enhances FSH mediated aromatisation in granulosa cells
    c. IGF-I is more prominent during embryogenesis
    d. IGF-II is more important in human ovarian follicle

11. Percentage of free estradiol and testosterone in women, respectively:
    a. 1, 1
    b. 1, 2
    c. 2, 1
    d. 2, 2

12. Conditions not associated with increase in SHBG levels:
    a. Hyperthyroidism
    b. Corticoids
    c. Pregnancy
    d. Estrogen

13. **Conditions associated with increase in SHBG levels:**
    a. Corticoids
    b. Androgens
    c. Progestins
    d. Hyperthyroidism

14. **Not true about SHBG:**
    a. Circulating levels directly related to body weight
    b. Synthesized in liver
    c. Marker for hyperinsulinemic insulin resistance
    d. Low levels predictor for development of type 2 diabetes mellitus

15. **All of the following are true for SHBG *except*:**
    a. A glycoprotein
    b. Heterodimer composed of two monomers
    c. Has single binding site for androgens and estrogens
    d. Dimerization is necessary to form single steroid binding site

16. **Major protein binding progesterone:**
    a. Albumin
    b. Transcortin
    c. SHBG
    d. Transferrin

17. **Estrogen in increasing order of their potency:**
    a. Estriol > Estradiol > Estrone
    b. Estradiol > Estrone > Estriol
    c. Estriol > Estrone > Estradiol
    d. Estrone > Estradiol > Estriol

18. **In the preovulatory phase in adult females, what are the blood levels of progesterone?**
    a. <1 ng/mL
    b. 1-2 ng/mL
    c. 3-5 ng/mL
    d. <1 mg/mL

19. **Which androgen is not secreted by ovary?**
    a. DHEA
    b. DHEA-S
    c. Androstenedione
    d. Testosterone

20. **In females, the majority of circulating DHT is derived from:**
    a. Androstenedione
    b. Testosterone
    c. Dehydroepiandrosterone
    d. Dehydroepiandrosterone sulphate

21. **Following are true about DHT in females, *except*:**
    a. Intracrine hormone
    b. Majority derived from testosterone
    c. 3α-androstanediol glucuronide is the major metabolite of DHT
    d. Hair follicles are sensitive to DHT

22. **All of the following tissues require DHT for development *except*:**
    a. External genitalia
    b. Urethra
    c. Prostate
    d. Seminal vesicles

23. **Active steroids and metabolites are excreted as sulfo-and glucuro-conjugates. Which of the following is not true regarding conjugation of a steroid?**
    a. Converts a hydrophilic compound into hydrophobic one
    b. Converts a hydrophobic compound into a hydrophilic one
    c. Decreases activity of a steroid
    d. Conjugation by liver and intestinal mucosa is essential for excretion into urine and bile

24. **Estrogen receptors are:**
    a. G protein coupled receptors
    b. Ion gate channels
    c. Intracellular receptors
    d. Receptors with intrinsic enzyme activity

25. **Receptors allowing entry into cell by process of internalization or endocytosis are all *except*:**
    a. Estrogen
    b. LDL receptor
    c. Growth hormone
    d. Prolactin

26. **When in the unbound state, following hormone reside in the cytoplasm and move into the nucleus after hormone-receptor binding:**
    a. Estrogen
    b. Mineralocorticoid
    c. Progesterone
    d. Androgen

27. **All, except one of the following are transferred across the nuclear membrane and bind to their receptors within the nucleus:**
    a. Glucocorticoid
    b. Estrogen
    c. Androgen
    d. Progesterone

28. **Conformational change of the hormone-receptor complex revealing or producing a binding site that is necessary in order for the complex to bind to the chromatin is known as:**
    a. Translocation
    b. Transformation
    c. Transcription
    d. Transregulation

29. **Not true about orphan receptors:**
    a. Number of orphan receptors is gradually increasing
    b. Specific ligands for these proteins have not been identified
    c. Part of nuclear receptor superfamily
    d. Share a common structure with the receptors for thyroid hormone

30. All of the following holds true for steroid hormone receptors, *except:*
    a. 48 nuclear receptors in the receptor superfamily
    b. Share a common structure with the receptors for thyroid hormone, 1, 25-dihydroxyvitamin D3, and retinoic acid
    c. Orphan receptors are not part of steroid hormone receptor superfamily
    d. Each receptor contains characteristic domains that are similar and interchangeable

31. What the ideal time to measure major sex steroids in females over the course of day?
    a. Anytime
    b. Early morning fasting
    c. Evening
    d. Midnight

32. Most potent androgen:
    a. Testosterone
    b. DHT
    c. Androstenedione
    d. DHEAS

33. Major circulatory androgen:
    a. Testosterone
    b. DHT
    c. DHEA
    d. DHEAS

34. Which of the following tissue development is under control of testosterone, not DHT?
    a. Urethra
    b. Prostate
    c. Muscle
    d. None of the above

35. Which of the following is not true for heat shock proteins?
    a. Proteins responsible for stabilization and protection of unbound receptor
    b. Help maintain a conformational shape that keeps the DNA binding region in an inactive state
    c. Produced in cells in response to stressful conditions
    d. HSPs are not present in cancerous cells

36. Most important factor for biologic activity of a steroid hormone:
    a. Half-life of hormone-receptor complex
    b. Amount of circulating hormone
    c. Elimination rate of hormone
    d. None

37. All of the following holds true for prolactin, *except:*
    a. Single-chain polypeptide
    b. Structure homologous to growth hormone and placental lactogen
    c. Macroprolactins are prolactins with greatest bioactivity
    d. Immunoassays do not always reflect the biologic situation

38. The critical determinant of circulating biologic half-life of a glycoprotein:
    a. Amount of sialic acid present
    b. Differences in amino acid sequences
    c. Carbohydrate component of glycoprotein
    d. Hydrophilicity of glycoprotein

39. Which carbohydrate component of the glycoproteins is responsible for prolonged biologic half-life of glycoprotein?
    a. Fructose
    b. Galactose
    c. Sialic acid
    d. Glucosamine

40. All of the following is true for glycoprotein hormones, *except:*
    a. Dimers composed of two glycosylated polypeptide subunits the a and b subunits
    b. hCG is minimally glycosylated glycoprotein hormone
    c. All of the glycopeptides share a common a chain
    d. Specific biologic activity of a glycopeptide hormone is determined by b subunit

41. Which of the following is pure antiestrogen?
    a. Fulvestrant
    b. Clomophene
    c. Ormiloxifene
    d. Raloxifene

42. The major biologic mechanism by which polypeptide hormones downregulate their own receptors and thus limit hormonal activity:
    a. Internalization
    b. Potocytosis
    c. Exteriorization
    d. Clustering

43. All steroid-producing organs can synthesize cholesterol from acetate, *except:*
    a. Ovary
    b. Placenta
    c. Adrenal gland
    d. Testes

44. Intrinsic bioactivity of gonadotropins to a great extent is determined by their degree of:
    a. Glycosylation
    b. Conjugation
    c. Hydroxylation
    d. Dehydrogenation

Answer with Explanations

1. **a. Paracrine communication**

   Ref: Speroff 8th/ed p 30

   Intercellular communication involving the local diffusion of regulating substances from a cell to nearby (contiguous) cells is known as **paracrine communication**.

2. **d. 21 carbon series**

   Ref: Speroff 8th/ed p 32

   - The sex steroids are divided into three main groups according to the number of carbon atoms they possess.
   - The 21-carbon series includes the corticoids as well as the progestins, and the basic structure is the **pregnane** nucleus.
   - The 19-carbon series includes all the androgens and is based on the **androstane** nucleus
   - The estrogens are 18-carbon steroids based on the **estrane** nucleus.

3. **b. Cortisol**

   Ref: Speroff 8th/ed p 36

   - Normal human ovary produces all three classes of sex steroids: estrogens, progestins, and androgens.

   The ovary differs from the testis in its fundamental complement of critical enzymes being deficient in **21-hydroxylase** and **11b-hydroxylase** reactions.

   Glucocorticoids and mineralocorticoids, therefore, are not produced in normal ovarian tissue.

4. **a. Dehydogenase enzymes**

   Ref: Kamini A Rao 2nd/ed p 113

Cytochrome P450

   - Generic term for a family of **oxidative** enzymes.
   - Termed 450 because of a pigment (450) absorbance shift when reduced.
   - P450 enzymes can metabolize many substrates; e.g. in the liver, *P450* enzymes metabolize toxins and environmental pollutants.
   - The human genome contains genes for 57 cytochrome *P450* enzymes, 7 in mitochondria and 50 in the endoplasmic reticulum (the major site for metabolic clearance).

5. **d. P450 scc**

   Ref: Kamini A Rao 2nd/ed p 113

   - Enzyme governing rate limiting step in steroidogenesis-P450 scc

   The **rate-limiting step** for the synthesis of all steroid hormones is cleavage of the side chain from cholesterol (C27) to yield pregnenolone (C21) which is catalyzed by P450 scc.

   The transfer of cholesterol from the outer mitochondrial membrane to the inner mitochondrial membrane where fully active P450 scc waits for substrate is the rate-limiting step in steroidogenesis.

6. **a. Steroidogenic acute regulator (StAR) protein**

   Ref: Speroff 8th/ed p 39

   Several proteins have been characterized and proposed as regulators of acute intracellular cholesterol transfer.

   - Sterol carrier protein 2 (SCP2) is able to bind and transfer cholesterol between compartments within a cell.
   - Another candidate is a small molecule, steroidogenesis activator polypeptide (SAP), and still another is peripheral benzodiazepine receptor (PBR), which affects cholesterol flux through a pore structure.
   - But the most studied and favored protein as a regulator of acute cholesterol transfer is **steroidogenic acute regulator (StAR) protein**. StAR messenger RNA and proteins are induced concomitantly with acute steroidogenesis in response to cyclic AMP stimulation. StAR protein increases steroid production and is imported and localized in the mitochondria.

7. **b. Found in mitochondria**

   Ref: Speroff 8th/ed p 37, Yen & Jaffe's 8th/ed p 85

   - Aromatase is an **endoplasmic reticulum** enzyme.

   Aromatase catalyzes three sequential hydroxylations of C19 substrate by using three molecules of NADPH and three molecular oxygen to produce one molecule of C18 steroid with a phenolic A ring.

   P450 arom mediates aromatization of androgens to estrogens and is found in the endoplasmic reticulum.

Enzyme	Cellular location	Reactions
P450 scc	Mitochondria	Cholesterol side chain cleavage
P450 c11	Mitochondria	11-hydroxylase, 18-hydroxylase, 19-methyloxidase
P450 c17	Endoplasmic reticulum	17-hydroxylase, 17,20-lyase
P450 c21	Endoplasmic reticulum	21-hydroxylase
P450 arom	Endoplasmic reticulum	Aromatase

8. **b. Estradiol to estrone**

Ref: Yen & Jaffe's 8th/ed p 89

The type-1 enzyme of HSD17β1 is referred to as the estrogenic 17β-HSD because it catalyzes the final step in estrogen biosynthesis by preferentially reducing the weak estrogen estrone to yield potent estrogen 17β-estradiol.

The 17β-hydroxysteroid dehydrogenase and 5α-reductase reactions are mediated by non-P450 enzymes. The 17β-hydroxysteroid dehydrogenase is bound to the endoplasmic reticulum and the 5α-reductase to the nuclear membrane. The 17β-hydroxysteroid dehydrogenase enzymes convert estrone to estradiol, androstenedione to testosterone, and DHEA to androstenediol, and vice versa.

9. **a. FSH receptors are induced by LH**

Ref: Speroff 8th/ed p 41

Two cell two gonadotropin theory
- FSH receptors are present on the granulosa cells.
- FSH receptors are induced by FSH itself.
- LH receptors are present on the theca cells and initially absent on the granulosa cells, but, as the follicle grows, FSH induces the appearance of LH receptors on the granulosa cells.
- FSH induces aromatase enzyme activity in granulosa cells.
- All these actions are modulated by autocrine and paracrine factors secreted by the theca and granulosa cells.

10. **c. IGF-I is more prominent during embryogenesis**

Ref: Speroff 8th/ed p 88

- IGF-II is more prominent during embryogenesis, whereas IGF-I is more active postnatally.

Insulin-like growth factor (IGF)
- Secreted by the **theca cells**.
- Also known as **Somatomedins**.
- **Single chain** polypeptides with structural and functional similarity to insulin and mediate growth hormone action.
- Enhances the LH stimulation of androgen production in the theca cells as well as FSH-mediated aromatization in the granulosa.
- Evidence indicates that the endogenous IGF in the human ovarian follicle is IGF-II in both the granulosa and the theca cells.
- Both IGF-I and IGF-II activities can be mediated by the type I IGF receptor, which is structurally similar to the insulin receptor.

11. **a. 1, 1**

Ref: Speroff 8th/ed p 43

While circulating in the blood, majority of the principal sex steroids, estradiol and testosterone, is bound to a protein carrier, known as sex hormone-binding globulin (SHBG) produced mainly in the liver. Another 30% is loosely bound to albumin, leaving only about 1% unbound and free. A very small percentage also binds to corticosteroid-binding globulin.

12. **b. Corticoids**

Ref: Yen & Jaffe's 8th/ed p 98; Cambridge. Infertility in Male 4th/ed p 201

Increased SHBG	Decreased SHBG
Estrogens	Androgens
Hyperthyroidism	Hypothyroidism
Aging	Growth hormone excess
Anticonvulsants	Obesity
Pregnancy	Glucocorticoid excess
	Progestins
	Hyperprolactinemia
	Postmenopausal
	Hyperinsulinemia

13. **d. Hyperthyroidism**

Ref: Yen & Jaffe's 8th/ed p 98; Cambridge. Infertility in Male 4th/ed p 201

Factors associated with decreased SHBG explained in previous answer.

14. **a. Circulating levels directly related to body weight**

Ref: Speroff 8th/ed p 43

- The circulating level of SHBG is inversely related to body weight and, thus, significant weight gain can decrease SHBG.

Increased insulin levels in the circulation lower SHBG levels, and this may be the major mechanism that mediates the impact of increased body weight on SHBG.

This relationship between the levels of insulin and SHBG is so strong that SHBG concentrations are a marker for hyperinsulinemic insulin resistance, and a low level of SHBG is a predictor for the development of type 2 diabetes mellitus.

15. b. Heterodimer composed of two monomers
Ref: Speroff 8th/ed p 44

SHBG
- It is a **glycoprotein**.
- It contains a single binding site for androgens and estrogens.
- It is a **homodimer** composed of two monomers.
- Its gene has been localized to the short arm (p12–13) of **chromosome 17**.
- 36 genetic studies have revealed that the SHBG gene also encodes the androgen-binding protein present in the seminiferous tubules, synthesized by the Sertoli cells.
- Dimerization is believed to be necessary to form the single steroid-binding site.

16. a. Albumin
Ref: Speroff 8th/ed p 44

Transcortin, also called corticosteroid-binding globulin, is a plasma glycoprotein that binds cortisol, progesterone, deoxycorticosterone, corticosterone, and some of the other minor corticoid compounds.

Progesterone circulates in the following percentages:
- 80% bound to albumin
- 18% bound to transcortin
- Less than 1% bound to SHBG
- 2% free

17. c. Estriol > Estrone > Estradiol
Ref: Speroff 8th/ed p 53; Yen & Jaffe's 8th/ed p 257

- A major factor in the potency differences among the various estrogens is rate of dissociation of steroid from its receptor.
- Estriol is a weak estrogen with 1% the potency of estradiol and 10% that of estrone, on weight basis.

- A major factor in the potency differences among the various estrogens (estradiol, estrone, estriol) is the **length of time** the estrogen-receptor complex occupies the nucleus.
- The higher **rate of dissociation** with the weak estrogen (estriol) can be compensated for by continuous application to allow prolonged nuclear binding and activity.

18. a. <1ng/mL
Ref: Speroff 8th/ed p 46

- In the preovulatory phase in adult females, in all prepubertal females, and in the normal male, the blood levels of progesterone are at the lower limits of immunoassay sensitivity: **less than 1 ng/mL.**
- After ovulation, i.e. during the luteal phase, progesterone ranges from 3 to 15 ng/mL.
- In congenital adrenal hyperplasia, progesterone blood levels can be as high as 50 times above normal.

19. b. DHEA-S
Ref: Speroff 8th/ed p 48

- DHEA-S are exclusively secreted by adrenal gland.
- The major androgen products of the ovary are dehydroepiandrosterone (DHEA) and androstenedione (and only a little testosterone), which are secreted mainly by stromal tissue derived from theca cells.
- With excessive accumulation of stromal tissue or in the presence of an androgen-producing tumor, testosterone becomes a significant secretory product.

20. a. Androstenedione
Ref: Speroff 8th/ed p 48

- In men, the majority of circulating DHT is derived from testosterone that enters a target cell and is converted by means of 5α-reductase to DHT.
- In women, because the production rate of androstenedione is greater than testosterone, blood DHT is primarily derived from androstenedione and partly from dehydroepiandrosterone. Thus, in women, the skin production of DHT is predominantly influenced by androstenedione.

21. b. Majority derived from testosterone
Ref: Speroff 8th/ed p 48

- Testosterone is the major circulating androgen.

DHT is largely metabolized intracellularly; hence, the blood DHT is only about **one-tenth** the level of circulating testosterone.

22. d. Seminal vesicles
Ref: Kamini A Rao 2nd/ed p 117

During fetal development, testosterone is essential for wolffian duct differentiation into following structures
- Epididymides
- Vasa deferentia
- Seminal vesicles

Testosterone is used as the intracellular mediator, whereas development of the urogenital sinus and urogenital tubercle into the male external genitalia, urethra, and prostate requires the conversion of testosterone to DHT.

23. a. Coverts hydrophilic compound into hydrophobic one

Ref: Biocatalysis and Biotransformation. 36:1-9

- Conjugation reaction involves covalent attachment of small hydrophilic endogenous molecule such as glucoronic acid, sulfate, or glycine to form water soluble compounds, that are more hydrophilic.
- Active steroids and metabolites are excreted as sulfo- and glucuro conjugates.
- Conjugation of a steroid converts a hydrophobic compound into a hydrophilic one and generally reduces or eliminates the activity of a steroid.
- Conjugation by liver and intestinal mucosa is a step in deactivation preliminary to, and essential for, excretion into urine and bile.

24. c. Intracellular receptors

Ref: Yen & Jaffe's 8th/ed p 117

Steroid hormone receptors are **intranuclear** receptors. Receptors within cells lead to transcription activation. Examples include the receptors for estrogen and thyroid hormones.

25. a. Estrogen

Ref: Yen & Jaffe's 8th/ed p 77

Numerous microvilli project from the plasma membrane on which lipoprotein-gathering receptors of the low-density lipoprotein receptor family are located (e.g. LDL receptors; LDL receptor-related protein, VLDL lipoprotein receptors, prolactin, growth hormone, and some of the growth factors). These receptors mediate lipoprotein uptake by endocytic mechanism that delivers the lipoprotein to lysosomes where apolipoproteins are degraded.

26. b. Mineralocorticoid

Ref: Yen & Jaffe's 8th/ed p 122

- Glucocorticoid and mineralocorticoid receptors, when in the unbound state, reside in the cytoplasm and move into the nucleus after hormone-receptor binding.
- Estrogens, progestins, and androgens are transferred across the nuclear membrane and bind to their receptors within the nucleus.

27. a. Glucocorticoid

Ref: Speroff 8th/ed p 53

28. b. Transformation

Ref: Speroff 8th/ed p 53

- Transformation refers to a conformational change of the hormone-receptor complex revealing or producing a binding site that is necessary in order for the complex to bind to the chromatin.
- In the unbound state, the receptor is associated with heat shock proteins that stabilize and protect the receptor and maintain a conformational shape that keeps the DNA binding region in an inactive state.
- Activation of the receptor is driven by hormone binding that causes a dissociation of the receptor-heat shock protein complex.

29. a. Number of orphan receptors is gradually increasing

Ref: Yen & Jaffe's 8th/ed p 117

- **Orphan receptor** is a protein that has a similar structure to other identified receptors but whose endogenous ligand has not yet been identified.
- If a ligand for an orphan receptor is later discovered, the receptor is referred to as an **"adopted orphan"**

Some nuclear receptors have defined natural ligands, such as steroid hormones, thyroid hormones, retinoids, or vitamin D, but others have no identified ligand and are called Orphan receptors. However, the number of orphan receptors is gradually diminishing (deorphaning).

30. c. Orphan receptors are not part of steroid receptor superfamily

Ref: Speroff 8th/ed p 55

- Steroid hormone receptors share a common structure with the receptors for thyroid hormone, 1,25-dihydroxyvitamin D3, and retinoic acid; thus, these receptors are called a superfamily.
- Each receptor contains characteristic domains that are similar and interchangeable. Therefore, it is not surprising that the specific hormones can interact with more than one receptor in this family.
- There are 48 nuclear receptors in the receptor superfamily.

31. a. Anytime

Ref: Speroff 8th/ed p 48

There is no circadian cycle of the major sex steroids in the female. However, short-term variations in the blood levels due to episodic secretion require multiple sampling for absolutely accurate assessment. Although frequent sampling is necessary for a high degree of accuracy, a **random sample** is sufficient for clinical purposes to determine whether a level is within a normal range.

32. b. DHT

Ref: Yen & Jaffe's 8th/ed p 291

DHT is most potent androgen that cannot be aromatized to estradiol. It is **nonaromatizable androgen**.

33. a. Testosterone
Ref: Kamini A Rao 2nd/ed p 159

- DHEA, DHEA-S and androstenedione are considered as pro-hormones as they do not bind to androgen receotors.
- DHT is largely metabolized intracellularly; hence, the blood DHT is only about one-tenth the level of circulating testosterone, and it is clear that testosterone is the major circulating androgen.

34. c. Muscle
Ref: Kamini A Rao 2nd/ed p 117

- The **most potent endogenous androgen DHT** is formed from testosterone by enzymatic action of 5α-reductase. This reaction is predominant in the epididymis and prostate where DHT plays an important role in maintaining sexual function.
- Muscle development is under the direct control of testosterone.

35. d. HSPs are not present in cancerous cells
Ref: Heat Shock Proteins and Cancer". Trends in Pharmacological Sciences. 38 (3): 226-56

- Heat shock proteins are the proteins that stabilize and protect the receptor and maintain a conformational shape that keeps the DNA binding region in an inactive state. Activation of the receptor is driven by hormone binding that causes a dissociation of the receptor-heat shock protein complex.
- Intracellular heat shock proteins are highly expressed in cancerous cells and are essential to the survival of these cell types due to presence of mutated and over expressed oncogenes. Hence, small molecule inhibitors of HSPs, especially HSP90 show promise as anticancer agent.

36. a. Half-life of hormone receptor complex
Ref: Speroff 8th/ed p 53

- Biologic activity is maintained only while the nuclear site is occupied with the hormone-receptor complex.
- The dissociation rate of the hormone and its receptor as well as the half-life of the nuclear chromatin-bound complex are factors in the biologic response because the hormone response elements are abundant and, under normal conditions, are occupied only to a small extent.
- Thus, an important clinical principle is the following: duration of exposure to a hormone is as important as dose.
- One reason only small amounts of estrogen need be present in the circulation is the long half-life of the estrogen hormone-receptor complex. Indeed, a major factor in the potency differences among the various estrogens (estradiol, estrone, estriol) is the length of time the estrogen-receptor complex occupies the nucleus.
- The higher rate of dissociation with the weak estrogen (estriol) can be compensated for by continuous application to allow prolonged nuclear binding and activity. Cortisol and progesterone must circulate in large concentrations because their receptor complexes have short half-lives in the nucleus.

37. c. Macroprolactins are prolactins with greatest bioactivity
Ref: Yen & Jaffe's 8th/ed p 895

- **Macroprolactinemia** may be an important clinical problem resulting in up to 10% of cases of misdiagnosed hyperprolactinemia.
- When macroprolactinemia is suspected (e.g. in patients with autoimmune diseases), polyethylene glycol precipitation should be carried out before immunoassay.
- Prolactin recovery <30% following PEG precipitation indicates the presence of macroprolactinemia.
- Variants of prolactin are the result of **posttranslational modifications**. Big prolactin has little biologic activity and does not cross-react with antibodies to the major form of prolactin. The so-called big variants of prolactin are due to separate molecules of prolactin binding to each other, either noncovalently or by interchain disulfide bonding. Some of the apparently larger forms of prolactin are prolactin molecules complexed to binding proteins.

38. a. Amount of sialic acid present
Ref: Speroff 8th/ed p 93

39. c. Sialic acid
Ref: Speroff 8th/ed p 93

- The carbohydrate components of the glycoproteins are composed of fructose, galactose, mannose, galactosamine, glucosamine, and sialic acid.
- Although the other sugars are necessary for hormonal function, sialic acid is the critical determinant of biologic half-life.
- Removal of sialic acid residues in hCG, FSH, and LH leads to **very rapid elimination** from the circulation.
- The higher content of sialic acid in FSH compared with LH accounts for the more rapid clearance of LH from circulation.

40. b. hCG is minimally glycosylated glycoprotein hormone

Ref: Speroff 8th/ed p 90

- β-hCG is the largest β subunit, containing a larger carbohydrate moiety and 145 amino acid residues, including a unique carboxyl-terminal tail piece of 29 amino acid groups.
- The extended sequence in the carboxy-terminal region of β-hCG contains four sites for glycosylation, the reason why hCG is glycosylated to a greater extent than LH, a difference that is responsible for the longer circulating half-life for hCG.

41. a. Fulvestrant

Ref: Yen & Jaffe's 8th/ed p 724

- **Fulvestrant** is a pure antiestrogen.
- It is FDA approved drug.
- Mechanism of action:
  - It inhibits estradiol mediated transcription by favoring of corepressors to the ER complex.
  - Increases the rate of degradation of the ER.
- It is also known as SERD, selective estrogen receptor down-regulator.
- The pure antiestrogens are derivatives of estradiol with long hydrophobic side chains at the 7 position.
- Binding with the pure antiestrogens prevents DNA binding.
- Because the site responsible for dimerization overlaps with the hormone-binding site, it is believed that pure antiestrogens sterically interfere with dimerization, and thus inhibit DNA binding.
- Fulvestrant, is used to treat metastatic breast cancer that has failed to respond to the usual endocrine therapy.

42. a. Internalization

Ref: Speroff 8th/ed p 95

- **Internalization** is the major biologic mechanism by which polypeptide hormones down-regulate their own receptors and thus limit hormonal activity.
- A similar process, called **potocytosis**, utilizes cholesterol-rich membrane invaginations called caveolae (far fewer in number and smaller in structure than the clathrin coated pits) for the internalization of small molecules and ions.

43. b. Placenta

Ref: Speroff 8th/ed p 34

- Cholesterol is the basic building block in steroidogenesis.

All steroid-producing organs except the placenta can synthesize cholesterol from acetate.

44. a. Glycosylation

Ref: Cambridge. Infertility in the Male 4th/ed p 19

- Beta subunit determine the functional specificity of gonadotropins, their intrinsic bioactivity is to a great extent is determined by their **degree of glycosylation**.
- Weekly glycosylated forms of hormones have short circulatory half-time and totally deglycosylated gonadotropins are unable to evoke generation of the second messenger signal.

CHAPTER 3

Neuroendocrinology

Multiple Choice Questions

1. Which of the following pituitary hormone is not under positive hypothalamic control unlike other hormones?
   a. Prolactin
   b. Growth hormone
   c. FSH
   d. ACTH

2. Which of the following is incorrect regarding GnRH?
   a. A total of 24 forms of GnRH have been identified
   b. GnRH localized to the hypothalamus is GnRH-I
   c. GnRH is decapeptide
   d. GnRH-II is the main form found in the brain

3. Prolactin gene expression is seen in all of the following tissues, *except*:
   a. Lactotropes of anterior pituitary gland
   b. Decidualised endometrium
   c. Hypothalamus
   d. Myometrium

4. Which of the following is incorrect regarding prolactin?
   a. Prolactin is highest in early morning hours
   b. Prolactin gene expression is stimulated by estrogen
   c. D2 type receptors are predominant in anterior pituitary gland
   d. TRH has stimulatory effect on prolactin secretion

5. Mode of inheritance of Kallmann's syndrome:
   a. X-linked
   b. Autosomal-dominant
   c. Autosomal-recessive
   d. All

6. All of the following is true regarding GnRH secretion, *except*:
   a. Cells that produce GnRH originate from olfactory placode
   b. Arcuate nucleus is key locus for GnRH secretion
   c. GnRH is nonapeptide
   d. Half life of GnRH is 2-4 minutes

7. Which of the following is true regarding feedback loops affecting GnRH secretion?
   a. Long feedback loop is due to effects of target gland hormones on hypothalamus and pituitary
   b. Short feedback loop is due to effects of pituitary hormones on hypothalamus
   c. Ultrashort feedback is inhibition by hypothalamic releasing hormone on its own synthesis
   d. All

8. Which of the following statement is correct regarding GnRH pulse frequency?
   a. The measurement of LH pulses is used as an indication of GnRH pulsatile secretion
   b. Pulsatile secretion is more frequent but lower in amplitude during the follicular phase
   c. During the luteal-follicular transition, pulse frequency increases approximately 4.5-fold
   d. All

9. Which of the following is incorrect regarding dopaminergic pathway?
   a. Dopamine directly suppress gonadotropin secretion
   b. Dopamine directly suppress arcuate GnRH activity
   c. Dopamine directly suppress pituitary prolactin secretion
   d. Dopamine directly suppress melanocyte-stimulating hormone

10. Which of the following is not true about major 'neurobiological brake'?
    a. Facilitates gonadotropin secretion in absence of estrogen
    b. Neuropeptide Y is a peptide
    c. It stimulates appetite
    d. Stimulates pulsatile release of GnRH

11. Which of the following is not true regarding intrapituitary autocrine paracrine system?
    a. Activin and inhibin are peptide members of the transforming growth factor-b family

b. Follistatin is secreted by granulosa cells
c. Inhibin and activin are secreted by granulosa cells
d. Activin stimulates follistatin production

12. Opiate production is regulated by gene transcription and the synthesis of precursor peptides. Which of the following is not the precursor peptide for opiates?
    a. Proopiomelanocortin (POMC)
    b. Proenkephalin A and B
    c. Prodynorphin
    d. All

13. How stress affects reproductive function?
    a. CRH directly inhibiting GnRH secretion
    b. Cortisol inhibits pituitary responsiveness to GnRH
    c. None of the above
    d. Both of the above

14. Which of the following is not correct for neuroendocrine hormones involved with reproduction?
    a. High levels of progesterone are responsible for the FSH surge at midcycle
    b. Lower GnRH pulse frequencies favor FSH secretion, and higher GnRH pulse frequencies favor LH secretion
    c. High levels of estrogen induce the LH surge at midcycle
    d. Pineal is the source of gonadal inhibiting substances

15. Catecholamines stimulating secretion of GnRH from hypothalamus:
    a. Dopamine
    b. Serotonin
    c. Norepinephrine
    d. Prostaglandins

16. Which of the following statement does not hold true for inhibin?
    a. Composed of two dissimilar peptides linked by covalent bonds
    b. Inhibin B peaks in follicular phase
    c. Inhibin A peaks is not detectable before puberty
    d. Inhibin has no effect on growth hormone, ACTH and prolactin production

17. Which of the following statement does not hold true for activin?
    a. Composed of two subunits identical to beta subunits of inhibin A and B
    b. Inhibin potentiates activin activity
    c. Activin inhibits growth hormone, ACTH and prolactin responses
    d. Derived from granulosa cells

18. A glycopeptide secreted by gonadotrophs, also called FSH—suppressing protein inhibiting FSH synthesis, secretion and FSH response to GnRH:
    a. Follistatin
    b. Inhibin A
    c. Inhibin B
    d. IGF-1

19. What is true regarding differential control of FSH and LH secretion?
    a. LH secretion is primarily regulated by GnRH, without involvement of the inhibin-activin-follistatin system
    b. Activin enhances and follistatin suppress GnRH activity
    c. Inhibin may enhance LH activity
    d. All

20. Which is incorrect regarding endogenous opioids and their effects on GnRH?
    a. Endorphins promote GnRH release
    b. B endorphins are 5-10 times more potent than morphine
    c. Ovarian sex steroids increase endorphin secretion
    d. Endorphin levels peak in luteal phase with nadir during menses

21. How does hyperprolactinemia affects female reproductive function?
    a. Disrupts normal follicular development
    b. Premature destruction of corpus luteum
    c. Inhibiting aromatase enzyme
    d. All

22. FSH is essential for follicular growth. Which of the following event is not related to FSH in menstrual cycle?
    a. Selection and maturation of dominant follicle
    b. Aromatization within granulosa cells
    c. Induction of LH surge
    d. Induction of FSH and LH receptors on granulosa cells

23. Luteinizing hormone should be present at concentrations within the LH window, which is over the threshold level and beneath the ceiling value. Which of the following effects is result of LH levels above ceiling value?
    a. Follicular premature luteinization
    b. Inadequate androgen and estrogen biosynthesis
    c. Absent paracrine signaling between granulosa and theca
    d. Optimum oocyte maturation

24. Which are the hormones not secreted by anterior pituitary?
    a. Prolactin
    b. FSH
    c. ACTH
    d. GnRH

25. Following is associated with corpus luteum of menstruation but not with corpus luteum of pregnancy:
    a. Corpus albicans
    b. hCG
    c. Estrogen
    d. Prolactin

26. Persistent high levels of which of the following hormone leads to positive feedback loop in hypothalamo-pituitary-ovary axis?
    a. Estradiol
    b. Estrone
    c. Testosterone
    d. Progesterone

27. Which of the following hormones stimulate growth of primary follicles?
    a. Activin
    b. Estrogen
    c. FSH
    d. Progesterone

28. Which of the following hormone produced by corpus luteum is low in follicular phase and maximal in luteal phase?
    a. Progesterone
    b. Estradiol
    c. LH
    d. Inhibin

29. Peptide hormone produced by testes responsible for suppression of FSH:
    a. Inhibin A
    b. Inhibin B
    c. Activin A
    d. Activin B

Answer with Explanations

1. **a. Prolactin**

   Ref: Kamini A Rao 2nd/ed p19

   - Hypothalamus has peptidergic neural cells that secrete releasing and inhibitory hormones.
   - These cells resemble both neurons and endocrine gland cells; respond to signals in the bloodstream, as well as to neurotransmitters within the brain in a process known as **neurosecretion**.
   - These neurotransmitters are secreted at the nerve terminal.
   - Neuroendocrine agents originating in the hypothalamus have positive stimulatory effects on growth hormone, TSH, ACTH, as well as gonadotropins.
   - An exception to the overall pattern of positive influence of hypothalamus on pituitary is the control of prolactin secretion.
   - Stalk secretion and transplantation cause release of prolactin from the anterior pituitary, implying a negative, inhibitory hypothalamic control. Furthermore, cultures of anterior pituitary tissue release prolactin in the absence of hypothalamic tissue or extracts.

2. **d. GnRH-II is main form found in the brain**

   Ref: Speroff 8th/ed p 160

   - GnRH-I is the main form found in the brain, whereas GnRH-II is widely distributed in other organs.

   ## Gonadotropin Releasing Hormone

   - Human GnRH-II expression is highest outside the brain.
   - An analysis of the evolution of GnRH indicates three major forms:
     1. Localized to the hypothalamus—GnRH-I
     2. Forms in midbrain nuclei and outside the brain—GnRH-II
     3. Forms in several fish species—GnRH-III
   - A total of **24 forms** of GnRH have been identified in multiple species, but GnRH-I and GnRH-II are the primary GnRHs in mammals.

3. **c. Hypothalamus**

   Ref: Yen & Jaffe's 8th/ed p 46

   Prolactin gene expression occurs in:
   - The lactotropes of the anterior pituitary gland
   - Decidualized endometrium
   - Myometrium

   The decidual mRNA is indistinguishable from pituitary prolactin mRNA except for four silent nucleotide differences and the decidual prolactin gene is 150 nucleotides longer in the 5' untranslated region.

4. **a. Prolactin is highest in early morning hours**

   Ref: Speroff 8th/ed p 162

   Prolactin levels are highest during sleep.

   Association of hyperprolactinemia with the elevation in TRH secretion that occurs with hypothyroidism is an important clinical manifestation.

5. **d. All**

   Ref: "Clinical genetic testing for Kallmann syndrome". JCEM. 98 (5): 1860-2

   The following inheritance pattern is documented:
   - X-linked
   - Autosomal-dominant
   - Autosomal-recessive

   The 5–7-fold increased frequency in males indicates that X-linked transmission is the most common.

6. **c. GnRH is a nonapeptide**

   Ref: Textbook of assisted reproductive techniques, Vol 2, 5th/ed p 513

   ## GnRH

   - GnRH is a **decapeptide** that is synthesized as part of a much larger precursor peptide, the **GnRH-associated peptide**, that has a 56-amino acid sequence.
   - The structure of GnRH is common to all mammals, including humans, and its action is similar in both males and females.
   - GnRH is a single-chain peptide comprising 10 amino acids.
   - In humans, the pulsatile release frequencies ranges from the shortest interpulse frequency of approximately 71 minutes in the late follicular phase to an interval of 216 minutes in the late luteal phase.
   - Native GnRH has a short plasma half-life and is rapidly inactivated by enzymatic cleavage.

7. **d. All**

   Ref: Speroff 8th/ed p 164

   The **long feedback loop** refers to the feedback effects of circulating levels of target gland hormones, and this occurs both in the hypothalamus and the pituitary.

The **short feedback loop** indicates a negative feedback of pituitary hormones on their own secretion, presumably via inhibitory effects on releasing hormones in the hypothalamus.

The **ultrashort feedback** refers to inhibition by the releasing hormone on its own synthesis.

8. **d. All**

   Ref: Yen & Jaffe's 8th/ed p 9

   - Pulsatile GnRH secretion is absolutely required for long-term stimulation of gonadotropin synthesis and secretion.
   - More frequent exposure to GnRH pulses can reduce gonadotropin responses to GnRH; continuous GnRH receptor stimulation leads to **desensitization** of gonadotropin synthesis and secretion.
   - The measurement of LH pulses is used as an indication of GnRH pulsatile secretion as the long half-life of FSH precludes its use for this purpose.

9. **a. Dopamine directly suppress Gonadotropin secretion**

   Ref: Speroff 8th/ed p 168

   - Dopamine is a neurohormone as it is directly secreted into the portal blood.
   - It does not exert a direct effect on gonadotropin secretion by the anterior pituitary; this effect is mediated through GnRH release in the hypothalamus.
   - Prolactin delivered to the intermediate lobe of the pituitary suppresses melanocyte-stimulating hormone release.

10. **a. Facilitates gonadotropin secretion in absence of estrogen**

    Ref: Yen & Jaffe's 8th/ed p 16

    - Neuropeptide Y is considered as major **neurobiologic brake**.

    In absence of estrogen, it inhibits gonadotropin secretion, while otherwise in presence of estrogen, it potentiates gonadotropin response to GnRH.

11. **b. Follistatin is secreted by granulosa cells**

    Ref: Speroff 8th/ed p 172

    - Follistatin is a peptide secreted by a variety of pituitary cells, including the gonadotropes.
    - Its main action: inhibition of FSH synthesis and secretion and the FSH response to GnRH, by binding to activin and in that fashion decreasing the activity of activin.
    - Activin stimulates follistatin production, and inhibin prevents this response.

12. **d. All**

    Ref: Kamini A Rao 2nd/ed p 23

    Opiate production is regulated by gene transcription and the synthesis of precursor peptides and at a post-translational level where the precursors are processed into the various bioactive smaller peptides.

    The endogenous opioids are three related families of naturally occurring substances produced in CNS that represent the natural ligands for opioid receptors.

    - *Proopiomelanocortin (POMC)*: The source of endorphins.
    - *Proenkephalin A and B*: The source of several enkephalins.
    - *Prodynorphin*: Yields dynorphins.

13. **d. Both of the above**

    Ref: Speroff 8th/ed p 177

    Corticotropin-releasing hormone (CRH) affects GnRH secretion by:
    1. Directly inhibiting hypothalamic GnRH secretion
    2. Augmenting endogenous opioid secretion.

    Besides the CRH-induced inhibition of GnRH release, the increase in cortisol generated by CRH stimulation of pituitary ACTH secretion also contributes to the suppression of reproduction; cortisol directly inhibits pituitary responsiveness to GnRH.

14. **a. High level of progesterone are responsible for the FSH surge at midcycle**

    Ref: Yen & Jaffe's 8th/ed p 18

    - Late follicular rise in progesterone begins approximately 12 hours before the LH surge may be important for the full expression of the midcycle gonadotropin surge.
    - Progesterone receptor antagonist mifepristone can delay the surge.
    - Low levels of progesterone acting at the level of the pituitary gland enhance the LH response to GnRH and are responsible for the FSH surge at midcycle.
    - Pineal gland is the source of gonadal inhibiting substances.

15. **c. Norepinephrine**

    Ref: Kamini A Rao 2nd/ed

    Catecholamines like norepinephrine, dopamine, serotonin and transmitters like opiates and prostaglandins appear to influence secretion of GnRH from hypothalamus.

    Norepinephrine seems to stimulate GnRH release, whereas dopamine, serotonin, endogenous opioids, and CRH appear capable of inhibiting or suppressing GnRH.

16. a. Composed of two dissimilar peptides linked by covalent bond
Ref: Kamini A Rao 2nd/ed p 23

- Inhibin is composed of two dissimilar peptides linked by **disulfide bonds**.

There are two forms of inhibin which are composed of one of the two inhibin beta subunits and a closely related alpha subunit to form inhibin A or inhibin B.

17. b. Inhibin potentiates activin activity
Ref: Kamini A Rao 2nd/ed p 23

Activin

- Derived from granulosa cells and pituitary gonadotrophs.
- Composed of two subunits identical to the b subunits of inhibin A and B.
- Augment FSH secretion but inhibit prolactin, ACTH, and growth hormone responses.
- Effects of activin are blocked by inhibin and follistatin.

18. a. Follistatin
Ref: Kamini A Rao 2nd/ed p 23

Follistatin

- Glycopeptide.
- Secreted by gonadotrophs.
- Also called FSH-suppressing protein involved in inhibiting FSH synthesis, secretion and FSH response to GnRH, by binding to and decreasing activity of activin.
- Activin stimulates follistatin production.

19. d. All
Ref: Speroff 8th/ed p 172

LH secretion is primarily regulated by GnRH, without involvement of the inhibin-activin-follistatin system, while FSH is controlled by other intrapituitary autocrine and paracrine system too apart from GnRH.

20. a. Endorphins promote GnRH release
Ref: Kamini A Rao 2nd/ed p 23

- Endorphins inhibit GnRH release within hypothalamus, resulting in inhibition of gonadotropin secretion but have no effect on pituitary response to GnRH.
- B endorphins are 5-10 times more potent than morphine
- Ovarian sex steroids increase central endorphin secretion, further depressing gonadotropin levels.
- Endorphin levels vary significantly throughout the menstrual cycle, with peak levels in the luteal phase and a nadir during menses.
- The dysphoria experienced by some women in the premenstrual phase of cycle may be related to a withdrawal of endogenous opiates.

21. d. All
Ref: Kamini A Rao 2nd/ed p 24

Effects of hyperprolactinemia on female reproductive function:
- Disrupts normal follicular development
- Atresia of dominant follicle
- Inhibits aromatase enzyme
- Inhibits progesterone synthesis by corpus luteum
- Premature destruction of corpus luteum
- Induces uterine adenomyosis

22. c. Induction of LH surge
Ref: Kamini A Rao 2nd/ed p 25

- LH surge is as a result of persistently raised estrogen levels.

Functions of FSH in menstrual cycle:
- Selection and maturation of dominant follicle
- Proliferation of granulosa cells
- Aromatization within granulosa cells
- Induction of FSH and LH receptors on granulosa cells
- Production of autocrine-paracrine factors- activin and inhibin
- FSH surge helps in ovulation
- Prevents germ cells from atresia in luteal- follicular transition

23. a. Follicular premature luteinization
Ref: Kamini A Rao 2nd/ed p 25, Textbook of assisted reproductive techniques, Vol 2, 5th/ed p 526

The amount of LH necessary to induce a response in the follicle varies from a minimum **"LH threshold"** to a maximum **"LH ceiling"**.

This amount has not been determined, but it has been suggested that **less than 1%** of follicular LH receptors need to be occupied in order to produce a steroidogenic response.

The LH dependent phase of menstrual cycle proceeds normally only if LH is present at concentrations within the LH window, which is over the threshold level and beneath the ceiling value.

The impact of different concentrations of LH on menstrual cycle is shown in the following table:

Effects below LH threshold	Effects within LH window	Effects above LH ceiling
Absent paracrine signalling between granulosa and theca	Normal follicular growth and development	Suppression of granulosa proliferation
Inadequate androgen and estrogen synthesis	Adequate granulosa proliferation and functional maturation	Follicular premature luteinisation

Contd...

Contd...

Effects below LH threshold	Effects within LH window	Effects above LH ceiling
Compromised oocyte maturation	Normal estrogen and androgen biosynthesis	Compromised oocyte development
	Optimum oocyte maturation	

24. d. GnRH

Ref: Textbook of assisted reproductive techniques, Vol 2, 5th/ed p 513

GnRH is secreted by hypothalamus, not anterior pituitary.

25. a. Corpus albicans

Ref: Kamini A Rao 2nd/ed p 35

Corpus luteum of nonpregnant cycle ultimately turns into corpus albicans.

26. a. Estradiol

Persistent high levels of estradiol are responsible for positive feedback loop in H-P-O axis leading to LH surge.

Low levels of estradiol inhibit FSH and LH.

27. c. FSH

Ref: Speroff 8th/ed p 202

FSH stimulates growth of primary follicle.

28. a. Progesterone

Ref: Speroff 8th/ed p 46

Progesterone is synthesized by corpus luteum.

Including the small contribution from the adrenal, the blood production rate of progesterone in preovulatory phase is less than 1 mg/day.

During luteal phase, production increases to 20-30 mg/day.

29. b. Inhibin B

Ref: Cambridge. Infertility in the male. 4th/ed p 23

- There is a reciprocal relationship between plasma FSH and inhibin B levels.

Inhibin is a glycoprotein hormone secreted by Sertoli cells composed of alpha subunit disulphide-linked to one of two beta subunits, to form inhibin A or B. Undetectable levels are seen in agonadal men and in men with testicular disorders, suggesting testicular origin.

CHAPTER 4

Endocrinology of Menstrual Cycle

Multiple Choice Questions

1. Maximum number of oocytes are seen at which stage of life?
   a. Early intrauterine life
   b. Late intrauterine life
   c. At birth
   d. At puberty

2. The total duration of time to achieve preovulatory status from secondary follicle state is:
   a. 14 days
   b. 85 days
   c. 28 days
   d. 120 days

3. The critical feature in rescuing a cohort of follicles from atresia eventually allowing a dominant follicle to emerge and pursue a path to ovulation:
   a. Increase in GnRH
   b. Increase in estrogen
   c. Increase in LH
   d. Increase in FSH

4. Fill in the blank: primordial follicle > .... > preantral follicle > preovulatory follicle:
   a. Primary follicle
   b. Antral follicle
   c. Ovulatory follicle
   d. None

5. The early visible signs of follicular development from primordial follicle stage:
   a. Increase in the size of the oocyte
   b. Granulosa cells becoming cuboidal
   c. Appearance of gap junctions
   d. All

6. Which of the following is most important inhibitor of primordial follicle growth?
   a. AMH   b. BMP
   c. Inhibin   d. Activin

7. Which of the following are promoters of primordial follicle growth?
   a. BMP
   b. Activin
   c. Neurotrophins
   d. All

8. Connexin expression in preovulatory follicles is up-regulated by FSH and down-regulated by LH. After ovulation, the gap junctions are important again in the corpus luteum, when their function is regulated by:
   a. Oxytocin
   b. Prolactin
   c. Estrogen
   d. Progesterone

9. Hormone produced by granulosa cells of preantral follicle:
   a. Estrogen
   b. Progesterone
   c. Androgen
   d. All

10. Aromatization is induced in granulosa cell through action of:
    a. FSH   b. LH
    c. Both a and b   d. Estrogen

11. The fate of the preantral follicle is in delicate balance between androgens and estrogens. Which of the following statement is not correct regarding this delicate balance?
    a. At low concentrations, androgens enhance their own aromatization
    b. At high concentrations, androgens are converted to more potent 5α-reduced androgens
    c. 5α androgens promote aromatase activity
    d. A successful follicle has estrogen-dominated microenvironment

12. **Premature elevation of LH in plasma and antral fluid leads to:**
    a. Decrease in mitotic activity in the granulosa cells
    b. Degenerative changes in follicle
    c. Rise in intrafollicular androgen levels
    d. All

13. **Antral follicles most likely to house a healthy oocyte have all of the following, except:**
    a. Highest estrogen concentrations
    b. Highest FSH receptors
    c. Lowest androgen concentrations
    d. High androgen/estrogen ratios

14. **Two cell two gonadotropin theory involves theca cell and granulosa cell. What is not correct for this theory?**
    a. Final stages of follicle maturation are optimised by FSH
    b. LH receptors are present only on the theca cells and FSH receptors only on granulosa cells
    c. Enzymes P450c17 is produced only in theca cells and P450arom only in granulosa cells
    d. Granulosa cells isolated from large antral follicles preferentially metabolize androgens to estrogens

15. **Which is correct regarding selection of dominant follicle?**
    a. Estrogen exerts a positive influence on FSH action within the maturing follicle
    b. Estrogen exerts negative feedback relationship with FSH at the hypothalamic-pituitary level
    c. First event in the process of atresia is a reduction in FSH receptors in the granulosa layer
    d. All

16. **Critical estradiol concentration and length of time during which estradiol elevation should be sustained for LH surge to occur?**
    a. 100 pg/mL, 50 hours
    b. 200 pg/mL, 50 hours
    c. 200 pg/mL, 30 hours
    d. 100 pg/mL, 30 hours

17. **Incorrect about the feedback system involved in endocrinology of menstrual cycle:**
    a. At low levels, estrogen exerts positive influence on LH
    b. At higher levels, estrogen exerts positive influence on LH
    c. At low levels, estrogen exerts negative influence on FSH
    d. At higher levels, estrogen exerts negative influence on FSH

18. **Relationship between inhibin and FSH is?**
    a. Inhibitory
    b. Stimulatory
    c. Reciprocal
    d. Synergistic

19. **Which is a wrong match?**
    a. Activin A: Alpha-Beta A
    b. Activin AB: Beta A-Beta B
    c. Inhibin-A: Alpha-Beta A
    d. Inhibin-B: Alpha-Beta B

20. **IGF-1 is synthesized in liver, mediated under influence of which hormone?**
    a. FSH
    b. Growth hormone
    c. LH
    d. ACTH

21. **Which of the following is not correct about autocrine-paracrine peptides?**
    a. Inhibin enhances LH stimulation of theca androgen synthesis
    b. Activin suppresses LH induced theca androgen synthesis
    c. Inhibin enhances aromatase activity
    d. Inhibin-B is the predominant inhibin in the follicular fluid of preantral follicles

22. **LH promotes luteinization of granulosa cells in dominant follicle. Which of the following is not correct regarding luteinization of preovulatory follicle?**
    a. High levels of preovulatory progesterone facilitates FSH surge
    b. Inhibits further cell growth by inhibiting granulosa cell mitosis
    c. Low levels of preovulatory progesterone facilitates LH surge
    d. LH stimulates P450scc and P450c17

23. **Ovulation occurs after .... hours of LH peak and .... hours of peak estradiol levels are attained:**
    a. 6, 24
    b. 10, 48
    c. 12, 36
    d. 24, 48

24. **LH Surge leads to all except:**
    a. Resumption of meiosis in oocyte
    b. Completion of meiosis in oocyte
    c. Cumulus expansion
    d. Prostaglandin production

25. **Progesterone-influenced midcycle rise in FSH leads to all *except*:**
    a. Cumulus expansion
    b. Inhibition of plasmin production
    c. LH receptors expression on granulosa cell
    d. Free the oocyte from follicular attachments

26. **Mechanisms responsible for shutting off of LH surge:**
    a. Loss of the positive stimulating action of estradiol
    b. Increasing negative feedback of progesterone
    c. Down-regulation of GnRH receptors
    d. All

27. **Cellular content of corpus luteum:**
    a. Luteal cells
    b. Endothelial cells
    c. Leukocytes
    d. All

28. **The luteal phase cannot be extended indefinitely even with progressively increasing LH exposure, indicating that the demise of the corpus luteum is due to an active luteolytic mechanism. Factors proposed to be responsible for luteolysis include all *except*:**
    a. Increased STARD1 expression
    b. PGF2α
    c. Endothelin-1
    d. TNF-α

29. **The rise in FSH at Luteal-follicular transition is attributed to decrease in all of the following hormones, *except*:**
    a. Inhibin A
    b. Inhibin B
    c. Progesterone
    d. Estrogen

30. **Which of the following is not the role of androgens in endocrinology of menstrual cycle?**
    a. Providing substrate for aromatization
    b. Enhancing atresia of less mature follicles
    c. Stimulating libido at periovulatory period
    d. Preovulatory progesterone rise

31. **Dominant follicle continues to grow even when FSH starts decreasing because of:**
    a. Greater FSH receptors
    b. High intrafollicular estrogen concentration
    c. Improved theca vasculature
    d. All

32. **Cyclooxygenase-2 inhibitors are associated with inhibition of ovulation by:**
    a. Blocking follicular rupture
    b. Inhibiting luteinization
    c. Inhibiting oocyte maturation
    d. Inhibiting cumulus expansion

Answer with Explanations

1. **a. Early intrauterine life**
   Ref: Yen & Jaffe's 8th/ed p 134; Kamini A Rao 2nd/ed p 29

   - Maximum number of oocytes is reached about **6–7 million** by **16–20 weeks** of gestation.
   - Rapid depletion occur before birth, resulting in **2 million oocytes at birth** and **3 lakhs at puberty**.
   - Out of these, about **400 follicles** will ovulate.

   ## Primordial Follicle Formation
   - Future components of mammalian ovary develop long before a distinct bipotential organ can be discerned.
   - During embryonic development, oocytes within the ovary are found as clusters, or germ cell cysts. These clusters form by both aggregation as well as clonal division.
   - Meiotic progression in oocytes ceases at the diplotene stage of prophase I when germ cells are enclosed by somatic cells into individual follicles called primordial follicles.
   - Oocytes in primordial follicles remain arrested until released to complete meiosis I during ovulation and form the "ovarian reserve", which is thought to ultimately determine reproductive lifespan.
   - The primordial germ cells originate in the **endoderm** of the yolk sac, allantois, and hindgut of the embryo, and by 5–6 weeks of gestation, they have migrated to the genital ridge.
   - A rapid mitotic multiplication of germ cells begins at 6–8 weeks of pregnancy, and by 16–20 weeks, the maximum number of oocytes is reached: a total of **6–7 million** in both ovaries.
   - The rate of decrease in follicle number is proportional to total number present, implying the most rapid decrease occurs before birth resulting in **2 million oocytes at birth** and **3 lakhs at puberty**. Out of these, about **400 follicles** will ovulate during a woman's reproductive years.

2. **b. 85 days**
   Ref: Kamini A Rao 2nd/ed p 30

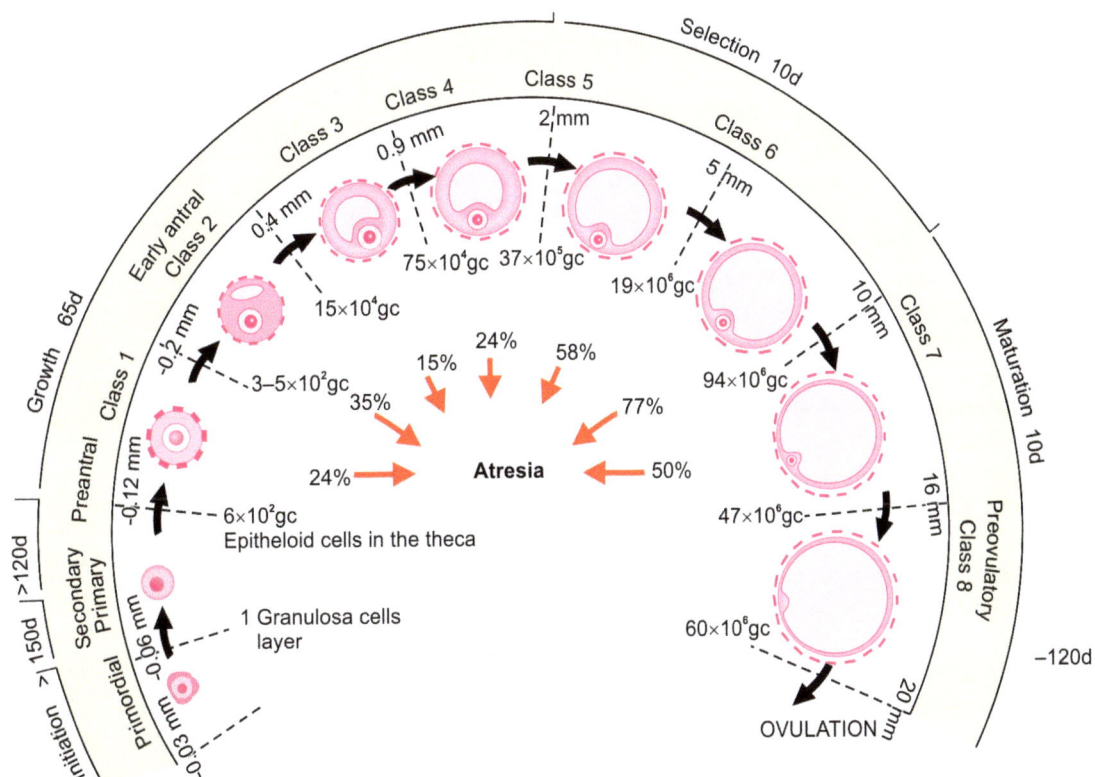

- The total duration of time to achieve preovulatory status is approximately **85 days**.

The early growth of follicles occurs over the time span of several menstrual cycles.

- The follicle destined to ovulate is one of a cohort recruited at the time of the **luteal-follicular transition**.
- Until follicle reaches **antral stage**, the growth is independent of hormonal regulation.
- Eventually, this cohort of follicles reaches a stage where, unless recruited or rescued by FSH, it is doomed toward apoptosis.

3. **d. Increase in FSH**

   Ref: Yen & Jaffe's 8th/ed p 149

- Normal reproductive function in women involves repetitive cycles of follicle development, ovulation and preparation of the endometrium for implantation should conception occur in that cycle.
- This pattern of regular ovulatory cycles is achieved through precise functional and temporal integration of stimulatory and inhibitory signals from the hypothalamus, the pituitary and the ovary.
- The reproductive system functions in a classic endocrine mode initiated by pulsatile secretion of GnRH from the hypothalamus into the pituitary portal venous system.
- GnRH regulates the synthesis and subsequent release of FSH and LH from the anterior pituitary into the circulation.
- FSH and LH stimulate ovarian follicular development, ovulation, and corpus luteum formation and the coordinated secretion of estradiol, progesterone, inhibin A, and inhibin B.
- A key component of this system is the modulatory effect of ovarian steroids and inhibins on gonadotropin secretion, acting either directly at the pituitary level or through alterations in the amplitude or frequency of GnRH secretion.
- Negative feedback restraint of FSH secretion is critical to the development of the single mature oocyte that characterizes human reproductive cycles.
- In addition to negative feedback controls, the menstrual cycle is unique among endocrine systems in its dependence on estrogen positive feedback to produce the preovulatory LH surge that is essential for ovulation.
- An increase in FSH is the critical feature in rescuing a cohort of follicles from atresia, the usual fate of most follicles, eventually allowing a dominant follicle to emerge and pursue a path to ovulation.
- In addition, maintenance of this increase in FSH for a critical duration of time is essential. Without the appearance and persistence of an increase in the circulating FSH level, the cohort is doomed to the process of apoptosis.
- So, both a critical level of FSH as well as a critical duration of FSH are mandatory for a dominant follicle to emerge.

4. **a. Primary follicle**

   Ref: Speroff 8th/ed p 200

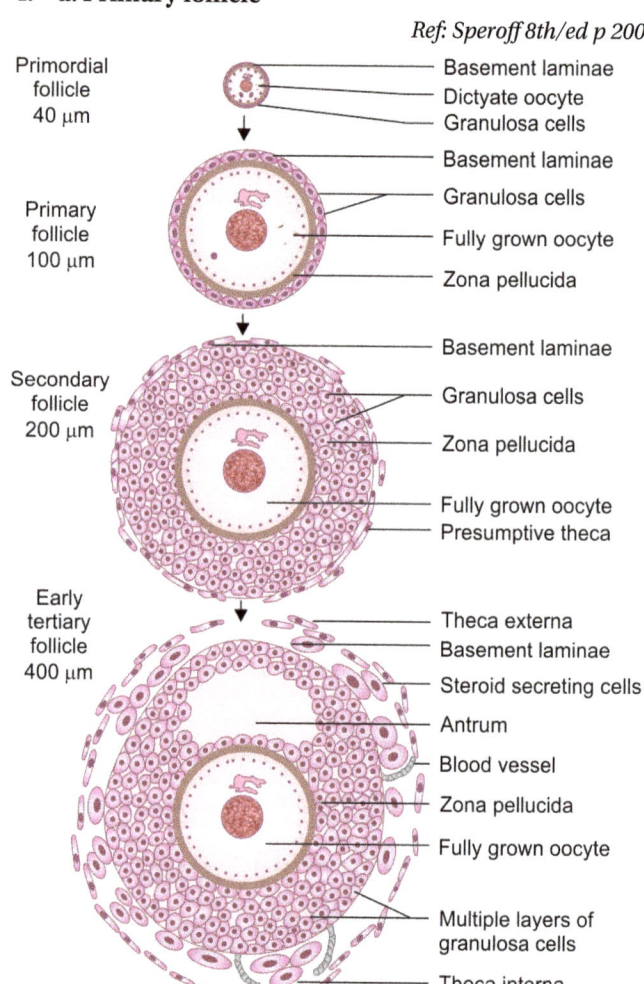

Stages of Follicle Development

Primordial follicle> primary follicle> secondary follicle> preantral follicle> antral follicle> preovulatory follicle > ovulatory follicle

5. **d. All**

   Ref: Speroff 8th/ed p 201

- The gap junctions serve as the pathway for nutritional, metabolite, and signal interchange between the granulosa cells and the oocyte.

The first visible signs of follicular development are:
- An increase in the **size** of the oocyte.
- Granulosa cells becoming **cuboidal** rather than squamous in shape.
- Appearance of **gap junctions** between granulosa cell and oocyte.

Gap Junction as Pathway for Maturation

- In one direction, inhibition of the final maturation of the oocyte (until the LH surge) is maintained by factors derived from the granulosa cells.
- In the other direction, the process of follicular growth is influenced by regulatory factors that originate in the oocyte.

These changes are better viewed as a process of maturation rather than growth.

6. a. AMH

Ref: Yen & Jaffe's 8th/ed p 136

Anti-Mullerian Hormone

- TGFβ family member
- Important as regulator of early follicle development, particularly for inhibition of primordial follicle activation.
- Involved in regression of the Müllerian duct during male reproductive tract development.
- In the ovary, AMH is expressed from granulosa cells of growing follicles until their development becomes dependent upon FSH at the later antral stages.
- AMH negatively regulates primordial follicle activation.
- Serum levels of AMH correlate with the number of antral follicles, and both decline with age.
- Thus, AMH has become a marker of ovarian reserve as well as reproductive disease in women.

7. d. All

Ref: Speroff 8th/ed p 202

Activins, inhibins, anti-Müllerian hormone (AMH) and bone morphogenetic proteins (BMPs) are members of the TGF-β family of proteins.

Activins promote and inhibins retard primordial follicle development, and their relative local concentrations in the fetal ovary during the time of follicle assembly may determine the size of the ovarian follicular pool.

AMH is an important inhibitor of primordial follicle growth, and BMPs exert the opposite effect.

Four mammalian neurotrophins involved in follicular development:
1. Nerve growth factor (NGF)
2. Brain-derived neurotropic factor (BDNF)
3. Neurotrophin-3 (NT-3)
4. Neurotrophin 4/5 (NT-4/5)

All of these exert their actions via binding to high-affinity transmembrane tyrosine kinase receptors.

8. a. Oxytocin

Ref: Speroff 8th/ed p 202

The Gap Junctions and Follicular Growth

- The gap junction is composed of channels formed by an arrangement of proteins known as connexins, and more recently as GJAs.
- The connexin gap junctions are essential for growth and multiplication of the granulosa cells, and for the nutrition and regulation of oocyte development.
- Connexin expression in ovarian follicles is up-regulated by FSH and down-regulated by LH.
- FSH maintains an open channel in the gap junctions, a pathway that is closed by LH.
- After ovulation, the gap junctions are important again in the corpus luteum, when their function is regulated by locally produced oxytocin.

9. d. All

Ref: Speroff 8th/ed p 203

- Preantral stage is reached when oocyte enlarges and is surrounded by a membrane, the zona pellucida.
- The granulosa cells undergo a multilayer proliferation as the theca layer continues to organize from the surrounding stroma.
- This growth is dependent upon gonadotropins and is correlated with increasing production of estrogen.
- Steroidogenesis in the ovarian follicle is mainly regulated by the gonadotropins.
- The granulosa cells of the preantral follicles have the ability to synthesize all three classes of steroids; however, significantly more estrogens than either androgens or progestins are produced.

10. a. FSH

Ref: Yen & Jaffe's 8th/ed p 76

- An aromatase enzyme system acts to convert androgens to estrogens and is a factor limiting ovarian estrogen production.
- Aromatization is induced or activated through the action of FSH.
- FSH act on granulosa cells to stimulate aromatization of androgens to estrogens.

11. c. 5α androgens promote aromatase activity

Ref: Speroff 8th/ed p 204

- The success of a follicle depends upon its ability to convert an androgen-dominated microenvironment to an estrogen-dominated microenvironment.

The fate of the preantral follicle is in delicate balance. At low concentrations, androgens enhance their own aromatization and contribute to estrogen production.

When exposed to an androgen-rich environment, preantral granulosa cells favor the conversion of androgens to more potent 5α-reduced androgens rather than to estrogens.

These androgens cannot be converted to estrogen and, in fact, inhibit aromatase activity. They also inhibit FSH induction of LH receptor formation.

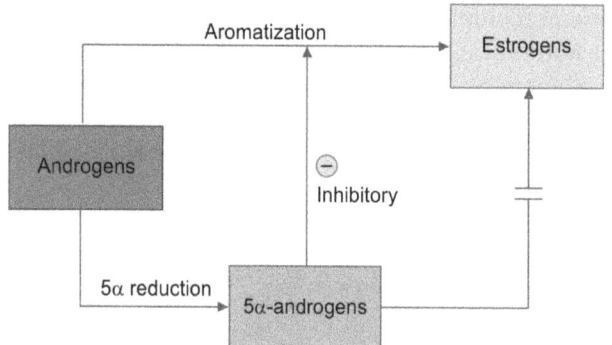

12. d. All

Ref: Speroff 8th/ed p 205

LH is not normally present in follicular fluid until the midcycle. Premature LH elevation in plasma and antral fluid leads to:
1. Decrease in mitotic activity in the granulosa cells
2. Degenerative changes in follicle
3. Rise in intrafollicular androgen levels

Therefore, the dominance of estrogen and FSH is essential for sustained accumulation of granulosa cells and continued follicular growth.

13. d. High Androgen/estrogen ratio

Ref: Speroff 8th/ed p 205; Kamini A Rao 2nd/ed p 30

Antral follicles most likely to house a healthy oocyte have:
- Highest estrogen concentrations
- Highest FSH receptors
- Lowest androgen/estrogen ratios

An androgenic milieu antagonizes estrogen-induced granulosa proliferation and, if sustained, promotes degenerative changes in the oocyte.

14. a. Final stages of follicular maturation are optimised by FSH

Ref: Speroff 8th/ed p 206; Kamini A Rao 2nd/ed p 32

Two Cell Two Gonadotropin Theory

This theory involves two cells as theca cell and granulosa cell and two gonadotropins as LH and FSH. The following concepts are very important regarding the theory:

- Final stages of follicle maturation are **optimised by** FSH is false as it is **LH** who is responsible for final maturation of oocyte increasing the amount of androgen substrate for estrogen production and promoting the growth of the dominant follicle while simultaneously hastening the regression of smaller follicles.
- LH receptors are present only on the theca cells and FSH receptors only on granulosa cells in early follicular phase.
- As the follicle emerges, the theca cells are characterized by their expression of P450c17, the enzyme step which is rate-limiting for the conversion of 21-carbon substrate to androgens. Granulosa cells do not express this enzyme and thus are dependent upon androgens from the theca in order to make estrogen. Increasing expression of the aromatization system (P450arom) is a marker of increasing maturity of granulosa cells.
- Granulosa cells from preantral and small antral follicles have tendency to convert androgen to the more potent 5α-reduced form.
- In contrast, granulosa cells isolated from large antral follicles preferentially metabolize androgens to estrogens.
- The conversion from an androgen microenvironment to an estrogen microenvironment is dependent upon a growing sensitivity to FSH brought about by the action of FSH and the enhancing influence of estrogen.

15. d. All

Ref: Speroff 8th/ed p 207; Kamini A Rao 2nd/ed p 32

- First event in the process of atresia is a reduction in FSH receptors in the granulosa layer.

This selection process is the result of two estrogen actions:
1. Local interaction between estrogen and FSH within the follicle—estrogen exerts a positive influence on FSH action within the maturing follicle
2. The effect of estrogen on pituitary secretion of FSH—estrogen exerts a negative feedback relationship with FSH at the hypothalamic-pituitary level which serves to withdraw gonadotropin support from the other less developed follicles.

The fall in FSH leads to a decline in FSH-dependent aromatase activity, limiting estrogen production in the less mature follicles.

The dominant follicle has two significant advantages:
a. A greater content of FSH receptors
b. High intrafollicular estrogen concentration.

16. b. 200 pg/mL, 50 hours
Ref: Speroff 8th/ed p 210; Kamini A Rao 2nd/ed p 33

- In women, the estradiol concentration necessary to achieve a positive feedback is more than 200 pg/mL, and this concentration must be sustained for approximately 50 hours.
- This level of estrogen essentially never occurs until the dominant follicle has reached a diameter of 15 mm.

The two critical features for LH surge to occur:
1. The **concentration** of estradiol and
2. The **length of time** during which the estradiol elevation is sustained.

The estrogen stimulus must be sustained beyond the initiation of the LH surge until after the surge actually begins. Otherwise, the LH surge is abbreviated or fails to occur at all.

17. a. At low levels, estrogen exerts positive influence on LH
Ref: Speroff 8th/ed p 210; Kamini A Rao 2nd/ed p 32

One should remember following points regarding '**The feedback system in endocrinology of menstrual cycle**':

- The secretion of FSH is very sensitive to the negative inhibitory effects of estrogen even at low levels.
- At higher levels, estrogen combines with inhibin for a suppression of FSH that is profound and sustained.
- In contrast, the influence of estrogen on LH release varies with concentration and duration of exposure.
- At **low levels**, estrogen imposes a **negative** feedback relationship with LH.
- At **higher levels**, however, estrogen exert a **positive** stimulatory feedback effect on LH release.

18. c. Reciprocal
Ref: Yen & Jaffe's 8th/ed p21

FSH stimulates the secretion of inhibin from granulosa cells and, in turn, is suppressed by inhibin—a reciprocal relationship.

Inhibins are heterodimer peptide members of TGF-β superfamily with two isoforms, inhibin A and B.

The chief function of both inhibins is to inhibit FSH release from pituitary gonadotropes.

19. a. Activin A: Alpha-Beta A
Ref: Yen & Jaffe's 8th/ed p21; Speroff 8th/ed p 213

Now this is an important concept regarding members of TGF-β superfamily:

- Inhibin consists of two dissimilar peptides (known as alpha- and beta-subunits) linked by disulfide bonds. They have identical alpha-subunit and distinct but related beta-subunits.

There are three subunits for inhibins: alpha, beta-A, and beta-B. Each subunit is a product of different messenger RNA, each derived from its own precursor molecule.

The 2 forms of inhibin:
- Inhibin-A: Alpha-Beta A
- Inhibin-B: Alpha-Beta B

- Activin, derived from granulosa cells, but present as well in the pituitary gonadotropes, contains two subunits that are identical to the beta subunits of inhibins A and B.

The 3 forms of activin:
- Activin A: Beta A-Beta A
- Activin AB: Beta A-Beta B
- Activin B: Beta B-Beta B

20. b. Growth hormone
Ref: Speroff 8th/ed p 214

A few facts you should remember about IGF:

- The insulin-like growth factors (also called somatomedins) are peptides that have structural and functional similarity to insulin
- The majority of circulating IGF-I is derived from growth hormone-dependent synthesis in the liver.
- IGF-II has little growth hormone dependence. It is believed to be important in fetal growth and development.
- IGF-II is produced in theca cells, granulosa cells, and luteinized granulosa cells. IGF-I receptors are not present on luteinized granulosa cells.
- IGF-II is the primary IGF in the human ovary.
- Laron-type dwarfism is characterized by a deficiency in IGF-I due to an abnormality in the growth hormone receptor.

21. c. Inhibin enhances aromatase activity
Ref: Speroff 8th/ed p 222

Following important points you must remember regarding autocrine-paracrine peptides:

- Inhibin enhances LH stimulation of theca androgen synthesis
- Activin suppresses LH induced theca androgen synthesis
- Inhibin can overcome the inhibitory action of activin on theca cells.
- Activin augments all FSH activities, especially aromatase activity. (Not inhibin)
- Activin suppresses androgen production, allowing the emergence of an estrogen microenvironment.
- Inhibin-B is the predominant inhibin in the follicular fluid of preantral follicles and inhibin-A increases when follicles become large and mature.

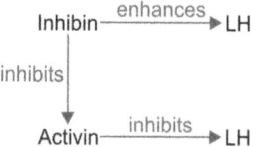

22. a. High level of preovulatory progesterone facilitates FSH surge
Ref: Speroff 8th/ed p 227; Yen & Jaffe's 8th/ed p 19

Acting through its own receptors, LH promotes luteinization of the granulosa in the dominant follicle, resulting in the production of progesterone. Following points must be kept in mind regarding preovulaory luteinization:

- It is the low levels of progesterone which facilitates FSH surge
- Preovulatory progesterone and progesterone receptor expression directly inhibit granulosa cell mitosis, limiting granulosa cell proliferation as these cells gain LH receptors.
- Low levels of preovulatory progesterone facilitates LH surge. High levels of progesterone blocks the midcycle LH surge.
- LH stimulates P450scc and P450c17, important enzymes for production of theca androgens, the substrate for granulosa estrogen.

23. c. 12, 36
Ref: Speroff 8th/ed p 228; Yen & Jaffe's 8th/ed p 189

Some data which should be remembered:
- Ovulation occur approximately **10-12 hours** after the LH peak and **24-36 hours** after peak estradiol levels are attained.
- The LH surge occur **34-36 hours** prior to follicle rupture.
- A threshold of LH concentration must be maintained for **14-27 hours** for full maturation of the oocyte to occur.
- Usually the LH surge lasts **48-50 hours**.
- Ovulation occurs more frequently in the **right ovary**.
- Oocytes from the **right ovary** have a higher potential for pregnancy.

24. b. Completion of meiosis in oocyte
Ref: Yen & Jaffe's 8th/ed p 130

The role of LH surge:
- Resumption of meiosis in the oocyte—meiosis is not completed until after the sperm has entered and the second polar body is released
- Terminal differentiation of the remaining granulosa and thecal cells to create corpus luteum
- Expansion of the cumulus; which is the production of a hyaluronan-rich extracellular matrix surrounding the oocyte, required for normal ovulation and fertilization.
- Synthesis of prostaglandins and other eicosanoids essential for follicle rupture.

25. b. Inhibition of plasmin production
Ref: Speroff 8th/ed p 232

The progesterone-influenced midcycle rise in FSH has following roles:
- Free the oocyte from follicular attachments
- Convert plasminogen to the proteolytic enzyme, plasmin
- Ensures that sufficient LH receptors are present to allow an adequate normal luteal phase
- Expansion and dispersion of the cumulus cells

26. d. All
Ref: Speroff 8th/ed p 232; Yen & Jaffe's 8th/ed p 164

The mechanism that shuts off the LH surge is unknown. However following theories are proposed:
- Loss of the positive stimulating action of estradiol
- Increasing negative feedback of progesterone
- Down-regulation of GnRH receptors
- Gonadotropin surge-inhibiting factor (GnSIF) originating in the granulosa cells of ovary

Gonadotropin surge-inhibiting factor (GnSIF), also known as Gonadotropin surge-Attenuating factor (GnSAF), is an ovarian factor that reduces GnRH-induced LH secretion.

27. d. All
Ref: Speroff 8th/ed p 234

- The nonsteroidogenic cells form the bulk, about 70%, of the total cell population.

The corpus luteum is not homogeneous. Besides the luteal cells, also present are endothelial cells, leukocytes, and fibroblasts.

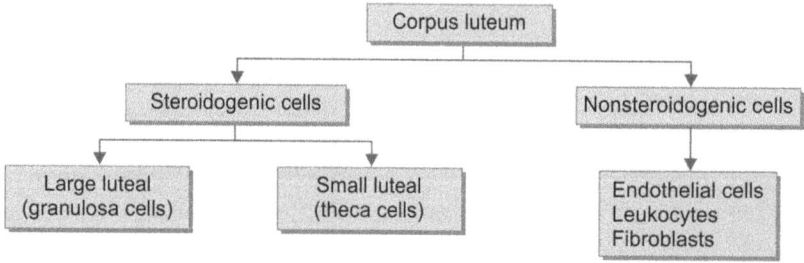

28. a. Increased STARD1 expression
Ref: Yen & Jaffe's 8th/ed p 195; Speroff 8th/ed p 236

- The functional life span of corpus luteum in a nonfertile cycle is normally 14+/−2 days.

Unless pregnancy occurs, the corpus luteum is transformed into an avascular scar referred to as the **corpus albicans**.

No definite luteolytic factor has been identified.

The morphological regression of luteal cells may be induced by the estradiol produced by the corpus luteum, mediated by nitric oxide.

Nitric oxide leads to:
- Prostaglandin synthesis
- Decreased progesterone production
- Luteal cells apoptosis

The final signal for luteolysis, however, is **prostaglandin $F_{2\alpha}$**, acting as physiological luteolysin.

Prostaglandin $F_{2\alpha}$ stimulates the synthesis of endothelin-1

Endothelin-1:
- Inhibits luteal steroidogenesis
- Stimulates prostaglandin production in luteal cells
- Stimulates the release of TNF-α, a growth factor known to induce apoptosis

A fall in STARD1 expression results in diminished progesterone production and hence luteolysis.

29. b. Inhibin B
Ref: Kamini A Rao 2nd/ed p 36

The selective rise in FSH at Luteal-follicular transition is attributed to 3 factors:
1. Demise of corpus luteum results in nadir in circulating levels of progesterone, estradiol and inhibin.
2. Decrease in negative feedback effect of luteal steroids and inhibin, particularly inhibin A. (Inhibin B is seen in follicular phase)
3. Change in pulsatile GnRH secretion toward an increasing pulse frequency which favors predominant FSH secretion. There is a 4.5-fold increase in GnRH pulse frequency with FSH pulse frequency rising to 3.5 fold and LH pulse frequency rising to 2 fold.

30. d. Preovulatory progesterone rise
Ref: Speroff 8th/ed p 228

Role of androgens in endocrinology of menstrual cycle:
i. Providing substrate for aromatization into estrogens within granulosa cells at low levels promoting estrogenic microenvironment
ii. Enhancing atresia of less mature follicles
iii. Systemic effect of stimulating libido at periovulatory period

31. d. All
Ref: Speroff 8th/ed p 208; Yen & Jaffe's 8th/ed p 171

Dominant follicle continues to grow even when FSH starts decreasing because dominant follicle is at advantage:
i. Greater content of **FSH receptors**.
ii. High **intrafollicular estrogen** concentration due to local autocrine-paracrine molecules.
iii. Improved theca **vasculature** allows preferential delivery of gonadotropins to dominant follicle.

32. a. Blocking follicular rupture
Ref: Speroff 8th/ed p 231

Role of prostaglandins in ovulation
- Prostaglandin synthesis is stimulated by interleukin-1b, implicating this cytokine in ovulation.
- Inhibition of cyclooxygenase-2 (COX-2) synthesis blocks follicle rupture without affecting the other LH-induced processes of luteinization and oocyte maturation.
- Prostaglandins act to free **proteolytic enzymes** within the follicular wall.

CHAPTER 5

Endocrinology of Pregnancy

Multiple Choice Questions

1. The massive amount of progesterone produced in pregnancy is derived from:
   a. Placental-maternal cooperation
   b. Placental-fetal cooperation
   c. Placenta produces its own progesterone
   d. Comes from corpus luteum

2. Major source of progesterone until about 10 weeks of gestation:
   a. Placenta   b. Fetus
   c. Corpus luteum   d. Adrenal gland

3. Major source of progesterone after 10 weeks of gestation:
   a. Corpus luteum   b. Placenta
   c. Fetus   d. Adrenal gland

4. Progesterone production by the placenta is largely dependent on:
   a. Maternal cholesterol
   b. Quantity of precursor available
   c. Uteroplacental perfusion
   d. Fetal well-being

5. The substrate for fetal adrenal gland production of glucocorticoids and mineralocorticoids:
   a. Estradiol   b. Androgens
   c. Cortisol   d. Progesterone

6. The vast majority of estrogen excreted in the maternal urine is derived from:
   a. Fetal androgens
   b. Maternal ovary
   c. Peripheral conversion
   d. Maternal androgens

7. Estrogen produced in greatest quantity during pregnancy:
   a. Estrone
   b. Estradiol
   c. Estriol
   d. Different trimesters have different levels

8. Adrenal gland from outer to inner is named as:
   a. Zona glomerulosa>zona fasciculata>zona reticularis
   b. Zona reticularis>zona fasciculata> zona glomerulosa
   c. Zona glomerulosa>zona reticularis>zona fasciculata
   d. Zona fasciculata>zona glomerulosa>zona reticularis

9. Screening for fetal aneuploidy utilizes which estrogen in the maternal circulation?
   a. Total blood estriol   b. Unconjugated estriol
   c. Estradiol   d. Estetrol

10. A family history of scaling in males as well as repeated postdate pregnancies and cesarean sections prompt which disorder?
    a. Placental sulfatase deficiency
    b. Placental aromatase deficiency
    c. Congenital adrenal hyperplasia
    d. Adrenal insufficiency

11. Which of the following is not correct for placental sulfatase deficiency?
    a. X-linked metabolic disease
    b. Preterm delivery
    c. Mostly males affected
    d. Ichthyosis

12. The characteristic steroid findings in placental sulfatase deficiency all *except:*
    a. High amniotic fluid DHEA and androstenedione
    b. Low maternal estriol levels
    c. Low maternal estetrol levels
    d. High amniotic fluid DHEAS levels

13. Extremely low levels of estriol are seen in all of the following *except:*
    a. Placental sulfatase deficiency
    b. Placental aromatase deficiency
    c. Diabetes mellitus
    d. Intrauterine death

14. Glycoprotein hormone with highest sialic acid content:
    a. FSH
    b. LH
    c. Human placental lactogen
    d. Human chorionic gonadotropin

15. Long half life of hCG is due to:
    a. Sialic acid
    b. Fructose
    c. Mannose
    d. Galactosamine

16. Which of the following is not true regarding human chorionic gonadotropin?
    a. Beta subunit has unique carboxyl terminal peptide
    b. Produced only by placenta
    c. Four sites of glycosylation
    d. Half life 24 hours

17. After how many weeks, removal of corpus luteum will not be followed by steroid withdrawal abortion?
    a. 7 weeks
    b. 10 weeks
    c. 14 weeks
    d. 20 weeks

18. Exogenous support for an early pregnancy until 10 weeks requires how much of progesterone daily?
    a. 50 mg
    b. 100 mg
    c. 200 mg
    d. 300 mg

19. There is virtual absence of which enzyme in the placenta?
    a. P450 c17
    b. P450 arom
    c. 3β-hydroxysteroid dehydrogenase
    d. P450 scc

20. Fetus supplies androgens to placenta in order to synthesize estrogens. What does fetus borrow from placenta?
    a. Estrogen
    b. Cholesterol
    c. Progesterone
    d. Androgen

21. Which of the following statements about human chorionic gonadotropin are not correct?
    a. The β subunit of hCG has multigenic expression
    b. Levels of hCG are lower in women carrying female fetuses
    c. DNA sequence of β-hCG genes and β-LH genes are 96% identical
    d. Synthesized in syncytiotrophoblast

22. Which of the following hormones are not secreted by placenta?
    a. Relaxin
    b. Somatostatin
    c. CRH
    d. TRH

23. Maternal circulating hCG concentration at the time of expected but missed periods:
    a. 50 IU/L
    b. 100 IU/L
    c. 200 IU/L
    d. 10 IU/L

24. Which of the following statements does not hold true for hCG?
    a. Hyperglycosylated hCG increases with gestation
    b. Synthesized mainly in the syncytiotrophoblast
    c. Maximal level of about 100,000 IU/L in the maternal circulation is reached at 8–10 weeks
    d. Can be detected in 8-cell stage embryo

25. Which statement is not true regarding hyperglycosylated hCG?
    a. Choriocarcinoma is associated with the increased hyperglycosylated hCG
    b. Maximum expression in 2nd trimester
    c. Plays a role in regulating trophoblastic invasion
    d. A low level may predict a failing pregnancy

26. The cholesterol utilized for progesterone synthesis enters trophoblast from maternal bloodstream as:
    a. LDL
    b. HDL
    c. VLDL
    d. Triglycerides

27. What is true about progestrone concentrations in pregnancy?
    a. Increase with advancing gestations
    b. Three times higher in myometrium
    c. Amniotic fluid concentrations are maximal between 10 and 20 weeks
    d. All

28. Which of the following are not correct for human placental lactogen?
    a. Secreted by cytotrophoblast
    b. Also known as human chorionic somatomammotropin
    c. Single chain polypeptide
    d. Similar in structure to growth hormone

29. True statement regarding hPL:
    a. Growth hormone-releasing hormone and somatostatin influence placental hPL secretion
    b. The level of hPL in the maternal circulation is correlated with fetal and placental weight
    c. Significant contribution in lactation in humans
    d. Improves insulin resistance in pregnancy

30. **Which of the following holds true regarding metabolic functions of hPL?**
    a. Stimulates lipolysis
    b. Stimulates insulin secretion
    c. Hypoglycemia promotes hPL secretion
    d. All

31. **Which of the following is incorrect regarding thyrotropic activity of hCG?**
    a. hCG is the only hormone released by placenta which has thyrotropic activity
    b. hCG has 1/4,000th of the thyrotropic activity of human TSH
    c. Hydatidiform mole can lead to hyperthyroidism
    d. Hyperemesis gravidarum patients may develop hyperthyroidism

32. **Incorrect statement about alpha fetoprotein:**
    a. Glycoprotein
    b. Derived from fetal liver and yolk sac
    c. In early pregnancy, amniotic fluid AFP comes from fetal liver
    d. Works as a protein carrier of steroid hormones in fetal blood

33. **Conditions associated with low alpha fetoprotein levels:**
    a. Trisomy 18
    b. Multiple pregnancy
    c. IUGR
    d. Neural tube defects

34. **All are associated with high alpha protein *except*:**
    a. Omphalocele
    b. Preeclampsia
    c. Preterm birth
    d. Down syndrome

35. **Which of the following statements is incorrect regarding relaxin?**
    a. Peptide hormone
    b. Levels keep on rising throughout pregnancy
    c. Produced by corpus luteum of pregnancy
    d. Helps in cervical ripening

36. **Decidualized endometrium secretes:**
    a. Renin
    b. Relaxin
    c. Prolactin
    d. All

37. **Which of the following is least likely to produce prolactin during pregnancy?**
    a. Fetal pituitary
    b. Fetal membranes
    c. Maternal pituitary
    d. Decidua

38. **Prolactin in amniotic fluid comes from:**
    a. Decidua
    b. Fetal membranes
    c. Maternal pituitary
    d. Fetal pituitary

39. **Schwangerschafts protein 1 is also known as:**
    a. Pregnancy-specific γ_1-glycoprotein (PSG)
    b. Pregnancy associated plasma protein-A (PAPP-A)
    c. Progesterone associated endometrial protein
    d. Placental protein 14

40. **Which of the following is incorrect regarding role of leptin in pregnancy?**
    a. The placenta is the principal source of leptin during pregnancy
    b. Leptin levels decline to normal nonpregnant values within 24 hours of delivery
    c. Leptin levels remain constant throughout pregnancy
    d. Abnormally high placental leptin production is associated with maternal diabetes mellitus and hypertension

Endocrinology of Pregnancy

Answer with Explanations

1. a. Placental-maternal cooperation
Ref: Speroff 8th/ed p 270

The placenta is an important endocrine organ. You must remember that placenta converts little, if any, acetate to cholesterol or its precursors. So, from where the progesterone comes from?

- Cholesterol and pregnenolone are obtained from the maternal bloodstream for progesterone synthesis.

The fetal contribution is negligible because progesterone levels remain high after fetal demise.

Thus, the massive amount of progesterone produced in pregnancy depends on **placental-maternal cooperation**, although some have argued that the fetal liver is an important source of cholesterol.

2. c. Corpus luteum
Ref: Yen & Jaffe's 8th/ed p 195

- In a cycle of conception, the corpus luteum is rescued from luteolysis by appearance of trophoblast-derived hCG.

In the corpus luteum of late pregnancy, hCG suppresses apoptosis, allowing structural maintenance of the gland and sustaining expression of the STARD1 gene.

- The progressively rising concentrations of this luteotropin, first detectable in peripheral blood **8 days** after ovulation, both stimulates steroidogenesis and prevents structural involution of the gland, which is major source of progesterone for first 10 weeks of gestation.

3. b. Placenta
Ref: Speroff 8th/ed p 271

- At term, progesterone levels range from 100 to 200 ng/mL.
- The term placenta produces about 250 mg/day.

After a transition period of shared function between the 7th week and 10th week, the placenta emerges as the major source of progesterone synthesis.

4. a. Maternal cholesterol
Ref: Speroff 8th/ed p 271

- The majority of placental progesterone is derived from maternal cholesterol that is readily available.

Progesterone production by the placenta is largely independent of:
- Quantity of precursor available
- Uteroplacental perfusion
- Fetal well-being

This is because the fetus contributes essentially no precursor.

5. d. Progesterone
Ref: Speroff 8th/ed p 273

- Progesterone serves as the substrate for fetal adrenal gland production of glucocorticoids and mineralocorticoids.
- The fetus lacks significant activity of the 3β-hydroxysteroid dehydrogenase, D^{4-5} isomerase system so produces steroids with a 3β-hydroxy-D^5 configuration like pregnenolone and DHEA, rather than 3-keto-D^4 products such as progesterone.
- Thus, the fetus must borrow progesterone from the placenta to circumvent this lack in order to synthesize the biologically important corticosteroids.
- In return, the fetus supplies what the placenta lacks: 19-carbon compounds to serve as precursors for estrogens.

So, one thing you should remember:
- Placenta lacks 17 hydroxylase system
- Fetus lacks 3β-HSD system
Based on this, you can solve many MCQs.

6. a. Fetal androgens
Ref: Yen & Jaffe's, 8th/ed p 256

- The fetal adrenals secrete more than 200 mg of DHEAS daily, about 10 times more than the mother.
- Estrogens are synthesized by **human placenta** from C19 steroids.
- The principal precursor used for placental estrogen formation is DHEA-S, supplied mainly by fetal adrenal glands.
- By the 20th week of pregnancy, the vast majority of estrogen excreted in the maternal urine is derived from fetal androgens.
- Approximately 90% of estriol excretion can be accounted for by DHEAS production by the fetal adrenal gland.
- The maternal contribution of DHEAS to total estrogen synthesis must be negligible because, in the absence

of normal fetal adrenal glands (as in an anencephalic infant), maternal estrogen levels and excretion are extremely low.

7. c. Estriol

Ref: Yen & Jaffe's 8th/ed p 256; Speroff 8th/ed p 276

Estriol in Pregnancy

- Estriol is the **major estrogen** produced in greatest quantity during pregnancy, which has an additional hydroxyl group at position 16.
- Estriol constitutes more than 90% of the estrogen in pregnancy urine, into which it is excreted as sulfate and glucuronide conjugates.
- Estriol is first detectable at 9 weeks when the fetal adrenal gland secretion of precursor begins.
- Estriol concentrations plateau at 31–35 weeks and then increase again at 35–36 weeks.
- Estriol concentrations increase with advancing gestation and range from 2 mg/24 hours at 26 weeks to 35-45 mg/24 hours at term.
- At term, the concentration of estriol in the maternal circulation is 8 to 13 ng/dL.
- In contrast, ovarian production of estriol in nonpregnant women is barely detectable.
- During pregnancy, estrone and estradiol production is increased about 100 times.
- The increase in maternal estriol excretion is about a thousand-fold.

8. a. Zona glomerulosa>zona fasciculata>zona reticularis

Ref: Inderbir Singh's Human embryology 11th/ed p 315

The adrenal gland consists of a superficial cortex and a deeper medulla.
- The cells of the cortex arise from coelomic epithelium.
- The cells of medulla derived from neural crest cells.

Fetal adrenal gland consists of:
1. Outer definitive zone, zona glomerulosa,
2. The transitional zone, zona fasciculata and
3. The zona reticularis.

(Remember it as GFR)

- Fetal adrenal gland begins to develop in the 5th week of intrauterine life.

9. b. Unconjugated estriol

Ref: Speroff 8th/ed p 298

Screening for fetal aneuploidy utilizes three markers in the maternal circulation:
1. Alpha fetoprotein,
2. Human chorionic gonadotropin
3. Unconjugated estriol

10. a. Placental sulfatase deficiency

Ref: Speroff 8th/ed p 282

Placental Sulfatase Deficiency

- **X-linked** metabolic disease
- Characterized by a **placental sulfatase deficiency** in the syncytiotrophoblasts and **postnatal ichthyosis**
- 1 in 2,000–3,000 newborn males

- Patients with the placental sulfatase disorder are unable to hydrolyze DHEAS or 16α-hydroxy-DHEAS; therefore, the placenta cannot form normal amounts of estrogen.
- A family history of scaling in males (as well as repeated postdate pregnancies and cesarean sections) should prompt a consideration for prenatal diagnosis.
- It is now recognized that steroid sulfatase deficiency is present in other tissues and can persist after birth.
- These children develop ichthyosis beginning between birth and 6 months of age, characterized by hyperkeratosis (producing scales on the neck, trunk, and palms) and associated with mild corneal opacities, pyloric stenosis, and cryptorchidism.
- This inherited disorder, thus, represents a single entity: placental sulfatase deficiency and X-linked ichthyosis, both reflecting a deficiency of microsomal sulfatase.
- A deficiency in placental sulfatase is usually discovered when patients **go beyond term** and are found to have extremely **low estriol levels** and no evidence of fetal distress.
- The patients usually fail to go into labor and require delivery by cesarean section.
- Most striking is the **failure of cervical softening** and dilation; thus, cervical dystocia occurs that is resistant to oxytocin stimulation.
- There are many case reports of this deficiency, almost all detected by finding low estriol levels.

The characteristic steroid findings are as follows:
- Extremely **low estriol and estetrol** levels in the mother
- Extremely **high amniotic fluid DHEAS** levels
- Normal amniotic fluid **DHEA** and androstenedione levels.

- The normal DHEA and androstenedione with a high DHEAS rule out congenital adrenal hyperplasia.

11. b. Preterm delivery

Ref: Speroff 8th/ed p 282; Yen & Jaffe's 8th/ed p 256

A deficiency in placental sulfatase is usually discovered when patients go beyond term and are found to have extremely low estriol levels and no evidence of fetal distress. (So, its post-term, not preterm).

Endocrinology of Pregnancy

12. a. High amniotic fluid DHEA and androstenedione
Ref: Speroff 8th/ed p 282

The normal DHEA and androstenedione with a high DHEAS rule out congenital adrenal hyperplasia.

13. c. Diabetes mellitus
Ref: Speroff 8th/ed p 284

Extremely low levels of estriol are seen in:
- Fetal demise
- Impending fetal demise
- Adrenal hypofunction
- Placental sulfatase deficiency
- Placental aromatase deficiency
- Some drugs

14. d. Human chorionic Gonadotropin
Ref: Yen & Jaffe's 8th/ed p 28; Speroff 8th/ed p 90
- The gonadotropins are trafficked from the endoplasmic reticulum to the cis-Golgi and undergo glycosylation as they traverse the Golgi reaching the trans-Golgi, to yield the mature hormones.
- The carbohydrate moieties appear to be important in subunit assembly and stabilization, secretion, and circulatory half-life.
- The particular type of glycosylation may influence biological activity.

Human Chorionic Gonadotropin
- A glycoprotein
- Half-life approximately **24 hours**
- Consists of two subunits, noncovalently linked by disulfide bonds, alpha and beta.
- The unique biologic activity as well as specificity in immunoassays is attributed to the molecular and carbohydrate differences in the β subunits.
- β-hCG is the largest β subunit, containing a larger carbohydrate moiety and 145 amino acid residues, including a **unique carboxyl terminal tailpiece** of 24 amino acid groups. It is this unique part of the hCG structure that allows the production of highly specific antibodies and the utilization of highly specific immunologic assays.
- It contains **four sites** for glycosylation, the reason why hCG is glycosylated to a greater extent than LH, a difference that is responsible for the longer circulating half-life for hCG.

15. a. Sialic acid
Ref: Speroff 8th/ed p 287
- The carbohydrate components of the glycoproteins are composed of fructose, galactose, mannose, galactosamine, glucosamine, and sialic acid.
- Although the other sugars are necessary for hormonal function, **sialic acid is the critical determinant** of biologic half-life.
- Removal of sialic acid residues in hCG, FSH, and LH leads to very rapid elimination from the circulation.

16. b. Produced only by placenta
Ref: Speroff 8th/ed p 287

All human tissues appear to make hCG, but the placenta is different in having the **ability to glycosylate** the protein, thus reducing its rate of metabolism and giving it biologic activity through a long half-life.

17. b. 10 weeks
Ref: Speroff 8th/ed p 289
- hCG takes over action of LH on about the **eighth day** after ovulation, 1 day after implantation, when β-hCG first can be detected in maternal blood.
- hCG has been detected at the 8-cell stage in the embryo using molecular biology techniques.
- Survival of pregnancy is dependent on steroids from the corpus luteum until the seventh week of pregnancy.
- From the seventh week to the tenth week, the corpus luteum is gradually replaced by the placenta.
- By the tenth week, removal of the corpus luteum will not be followed by steroid withdrawal abortion.

18. b. 100 mg
Ref: Speroff 8th/ed p 270

Exogenous support for an early pregnancy (until 10 weeks) requires 100 mg of progesterone daily, associated with a maternal circulating level of approximately 10 ng/mL.

19. a. P450 c17
Ref: Speroff 8th/ed p 273

There is a virtual absence of 17α-hydroxylation and 17-20 desmolase (lyase) activity (P450 c17) in the human placenta. This has 2 consequences:
1. The 21-carbon products (progesterone and pregnenolone) cannot be converted to 19-carbon steroids (androstenedione and dehydroepiandrosterone).
2. Like progesterone, estrogen produced by the placental aromatase (P450 arom) enzyme system must derive precursors from outside the placenta.

20. c. Progesterone
Ref: Speroff 8th/ed p 273; Yen & Jaffe's 8th/ed p 256

(Just remember one simple thing: placenta lacks 17a hydroxylase, fetus lacks 3β-hydroxysteroid dehydrogenase)
- The fetal zone in the adrenal gland is extremely active but produces steroids with a 3β-hydroxy-D^5 configuration

like pregnenolone and dehydroepiandrosterone (DHEA), rather than 3-keto-D^4 products such as progesterone.
- The fetus, therefore, lacks significant activity of the 3β-hydroxysteroid dehydrogenase, D^{4-5} isomerase system.
- Thus, the fetus must borrow progesterone from the placenta to circumvent this lack in order to synthesize the biologically important corticosteroids.
- In return, the fetus supplies what the placenta lacks: 19-carbon compounds to serve as precursors for estrogens.

21. **b. Levels of hCG are lower in women carrying female fetuses**

Ref: Speroff 8th/ed p 289

Its otherwise, hCG levels close to term are higher in women carrying **female fetuses.** This is true of serum levels, placental content, urinary levels, and amniotic fluid concentrations. The mechanism and purpose of this difference is not known.

22. **a. Relaxin**

Ref: Yen & Jaffe's 8th/ed p 195, 220

- Relaxin is produced by the large luteal cells of corpus luteum.
- Relaxin is produced exclusively in pregnancy.

Relaxin

- Plays role in **facilitating decidualization** of the endometrium, suppression of myometrial contractile activity, and the maternal adaptation to pregnancy.
- The highest circulating levels are achieved in the **first trimester**, and then decrease by 20% and remain constant throughout pregnancy.
- Relaxin has also been implicated as a stimulus for **glycodelin** expression.

Hypothalamic-Like Hormones

- GnRH
- CRH
- TRH
- Somatostatin
- GHRH
- Neuropeptide Y

23. **b. 100 IU/L**

Ref: Speroff 8th/ed p 289

- The maternal circulating hCG concentration is approximately **100 IU/L** at the time of the expected but missed menses.

A maximal level of about 100,000 IU/L in the maternal circulation is reached at 8-10 weeks of gestation.

hCG levels decrease to about 10,000-20,000 IU/L by 18-20 weeks and remain at that level to term.

24. **a. Hyperglycosylated hCG increases with gestation**

Ref: Speroff 8th/ed p 289

Human Chorionic Gonadotropin

- hCG levels decrease to about 10,000-20,000 IU/L by 18-20 weeks and remain at that level to term.
- Advancing gestation is associated with increasing amounts of **"nicked" hCG** molecules in the maternal circulation.
- These molecules are missing a peptide linkage on the b-subunit, and, therefore, they dissociate into free a and b subunits.
- At any one point in time, the maternal circulation contains hCG, nicked hCG, free subunits, and fragments of hCG.
- **Hyperglycosylated hCG**—The carbohydrate content of hCG varies throughout pregnancy, with more glycosylation present in early pregnancy.

25. **b. Maximum expression in 2nd trimester**

Ref: Speroff 8th/ed p 290

Hyperglycosylated hCG

- Hyperglycosylated hCG detected in mothers in the first week of normal pregnancies is the major circulating form of hCG, but the levels decrease rapidly to be replaced by the usual hCG isoform by the second trimester.
- Choriocarcinoma is associated with the increased secretion of β-hCG that is glycosylated to a greater degree, so-called hyperglycosylated hCG, sometimes called **invasive trophoblast antigen.**
- These findings suggest that hyperglycosylated hCG plays a role in regulating trophoblastic invasion.
- Hyperglycosyalted hCG is mainly autocrine in its activity, whereas regular hCG functions as a classic hormone in maintaining the corpus luteum.
- Measurement of hyperglycosylated hCG in the first weeks of pregnancy may have a role in screening for Down syndrome.
- Some of the inaccuracy associated with routine pregnancy testing, especially home pregnancy tests, can be attributed to the variability in detecting hyperglycosylated hCG.
- Low levels in early weeks of pregnancy may predict a failing pregnancy.

26. a. LDL

Ref: Yen & Jaffe's 8th/ed p 77

The cholesterol utilized for progesterone synthesis enters trophoblast from maternal bloodstream as LDL cholesterol by means of the process of endocytosis (internalization).

27. d. All

Ref: Speroff 8th/ed p 272

Amniotic fluid progesterone concentration is maximal between 10 and 20 weeks and then decreases gradually.

Myometrial levels are about **3 times higher** than maternal plasma levels in early pregnancy, remain high, and are about equal to the maternal plasma concentration at term.

At term, progesterone levels range from 100 to 200 ng/mL, and the placenta produces about 250 mg/day.

28. a. Secreted by cytotrophoblast

Ref: Speroff 8th/ed p 291; Yen & Jaffe's 8th/ed p 265

Human Placental Lactogen

- Also called human chorionic somatomammotropin.
- Secreted by the syncytiotrophoblast.
- Single-chain polypeptide of 191 amino acids held together by 2 disulfide bonds.
- There is high degree of sequence homology to both human growth hormone (hGH) and prolactin, but has only 3% of hGH somatotropin activity.
- HCS binds with high affinity to prolactin receptors, but with low affinity to GH receptors, suggesting that it functions largely as a lactogen rather than a somatogen in pregnancy.
- The growth hormone-hPL gene family consists of 5 genes on chromosome 17q22–q24.
- The half-life of hPL is about **15 minutes**; hence its appeal as an index of placental problems.
- There is **no circadian variation**, and only minute amounts of hPL enter the fetal circulation.

29. b. The level of hPL in maternal circulation is correlated with fetal and placental weight

Ref: Speroff 8th/ed p 291; Yen & Jaffe's 8th/ed p 265

- The level of hPL in the maternal circulation is correlated with fetal and placental weight, steadily increasing until plateauing in the last 4 weeks of pregnancy (5–10 mg/mL).
- Very high maternal levels are found in association with multiple gestations.
- Although hPL is similar in structure to growth hormone, neither growth hormone-releasing hormone nor somatostatin influence placental hPL secretion.
- Although hPL has about 50% of the lactogenic activity of sheep prolactin in certain bioassays, its lactogenic contribution in human pregnancy is uncertain.
- In the mother, hPL stimulates insulin secretion and IGF-I production and induces insulin resistance and carbohydrate intolerance. However, the well-recognized insulin resistance in pregnancy is not solely an effect of hPL.

30. d. All

Ref: Speroff 8th/ed p 294; Yen & Jaffe's 8th/ed p 265

Metabolic Role of hPL

- In the mother, hPL stimulates insulin secretion and IGF-I production and induces insulin resistance and carbohydrate intolerance.
- hPL is elevated with hypoglycemia and depressed with hyperglycemia.
- hPL mobilize lipids as free fatty acids, stimulates lipolysis.

Conditions associated with low maternal levels of HCS:
- Hypertension
- Preeclampsia
- IUGR

Conditions associated with high maternal levels of HCS:
- Gestational diabetes
- Pregnancies with macrosomic babies

31. a. hCG is only hormone released by placenta which has thyrotropic activity

Ref: Speroff 8th/ed p 295

The human placenta contains two thyrotropic substances. (hCG is not the only one):

- One is called human chorionic thyrotropin (hCT), which is similar in size and action to pituitary TSH. (The content in the normal placenta is very small, and it is unlikely that it has any physiologic importance)
- hCT differs from the other glycoproteins in that it does not appear to share the common a subunit.
- hCG has intrinsic thyrotropic activity, indicating that **hCG is the second placental thyrotropic substance**.
- It has been calculated that hCG contains approximately1/4,000th of the thyrotropic activity of human TSH.
- In conditions with very elevated hCG levels, such as hydatidiform mole, the thyrotropic activity can be sufficient to produce hyperthyroidism.
- Hyperemesis gravidarum is usually associated with very high hCG levels, and some of these patients develop hyperthyroidism as well.

32. c. In early pregnancy amniotic fluid AFP comes from fetal liver

Ref: Speroff 8th/ed p 297

Alpha-Fetoprotein (AFP)

- Unique glycoprotein (590 amino acids and 4% carbohydrate)
- Derived largely from **fetal liver** and partially from the **yolk sac** until it degenerates at about 12 weeks.
- In early pregnancy (5-12 weeks), amniotic fluid AFP is mainly from **yolk sac origin**, whereas maternal circulating AFP is mainly from the fetal liver.
- Its function is unknown, but it is comparable in size to albumin and contains 39% sequence homology; it may serve as a protein carrier of steroid hormones in fetal blood.
- Peak levels of AFP in the fetal blood are reached at the end of the first trimester; then levels decrease gradually until a rapid decrease begins at 32 weeks.
- Maternal blood levels are much lower than fetal levels, rising until week 32 and then declining.

33. a. Trisomy 18

Ref: Speroff 8th/ed p 298

Trisomy 18 is associated with low alpha fetoprotein levels. All three markers used for aneuploidy screening (AFP, β-hCG, and unconjugated estriol) are low.

34. d. Down syndrome

Ref: Speroff 8th/ed p 298

Down syndrome is associated with low alpha fetoprotein and low unconjugated estriol but high hCG level.

Conditions associated with high AFP levels:
- Open neural tube defects
- Anterior abdominal wall defects
- Multiple pregnancies

High levels of AFP run risk for:
- Spontaneous miscarriage
- Stillbirth
- Preterm birth
- Preeclampsia
- Neonatal death
- Low birth weight

35. b. Levels keep on rising throughout pregnancy

Ref: Yen & Jaffe's 8th/ed p 195; Speroff 8th/ed p 299

Relaxin

- Peptide hormone
- Produced by the corpus luteum of pregnancy
- Not detected in the circulation of men or nonpregnant women
- Similar in structure to insulin, composed of two short peptide chains linked by disulfide bridges.
- The maternal serum concentration rises during the first trimester when the corpus luteum is dominant and declines in the second trimester.
- This suggests a role in maintaining early pregnancy, but its function is not really known.
- In animals, relaxin softens the cervix (ripening), inhibits uterine contractions, and relaxes the pubic symphysis.

36. d. All

Ref: Speroff 8th/ed p 300

Following ovulation, the endometrium becomes a secretory organ.

Decidualized endometrium secretes:
- Renin, which may be involved in the regulation of water and electroytes in the amniotic fluid.
- Relaxin, which may influence prostaglandin production in the membranes.
- Prolactin is synthesized by endometrium during a normal menstrual cycle, but this synthesis is not initiated until histologic decidualization begins about day 23.

37. b. Fetal membranes

Ref: Speroff 8th/ed p 300

- The prolactin in the fetal circulation is derived from the fetal pituitary.

During pregnancy, prolactin secretion is limited to the fetal pituitary, the maternal pituitary, and the uterus.

Neither trophoblast nor fetal membranes synthesize prolactin, but both the myometrium and endometrium can produce prolactin.

38. a. Decidua

Ref: Speroff 8th/ed p 301

Prolactin derived from the decidua is the source of prolactin found in the amniotic fluid.

The maternal and fetal blood levels of prolactin are derived from the respective pituitary glands, and, therefore, dopamine agonist suppression of pituitary secretion of prolactin throughout pregnancy produces low maternal and fetal blood levels, yet there is normal fetal growth and development, and amniotic fluid levels are unchanged.

Fortunately, decidual secretion of prolactin is unaffected by dopamine agonist treatment because decidual prolactin is important for fluid and electrolyte regulation of the amniotic fluid.

39. a. Pregnancy specific γ₁-glycoprotein (PSG)

Ref: Speroff 8th/ed p 304

- Pregnancy-specific γ_1-glycoprotein (PSG) was previously known as Schwangerschafts protein 1.
- The physiologic function of PSG produced by the placenta is unknown, but it has been used as a test for pregnancy and a marker for malignancies, including choriocarcinoma.
- Molecular studies have revealed that PSG consists of a family of glycoproteins encoded by genes on chromosome 19.
- The PSG family is closely related to the carcino-embryonic antigen (CEA) proteins.
- Pregnancy-associated plasma protein-A (PAPP-A) is a placental protein that is similar to a macroglobulin in the serum. Low levels of PAPP-A in the first trimester are associated with adverse obstetrical outcomes.
- Progesterone-associated endometrial protein, previously called placental protein 14, is now recognized to originate in secretory endometrium and decidua.

40. c. Leptin levels remain constant throughout pregnancy

Ref: Yen & Jaffe's 8th/ed p 267

Leptin and Pregnancy

- The placenta is the principal source of leptin during pregnancy.
- Most of the leptin produced by the placenta is secreted into the maternal circulation, and as a consequence leptin levels are elevated during pregnancy.
- In the first trimester, maternal plasma leptin levels are double non-pregnant values and **continue to increase** during the second and third trimesters.
- In the second and third trimesters, leptin is also expressed by the chorion and amnion.
- The proportion of placental leptin directed to the fetus is uncertain and its role in fetal development is unknown.
- Leptin levels decline to normal nonpregnant values **within 24 hours** of delivery.
- The abnormally high placental leptin production is associated with maternal diabetes mellitus and hypertension and umbilical leptin levels correlate with fetal adiposity.
- Interestingly, leptin levels during pregnancy do not correlate with body mass index as they do in the nonpregnant state.
- Pregnancy appears to be a state of hyperleptinemia and leptin resistance, with uncoupling of eating behavior, satiety, and metabolic activity.
- Leptin is lipolytic and favors fatty acid mobilization from adipose tissue.
- Based on its actions in the hypothalamus, leptin may regulate satiety and maternal energy expenditure during pregnancy.
- It also may act in the liver, pancreas, and muscle to decrease insulin sensitivity and mobilize glucose. Thus, leptin appears to be another hormone utilized by the placenta to modulate maternal metabolism and partition energy supplies to the fetus.

CHAPTER 6

Normal and Abnormal Sexual Development

Multiple Choice Questions

1. Primary genetic signal determining the direction of gonadal differentiation in mammals:
   a. SF1
   b. SRY
   c. WT1
   d. GATA4

2. Nuclear receptor activating SRY promoter:
   a. WT1
   b. GATA4
   c. SF1
   d. SOX

3. Genes involved in regulation of SRY gene are all except:
   a. INSL3
   b. SF1
   c. WT1
   d. GATA4

4. SRY target gene most likely involved in promotion of testis development?
   a. WNT4
   b. RSPO1
   c. DAX1
   d. SOX9

5. Genes involved in testis development:
   a. FGF 9
   b. FOXL2
   c. RSPO1
   d. DAX1

6. Genes not associated with ovary development:
   a. FOXL2
   b. FGF9
   c. RSPO1
   d. DAX1

7. Putative meiosis inducing factor produced in mesonephros leading male germ cell to enter mitotic arrest and oogonia to proliferate further is:
   a. Retinoic acid
   b. CYP26B1
   c. NANOS2
   d. DMC1

8. All of the following is true about testis differentiation and development, except:
   a. Sertoli cell precursors express SRY
   b. SOX9 is a reliable marker for developing Sertoli cells
   c. Leydig cells differentiate from cells already within the gonad
   d. FGF9 and PGD_2 play important roles in testis differentiation

9. All of the following is true about ovary differentiation and development, except:
   a. Bipotential gonad begins to differentiate into an ovary about 2 weeks earlier than testis development
   b. Normal ovarian differentiation requires the presence of germ cells
   c. WNT4 and RSPO1 genes play an important role in ovarian differentiation
   d. Ovary achieves mature compartmentalization by 20 weeks of intrauterine life

10. All of the following are members of transforming growth factor β (TGF-β) superfamily of proteins, except:
    a. Brain derived neurotropic factor
    b. Anti-Müllerian hormone
    c. Activin
    d. Bone morphogenetic protein

11. Which one of the following is not the derivative of Wolffian duct?
    a. Vas deferens
    b. Epididymis
    c. Vas efferens
    d. Seminal vesicles

12. Which one of the following is not the derivative of Müllerian duct?
    a. Fallopian tubes
    b. Ovary
    c. Uterus
    d. Upper portion of the vagina

13. Fetal testes start secreting testosterone by how many weeks?
    a. 8 weeks
    b. 18 weeks
    c. 28 weeks
    d. Only after birth

14. Which of the following is dependent on DHT for its development?
    a. Seminal vesicles
    b. Epididymis
    c. Vas deferens
    d. Penis

15. Most important factor for Wolffian duct differentiation:
    a. Local testosterone levels
    b. Circulating testosterone levels
    c. Local DHT levels
    d. Circulating DHT levels

16. Transcriptional regulators of patterning, important for the differentiation of the vasal duct into its morphologically and functionally distinct segments:
    a. SOX9
    b. inhibin beta A
    c. TGF
    d. HOX genes

17. Why abnormalities in the renal system are highly associated with abnormalities in development of the fallopian tubes, uterus, and upper vagina?
    a. Wolffian ducts act like migrational template for Müllerian ducts
    b. Müllerian ducts are derived from Wolffian ducts
    c. Woffian ducts and Müllerian ducts have same origin
    d. Both A and B

18. AMH leads to regression of Müllerian ducts around what gestational age?
    a. 8 weeks
    b. 18 weeks
    c. 28 weeks
    d. 20 weeks

19. Which of the following is not a correct derivative?
    a. Genital tubercle: penis and clitoris
    b. Genial folds: ventral aspect of penis and labia minora
    c. Genital swellings: scrotum and labia minora
    d. Urogenital sinus: penile urethra and vestibule

20. Leydig cell testosterone production maximises at:
    a. 8 weeks
    b. 18 weeks
    c. 28 weeks
    d. 38 weeks

21. DHT is required for development of one of the following:
    a. Epididymis
    b. Vas deferens
    c. Vas efferens
    d. Prostate

Congenital Adrenal Hyperplasia

22. Most common enzyme defect in CAH:
    a. 17α-hydroxylase
    b. 11β-hydroxylase
    c. 3β-hydroxylase
    d. 21-hydroxylase

23. Most frequent cause of sexual ambiguity in neonate:
    a. 21-hydroxylase
    b. 11β-hydroxylase
    c. 3β-hydroxylase
    d. 17α-hydroxylase

24. Most common endocrine cause of neonatal death:
    a. Simple virilizing classical 21-hydroxylase deficiency
    b. Salt wasting Classical 21-hydroxylase deficiency
    c. Hypothyroidism
    d. Nonclassical 21-hydroxylase deficiency

25. Mode of inheritance of CAH:
    a. Autosomal recessive
    b. Autosomal dominant
    c. X linked recessive
    d. X linked dominant

26. Which of the following phenotype of CAH are not at risk of having child with classical CAH?
    a. Compound heterozygotes with one classic and other variant allele
    b. One classic and one normal allele
    c. Compound heterozygotes with both variant alleles
    d. Both classic alleles

27. A 22-year-old woman presents with oligomenorrhea and irregular menstrual cycle. On examination, she is a hirsute with Ferriman-Gallwey score 10, Tanner stage 4 breast development, local examination showed clitoral length 1.8 cm. Serum testosterone levels 90 ng/dL. DHEAS levels are normal. What is the next step in evaluation?
    a. 17 hydroxy progesterone levels
    b. Serum LH
    c. Serum androstenedione
    d. ACTH stimulation test

28. Same woman presents with report of 17OHP as 450 ng/dL. What is the next step in evaluation?
    a. ACTH stimulation test
    b. 17 hydroxy progesterone levels
    c. Serum LH
    d. Serum androstenedione

29. A neonate presents with ambiguous genitalia and hypertension. Serum electrolyte report shows hypokalemia. Which enzyme defect is most likely cause of such condition?
    a. 21 hydroxylase deficiency
    b. 3β-hydroxysteroid dehydrogenase deficiency
    c. 11β-hydroxylase deficiency
    d. 18-hydroxylase deficiency

30. A 20-year-old woman presents with oligomenorrhea and irregular menstrual cycle. On examination, she is a hirsute with Ferriman-Gallwey score 16, Tanner stage 4 breast development, local examination showed clitoris length 2.0 cm. Serum testosterone levels 97 ng/dL. DHEAS levels mildly elevated. Serum 17OHP levels 50 ng/dL and stimulated levels 100 ng/dL. What is the next step in evaluation?
    a. 17α-hydroxypregnenolone concentration after ACTH stimulation
    b. Pregnenolone concentration after ACTH stimulation
    c. DHEAS concentration after ACTH stimulation
    d. DHEA concentration after ACTH stimulation

31. Dexamethasone treatment for prevention of virilization of female fetus in case of CAH should be started for maximal effectiveness by which week of gestation?
    a. 5–6 weeks
    b. 4–5 weeks
    c. 6–9 weeks
    d. After 9 weeks

32. Children with CAH are at increased risk of all of the following, *except:*
    a. Delayed puberty
    b. Short stature
    c. Hypertension
    d. Obesity

33. What is the best time of the day to give dexamethasone in patients with CAH?
    a. Early morning
    b. Bedtime
    c. Irrespective of the daytime
    d. Evening

34. Which of the following does not hold true for CAH management in pregnancy?
    a. Increased risk of decreased fertility in classical CAH due to chronic anovulation
    b. Small pelvis might result if bone age is advanced to age 13–14 before treatment started, thus high risk for cesarean section
    c. High capacity of placental aromatase activity effectively protects the fetal female genitalia from virilization
    d. Hydrocortisone treatment should be replaced by dexamethasone treatment in pregnancy as placenta can metabolize dexamethasone

35. Non-steroidogenic enzyme resulting in CAH:
    a. P450 Oxidoreductase deficiency
    b. 21 hydroxylase deficiency
    c. 17-20 lyase deficiency
    d. 17 hydroxylase deficiency

36. Which does not hold true for P450 Oxidoreductase deficiency as cause of CAH?
    a. It affects the activity of multiple P450 enzymes involved in steroidogenesis
    b. Newly described steroidogenic enzyme as a cause of CAH
    c. POR serves as the electron donor in the activation of all microsomal P450 enzymes
    d. Females with POR deficiency frequently become virilized in utero

37. Aromatase enzyme is found in all of the following tissues *except:*
    a. Liver
    b. Gonads
    c. Brain
    d. Placenta

38. Which of the following statements is not true regarding aromatase enzyme?
    a. Encoded by the CYP19A1 gene, located on chromosome 15
    b. The enzyme is active in the gonads, the placenta, the brain, and in adipose
    c. Catalyzes conversion of 21-carbon compounds to 18-carbon compounds
    d. Aromatase deficiency is a rare autosomal recessive leading to female fetal virilization and maternal hirsutism

39. Inadvertent exposure of danazol in 3rd trimester of pregnancy will lead to:
    a. Clitoromegaly
    b. Labioscrotal fusion
    c. Both a and b
    d. None as if given in 1st trimester only does danazol affects female fetus

40. Gestational hyperandrogenism can result from:
    a. Maternal drug ingestion
    b. Pregnancy luteoma
    c. Theca lutein cysts
    d. All

41. A 20-year-old pregnant woman presenting with signs and symptoms of virilization at 12 weeks. Ultrasonography is suggestive of molar pregnancy with bilateral theca lutein cysts 10 × 10 cm each side. Which of the following does not hold true regarding her condition?
    a. Associated with increased maternal serum hCG concentrations
    b. High risk of female child becoming virilized
    c. May persist long after evacuation of molar pregnancies despite rapid decrease in serum hCG levels
    d. Approximately 30% of pregnant women become hirsute or virilize

42. A 16-year-old girl presents with her mother in OPD complaining lack of onset of menarche. On examination, she has tanner stage 4 breast development and pubic hair. On local examination, she has a blind vaginal pouch. Ultrasonography reveals absence of uterus. Her karyotype is 46XX. Which of the following statement is most unlikely for present situation?
    a. Ovaries may be normal, undescended, hypoplastic, or associated with an inguinal hernia.
    b. Affected patients often also have urologic anomalies
    c. Affected patients often have cardiac anomalies
    d. Affected patients might have skeletal malformations

43. A 15-year-old girl presents with primary amenorrhea. On examination, she has prepubertal breast development. Tanner stage 3 pubic hair. Ultrasonography revealed normal uterus, cervix and vagina. Gonads appeared streak. Hormonal assays reveals hypergonadotropic hypogonadism. Karyotype comes 46XY. Most probable diagnosis:
    a. Androgen insensitivity syndrome
    b. Swyer syndrome
    c. Testicular regression syndrome
    d. Steroid 5α reductase deficiency

44. A 13-year-old girl presents with her mother with progressive signs of virilization. On examination, breasts prepubertal, pubic hair sparse. There is evidence of short blind vaginal pouch. Ultrasonography revealed absence of uterus, with testes localized in inguinal canal. Hormonal assays show normal serum testosterone levels in male range. Karyotype reveals 46XY. Most probable diagnosis?
    a. Steroid 5α reductase deficiency
    b. Swyer syndrome
    c. Androgen insensitivity syndrome
    d. Testicular regression syndrome

45. A 15-year-old girl presents with primary amenorrhea. On examination, she has prepubertal breast development. Tanner stage 2 pubic hair. There is evidence of blind pouch of vagina. She is hypertensive. Serum electrolytes show hypernatremia with hypokalemia. Hormonal assays reveals hypergonadotropic hypogonadism. Karyotype comes 46XY. Most probable diagnosis:
    a. Swyer syndrome
    b. Androgen insensitivity syndrome
    c. 17α-hydroxylase deficiency
    d. Steroid 5α-reductase deficiency

46. Rarest and most severe form of CAH:
    a. P450 oxidoreductase deficiency
    b. 21-hydroxylase deficiency
    c. Congenital lipoid adrenal hyperplasia
    d. 17-hydroxylase deficiency

47. Congenital lipoid adrenal hyperplasia results from mutations in:
    a. Steroidogenic acute regulatory (StAR) protein
    b. 21-hydroxylase
    c. 17-hydroxylase
    d. P450 oxidoreductase

48. Disorder resulting in global deficiency of steroid hormones with progressive cellular damage due to accumulation of cholesterol:
    a. Congenital lipoid adrenal hyperplasia
    b. P450 oxidoreductase deficiency
    c. 21-hydroxylase deficiency
    d. 17-hydroxylase deficiency

49. Only inherited disorder of steroidogenesis not caused by a defect in one of the steroidogenic or nonsteroidogenic enzymes:
    a. P450 oxidoreductase deficiency
    b. 21-hydroxylase deficiency
    c. 17-hydroxylase deficiency
    d. Mutation of StAR gene

50. Which tissue will show lowest 17-hydroxylase enzyme activity?
    a. Ovarian theca cell
    b. Testicular leydig cells
    c. Adrenal reticularis
    d. Ovarian granulosa cell

51. Which of the following is non-P450 enzyme involved in steroid synthesis pathway?
    a. 17-hydroxylase
    b. 17β-hydroxysteroid dehydrogenase
    c. 17,20-lyase
    d. 19-methyloxidase

Androgen Insensitivity Syndrome

52. Which of the following inherited disorder of sexual development show X-linked recessive pattern of inheritance?
    a. Complete androgen insensitivity syndrome
    b. Congenital adrenal hyperplasia
    c. Klinefelter syndrome
    d. Kallmann syndrome

53. Which of the following statement is incorrect for AIS?
    a. Result from a wide variety of inactivating mutations in the AR gene
    b. X-linked recessive pattern of inheritance
    c. AIS always follow Mendelian inheritance pattern
    d. 40% of patients represent de novo mutations

54. A 15-year-old girl presents with primary amenorrhea. On examination, she has stage 5 breast development. Tanner stage 2 pubic hair. There is evidence of blind pouch of vagina. Hormonal assays reveals serum testosterone concentrations in normal male range, LH levels are increased, and the serum FSH in the normal range. Ultrasonography revealed absent uterus with gonads in inguinal canal. Karyotype 46XY. Most probable diagnosis:
    a. Complete androgen insensitivity syndrome
    b. Congenital adrenal hyperplasia
    c. Swyer syndrome
    d. Müllerian agenesis

55. For the above patient, which of the following statements is incorrect regarding time to perform gonadectomy?
    a. Gonadectomy is indicated soon after diagnosis due to significant risk of germ cell tumors in occult testicular elements (20–30%) in case of Swyer syndrome
    b. Overall risk for tumor development is quite low (5–10%), particularly before puberty
    c. Gonadectomy is indicated soon after diagnosis due to significant risk of germ cell tumors in AIS
    d. Gonadectomy generally is best delayed until after puberty is completed

56. Fill in the blank for phenotypic spectrum of Androgen insensitivity syndromes:
    Complete AIS > Incomplete AIS >..........> Infertile male
    (From phenotypic female to phenotypic male)
    a. Reifenstein syndrome
    b. Partial androgen insensitivity syndrome
    c. Noonan syndrome
    d. Kennedy syndrome

57. Reifenstein syndrome is another name for which condition?
    a. Complete AIS
    b. Incomplete AIS
    c. LH/ HCG receptor defect
    d. Uterine hernia syndrome

58. A 14-year-old girl presents with primary amenorrhea. On examination both breast development and pubic hair absent. Hormonal assays show raised LH, normal FSH, low testosterone levels. Ultrasonography shows absence of uterus. Karyotype comes out to be 46XY. Most likely diagnosis?
    a. LH receptor defects
    b. Swyer syndrome
    c. Complete androgen insensitivity syndrome
    d. MRKH syndrome

59. A 25-year-old male presents with primary infertility. On examination, normal androgenization. Normal scrotal development. Bilateral testes seems absent. Evidence of bilateral inguinal masses. Ultrasonography reveals Müllerian duct structures in inguinal masses. Karyotype comes out as 46XY. Most likely diagnosis:
    a. LH receptor defects
    b. Uterine hernia syndrome
    c. Swyer syndrome
    d. Complete androgen insensitivity syndrome

Turner Syndrome

60. The sine qua non of Turner syndrome, i.e, only abnormality present in virtually all patients:
    a. Shield chest   b. Cubitus valgus
    c. Horse shoe kidney d. Short stature

61. Synonyms of Turner syndrome:
    a. Bonnevie-Ullrich syndrome
    b. Monosomy X
    c. Ullrich-Turner syndrome
    d. All

62. Inheritance of Turner syndrome:
    a. Autosomal dominant
    b. Autosomal recessive
    c. X linked dominant
    d. Sporadic

63. Which syndrome is designated as 'Male turner syndrome'?
    a. Noonan syndrome   b. Klinefelter syndrome
    c. Kallmann syndrome d. Aarskog syndrome

64. Which patients with Turner syndrome present with severe mental retardation:
    a. Small X-ring chromosome
    b. Isochromosome
    c. Terminal deletion
    d. All turner syndrome patients present with mental retardation

65. Turner syndrome patient who require gonadectomy:
    a. 45,XO/46,XO
    b. 45,XO/46,XX
    c. 45,XO/45,XY
    d. All require gonadectomy once pubertal development is complete

66. Most common congenital cause of hypogonadism in males:
    a. 47, XXXY
    b. 48, XXY
    c. 46, XY/ 47, XXY
    d. 46, XY/ 48, XXXY

67. Which of the following is most likely to be present in patient with congenital bilateral absence of vas deferens?
    a. Caput epididymidis
    b. Seminal vesicles
    c. Ejaculatory duct
    d. Cauda epididymidis

68. Which of the following systems is least likely to be involved in cystic fibrosis?
    a. Pancreatic system
    b. Nervous system
    c. Reproductive system
    d. Respiratory system

69. Syndromes affecting extratesticular ductal system, leading to male infertility:
    a. CBAVD
    b. Failure of mesonephric duct differentiation
    c. Young syndrome
    d. All

70. The US Food and Drug Administration classifies Dexamethasone as which category drug:
    a. A
    b. B
    c. C
    d. D

Answer with Explanations

1. b. SRY

Ref: Yen & Jaffe's 8th/ed p 142, Speroff 8th /ed p 333

- Individuals carrying Y chromosomes are considered genetically males
- The SRY gene is located on **Y chromosome**
- It has been shown to be essential for gonad to differentiate into testes.

SRY is required for activation of SRY-box containing gene (SOX9) expression, and SOX9 and steroidogenic factor 1 (SF1) have been shown to cooperate in regulation of AMH transcription.

- In the testis, regulation of transcription factor SOX9 by testis-determining factor, sex determining region on chromosome Y (SRY) is required for Sertoli cell differentiation.
- In humans, **46, XX male sex reversal** occurs when pairing between the X and Y chromosomes during male meiosis extends abnormally into adjacent non-homologous regions, allowing inappropriate recombination and transfer of Y-specific DNA onto the X chromosome.
- SRY now is generally established as the **primary genetic signal** determining the direction of gonadal differentiation in mammals.

2. c. SF1

Ref: Speroff 8th /ed p 333

- The nuclear receptor SF1 (Steroidogenic Factor 1) has emerged as a likely and important activator of SRY gene. SF1 binds to and activates the SRY promoter.
- In humans, SF1 haploinsufficiency is a known cause of **XY female sex reversal**.
- SF1 polymorphism that reduces transactivation function by approximately 20% is recognized as a susceptibility factor for the development of micropenis and cryptorchidism.

3. a. INSL3

Ref: Speroff 8th /ed p 333; Yen & Jaffe's 8th/ed p 377

Genes involved in regulation of SRY gene:
1. Steroidogenic factor 1: described above
2. Splice variants of Wt1 (Wilms tumor 1) and GATA4 (GATA binding protein 4) also may be involved in the regulation of SRY expression; both are transcription factors containing **zinc-finger motifs** that can interact and synergistically activate the promoter of human SRY.
3. WT1 mutations are associated with gonadal dysgenesis and ambiguous genitalia in males.

- Insulin-like factor (INSL3) is a Leydig cell-derived peptide, involved in development of gubernacular ligaments, and prevention of cryptorchidism.

4. d. SOX9

Ref: Speroff 8th /ed p 334

SRY appears to activate number of genes that promote testis development. The 204 amino acid protein product of SRY (SRY) contains a 79 amino acid domain very similar to that in a recognized family of transcription factors known as the **high mobility group** (HMG), which bind to DNA and regulate gene transcription.

Members of the related SRY HMG box (SOX) protein family of transcription factors play a crucial role in the cascade of events that drives testis differentiation, and most of the SRY point mutations identified in sex-reversed patients translate to abnormalities in the amino acid sequence of SOX proteins.

- Substantial evidence now indicates that SOX9 is the most likely SRY target gene.

5. a. FGF9

Ref: Speroff 8th /ed p 335

The developmental consequences of activating and inactivating mutations in SOX9 resemble those of similar mutations in SRY, implying not only that SOX9 is required for testis differentiation, but also that SRY activation of SOX9 may be all that is necessary to activate other genes important to testis development, such as FGF9 (fibroblast growth factor 9), repress genes that induce ovary development.

6. b. FGF9

Ref: Speroff 8th /ed p 334.

Genes involved in ovarian development:
- WNT4 (a member of the wingless family of genes)
- RSPO1 (R-spondin 1)

- DAX1 (dosage-sensitive sex reversal, adrenal hypoplasia critical region, on chromosome X, gene 1)
- FOXl2 (forkhead box L2).

7. **a. Retinoic acid**

Ref: Speroff 8th /ed p 336, Cambridge, infertility in the male, 4th/ed p 65

Retinoic Acid

Putative meiosis inducing or inhibiting factors have focused attention on retinoic acid, which is produced in the mesonephros.

Local levels of retinoic acid may regulate germ cell differentiation in the developing gonad, with retinoic acid diffusing from the adjacent mesonephros acting as the **functional meiosis inducing factor** in female germ cells, and with CYP26B1 produced by Sertoli cells in the developing testis cords acting as the functional meiosis inhibiting factor in male germ cells.

NANOS2, a gene expressed exclusively in male germ cells, may also act as a specific meiosis inhibiting factor.

> Retinol (vitamin A) is centrally important to spermatogenesis:
> - It helps to maintain the **blood–testis barrier**
> - Enhances the effects of testosterone on the **Sertoli cell**
> - Helps enable **adhesion** of spermatogonia
> - Involved in proper **spermiation**

8. **c. Leydig cells differentiate from cells already within the gonad**

Ref: Speroff 8th /ed p 336, Cambridge; infertility in the male, 4th/ed p 30

A few points about testis development to be kept in mind:
- Sertoli cell precursors express SRY.
- The subset of somatic cells expressing SRY immediately also begins to express SOX9, a reliable marker for developing Sertoli cells.
- In turn, SOX9-positive Sertoli cell precursors secrete other paracrine signaling molecules such as FGF9 and prostaglandin D_2 (PGD_2), which also play important roles in testis differentiation.
- Under the control of SRY, Sertoli cells also secrete a factor that induces a migration of cells from the adjacent mesonephros.
- The developing testis enlarges rapidly with the influx of migrating cells, which differentiate into endothelial cells and Leydig cells upon their arrival in the developing gonad.
- Male-specific peritubular myoid cells appear to differentiate from cells already within the gonad.
- The **origin of the fetal Leydig cells is a subject of ongoing debate**. The following theories are proposed:
  - Mesenchymal cells of the **mesonephros** migrating into the testis.
  - Stem cells moving in from the **coelomic epithelium** overlying the developing gonad.
  - **Neural crest cells**.

The neural crest is an ephemeral body that extends along the rostrocaudal axis of the developing vertebrate embryo. Formed during neurulation, the migratory neural crest cells give rise to most of the peripheral nervous system, facial skeleton, and numerous other derivatives throughout the embryo, including neuroendocrine cells and possibly fetal Leydig cells.

9. **a. Bipotential gonad begins to differentiate into an ovary about 2 weeks earlier than testis development**

Ref: Speroff 8th /ed p 338

Just like in male, you should remember following points regarding development of ovary:
- In females lacking a Y chromosome and SRY, the bipotential gonad begins to differentiate into an ovary about **2 weeks later** than testis development begins in the male.
- Normal ovarian differentiation requires the presence of germ cells; in their absence, the gonadal somatic cells fail to differentiate, indicating some form of communication between germ cells and somatic cells.
- WNT4 and RSPO1 are two genes that play an important role in ovarian differentiation.
- By 20 weeks of gestation, the ovary achieves mature compartmentalization, consisting of an active cortex containing follicles exhibiting early stages of maturation and atresia, and a developing stroma.

10. **a. Brain derived neurotropic factor**

Ref: Speroff 8th /ed p 202

Molecular events that regulate primordial follicle formation:
- Members of the transforming growth factor β (TGF-β) superfamily of proteins:
  A. Activins
  B. Inhibins
  C. Anti-müllerian hormone (AMH) and
  D. Bone morphogenetic proteins (BMPs)

- Activins promote and inhibins retard primordial follicle development.
- Their relative local concentrations in the fetal ovary during the time of follicle assembly may determine the size of the ovarian follicular pool.
- AMH appears to be an important **inhibitor** of primordial follicle growth, and BMPs exert the opposite effect.

Neurotropins play a role in ovarian development.

Four mammalian neurotropins have been identified:
A. Nerve growth factor (NGF)
B. Brain-derived neurotropic factor (BDNF)
C. Neurotropin-3 (NT-3)
D. Neurotropin 4/5 (NT-4/5), all of which exert their actions via binding to high-affinity transmembrane tyrosine kinase receptors encoded by members of the trk proto-oncogene family.

11. c. Vas efferens

Ref: Cambridge, infertility in the male, 4th/ed p 11

Development of Vas Efferens

- The most cranial portion of the Wolffian duct disintegrates leaving the remnant tissue called the **appendix epididymis**.
- The mesonephric tubules (**not ducts**) that grow near the developing testes, become incorporated into the testis–epididymis structure as efferent ductules.
- **These tubules (now efferent ductules) empty into the Wolffian duct.**
- The more distal ends of the testis cords form the tubuli recti and the rete testis.

12. b. Ovary

Ref: Speroff 8th/ed p 341, Cambridge, infertility in the male, 4th/ed p 91

- The Wolffian duct develops first, differentiates into the:
  - Epididymis
  - Vas deferens
  - Seminal vesicles
- The Wolffian ducts regresses in females
- The Müllerian duct develops later, even after the beginning of sex determination, differentiates into:
  - Fallopian tubes
  - Uterus
  - Upper portion of the vagina in females
- The Müllerian duct regresses in males.

Ovaries are derived from **genital ridge**.

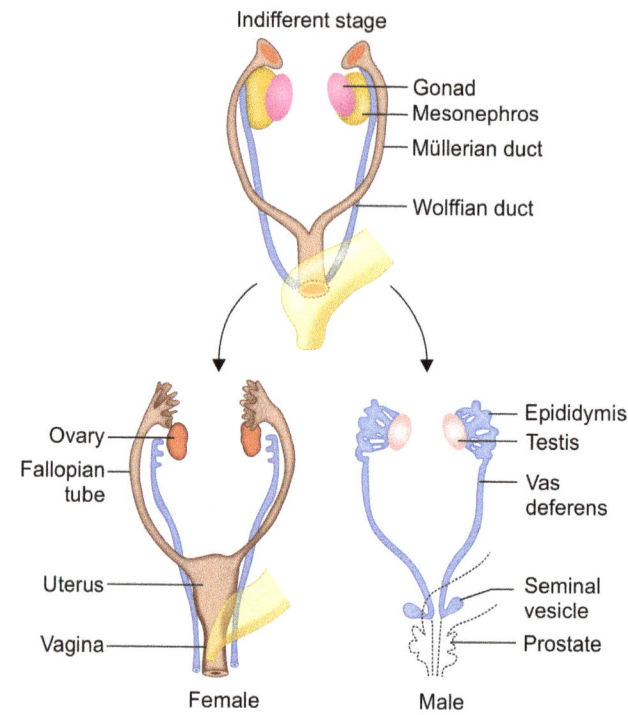

13. a. 8 weeks

Ref: Speroff 8th/ed p 343

- In the male, the Leydig cells of the fetal testis begin to secrete testosterone at **8–9 weeks** of gestation.
- Masculinization of the external genitalia begins at **10 weeks**.
- The process typically is completed by **12 to 14 weeks** of gestation.
- Testosterone rises rapidly to peak concentrations at **15–18 weeks**.

Fetal Testosterone Production

- Fetal testosterone stimulates development of the Wolffian duct system, from which the epididymis, vas deferens, and the seminal vesicles derive.
- As maternal hCG levels decline, beginning at approximately 20 weeks gestation, Leydig cell testosterone secretion comes under the control of fetal pituitary luteinizing hormone (LH).
- In the absence of LH, as in males with anencephaly and other forms of congenital hypopituitarism, Leydig cells all but disappear and the internal and external genitalia do not develop fully.

14. d. Penis

Ref: Speroff 8th/ed p 343

- The process of male external genitalia development typically is completed by **12 to 14 weeks** of gestation.

Thereafter, the principal change is in the growth and length of the penis.
- Complete development of the male external genitalia and differentiation of the prostate requires the conversion of testosterone to dihydrotestosterone (DHT), via the action of the intracellular enzyme 5α-reductase.
- The genital tubercle and the labioscrotal swellings are highly sensitive to DHT, being rich in both androgen receptors and 5α-reductase activity.

15. **a. Local testosterone levels**

Ref: Speroff 8th/ed p 339

Local Testosterone

- High local concentrations of testosterone stimulate the ipsilateral Wolffian duct to differentiate into the epididymis, vas deferens, and seminal vesicle.
- Duct system differentiation proceeds, therefore, according to the nature of the adjacent gonad.
- High concentrations of testosterone are required because the ducts do not have the ability to convert testosterone to dihydrotestosterone (DHT).

16. **d. HOX genes**

Ref: Cambridge, infertility in the male, 4th/ed p 91, Speroff 8th/ed p 340

- The mesonephric duct becomes the epididymis and vas deferens, and the residual mesonephric tubules form the efferent ducts.
- The efferent ducts unite with the rete testis, thus making the connection between the separately developing testis and the excurrent duct system.
- Mesonephric tubules failing to connect with the rete testis typically atrophy, but a few may persist as paraepididymides or appendices of the epididymis.
- Gene expressions necessary for epididymal development at these early stages include members of the WNT family, e.g. WNT4, WNT7 α, a number of **homeobox genes**, e.g. HOXA10, HOXA11, HOXA13, and so-called **paired-box genes**, e.g. PAX2 and PAX8.
- Region-specific expression of homeobox (HOX) genes are transcriptional regulators of patterning. They appear important for the differentiation of the duct into its morphologically and functionally distinct segments (caput, corpus, and caudal regions).

17. **a. Wolffian ducts act like migrational template for Müllerian ducts**

Ref: Speroff 8th/ed p 341

- Abnormalities in the renal system are highly associated with abnormalities in development of the fallopian tubes, uterus, and upper vagina.

The Wolffian ducts make no direct contribution to the müllerian ducts, but are essential for normal müllerian development, serving as a guide or **migrational template**. If the Wolffian ducts do not form, müllerian duct development also fails.

18. **a. 8 weeks**

Ref: Cambridge, infertility in the male, 4th/ed p 8

- By the sixth week of development, if the embryo is chromosomally XY, cells in the sex cords in the medulla will grow and become Sertoli cells, under the influence of SRY, and the cortex will disappear.
- The Sertoli cells will start to produce AMH, which will halt the development of the paramesonephric ducts and eventually cause rapid regression during the eighth to tenth week of development.

Remnants in the males include:
- Appendix testis
- Prostatic utricle

Rarely, a genetic male due to an AMH malfunction will have persistence of the Müllerian ducts (and thus a uterus and fallopian tubes will develop), a condition called **hernia uteri inguinale**.

19. **c. Genital swellings: scrotum and labia minora**

Ref: Cambridge, infertility in the male, 4th/ed p 11

Embryological derivatives	
1. Genital tubercle	Penis and clitoris
2. Genial folds	Ventral aspect of penis and labia minora
3. Genital swellings	Scrotum and labia majora
4. Urogenital sinus	Penile urethra and vestibule

20. **b. 18 weeks**

Ref: Speroff 8th/ed p 339

Testosterone is secreted by the fetal testes soon after Leydig cell formation at around 8 weeks gestation and rises rapidly to peak concentrations at 15–18 weeks.

Fetal testosterone stimulates development of the Wolffian duct system, from which the epididymis, vas deferens, and the seminal vesicles derive.

Testosterone levels in the male fetus correlate with:
- Leydig cell development
- Overall gonadal weight
- 3β-hydroxysteroid dehydrogenase activity
- hCG concentrations

As maternal hCG levels decline, beginning at approximately 20 weeks gestation, Leydig cell testosterone secretion comes under the control of fetal pituitary luteinizing hormone (LH).

21. d. Prostate

Ref: Cambridge, infertility in the male, 4th/ed p 91, 257; Speroff 8th/ed p 343

Role of DHT in Development of External Genitalia

- Complete development of the male external genitalia and differentiation of the prostate requires the conversion of testosterone to dihydrotestosterone (DHT), via the action of the intracellular enzyme **5α-reductase**.
- The genital tubercle and the labioscrotal swellings are highly sensitive to DHT, being rich in both androgen receptors and 5α-reductase activity.
- Testosterone and DHT are the major steroids that bind to the androgen receptor (AR).
- In some target organs, such as the prostate, the main androgen bound to the AR is DHT, while in other tissues, such as the Wolffian duct or testis, testosterone is the preferred ligand.

- Testosterone–androgen receptor complexes mediate fetal Wolffian duct virilization.
- DHT–androgen receptor complexes mediate differentiation of the male external genitalia.
- This could explain why patients with 5α-reductase deficiency and the inability to convert testosterone to DHT have normally virilized internal genitalia, but predominately female external genitalia.
- On the other hand, patients with a disorder of the androgen receptors, such as those with testicular feminization, fail to develop Wolffian structures and appear as phenotypic females.

22. d. 21-hydroxylase

Ref: Yen & Jaffe's 8th/ed p 87; Endocrine society guidelines on CAH. J Clin Endocrinol Metab 103: 4043–4088, 2018

- 21-hydroxylase deficiency is **most common** cause of autosomal recessive congenital adrenal hyperplasia.

Congenital Adrenal Hyperplasia

- P450c21 is an adrenal **endoplasmic reticulum enzyme** that catalyzes 21-hydroxylation of progesterone and 17α-hydroxyprogesterone in the pathway of mineralocorticoid and glucocorticoid synthesis.
- Affected females are virilized by excess production of adrenal androgens driven by elevated ACTH levels.
- The sign and symptoms of CAH caused by 21-hydroxylase deficiency reflect deficits in cortisol and aldosterone, along with accumulation of adrenal androgens that result from elevated ACTH levels, due to the absence of cortisol-negative feedback on hypothalamic-corticotrophin axis.

23. a. 21-hydroxylase

Ref: Cambridge. Infertility in the male. 4th/ed p 262

- Congenital adrenal hyperplasia (CAH) accounts for about 80% of the masculinized females and 90% of these result from a 21-hydroxylase deficiency.
- CAH is of particular concern because of the possibility of salt-wasting and low glucocorticoid and mineralocorticoid levels.

Less common causes of CAH include defects in:
- 11β-hydroxylase
- 3β-HSD
- P450 aromatase

As a result of the deficiency, the androgenic steroid precursors accumulate, and masculinization of the female occurs.

24. b. Salt wasting classical 21-hydroxylase deficiency

Ref: Yen & Jaffe's 8th/ed p 87, Speroff 8th/ed p 349

CAH Clinical Phenotypes

- The clinical phenotypes are variable and dependent on the severity of the 21-hydroxylase deficiency.
- Three forms:
  1. Non-salt wasting
  2. Salt wasting
  3. Non-classic forms
- Salt wasting form is associated with severe enzyme deficiency.
- CAH due to 21-hydroxylase deficiency is the **most frequent cause** of sexual ambiguity and the most common endocrine cause of neonatal death.
- The more serious **"salt-wasting" variety** of classical 21-hydroxylase deficiency is characterized by severe deficiencies of both cortisol and aldosterone, resulting in salt-wasting and dehydration in addition to virilization.
- In the **less severe "simple virilizing" form** of the disorder, elevated levels of ACTH are able to drive sufficient glucocorticoid and mineralocorticoid production to prevent circulatory collapse, but excess androgen production in utero results in masculinization of the external genitalia.
- The third and **least severe "nonclassical" form** of 21-hydroxylase deficiency generally does not become

apparent until adolescence or early adulthood, when abnormally high androgen levels cause hirsutism and menstrual irregularities.

25. **a. Autosomal recessive**

Ref: Speroff 8th/ed p 351

- All forms of CAH, including 21-hydroxylase deficiency, are transmitted as autosomal recessive disorders.

Inheritance of CAH

- Humans have 2 CYP21A genes; one is a nonfunctional **pseudogene** (CYP21A1, also designated CYP21P, encoding an inactive form of the enzyme), and the other is the **active gene** (CYP21A2).
- The 2 genes have greater than 90% homology and reside in the same region within the HLA histocompatibility complex on the short arm of chromosome 6 (6p21.3), which provides ample opportunity for recombination during meiosis.
- Women who carry a **classic mutation** are at risk for having a child with the severe form of the disorder.
- They may be asymptomatic, having one classic mutation and one normal allele, or exhibit the nonclassical form of CAH, having one classic mutation and a variant allele associated with mild enzyme deficiency (compound heterozygote).
- Compound heterozygotes having two variant alleles can exhibit the features of nonclassical CAH but are not at risk for having a child with classical CAH.

26. **c. Compound heterozygotes with both variant alleles**

Ref: Speroff 8th/ed p 351

Compound heterozygotes having two variant alleles can exhibit the features of nonclassical CAH but are not at risk for having a child with classical CAH.

27. **a. 17- hydroxyprogesterone levels**

Ref: Speroff 8th/ed p 352; Endocrine society guidelines on CAH. J Clin Endocrinol Metab 103: 4043–4088, 2018

- The diagnosis of 21-hydroxylase deficiency is based on high serum concentrations of 17-OHP, primary substrate for the enzyme.

Diagnosis of Late Onset CAH

- In the late-onset nonclassical form of 21-hydroxylase deficiency, serum 17OHP concentrations often are only slightly elevated, especially late in the day.
- The serum dehydroepiandrosterone sulfate (DHEAS) concentration usually is normal.

- In adult women, morning values less than 200 ng/dL (obtained during the early follicular phase of the cycle) exclude the diagnosis, levels over 800 ng/dL are virtually diagnostic, and intermediate results require additional evaluation with an ACTH stimulation test; in most patients with nonclassical 21-hydroxylase deficiency, the stimulated 17OHP level will exceed 1,500 ng/dL.

28. **a. ACTH stimulation test**

Ref: Speroff 8th/ed p 352; Endocrine society guidelines on CAH. J Clin Endocrinol Metab 103: 4043–4088, 2018

- When the diagnosis is suspected but uncertain, it can be confirmed by performing an ACTH stimulation test, obtaining blood samples before and 60 minutes after administering cosyntropin (synthetic ACTH 1–24; 1 mg/m^2 or 0.25 mg);
- Stimulated 17OHP levels typically exceed 1,500 ng/dL.
- Diagnosis also can be confirmed by genotyping, which can detect approximately 95% of mutations.

29. **c. 11β-hydroxylase deficiency**

Ref: Yen & Jaffe's 8th/ed p 89; Speroff 8th/ed p 353

- Like 21-hydroxylase deficiency, 11β-hydroxylase deficiency has severe salt-wasting and simple virilizing forms, and a milder late-onset form.

Mutations that inactivate HSD11B2 produce a syndrome of apparent mineralocorticoid excess which leads to hypertension, hypokalemia, and renal structural abnormalities.

- Whereas both 21-hydroxylase deficiency and 11β-hydroxylase deficiency may result in salt-wasting, approximately two-thirds of patients with 11β-hydroxylase deficiency exhibit hypertension due to an increased production of mineralocorticoids.
- Hypokalemia also may be observed and plasma renin activity often is low. These effects generally have been attributed to excess production of 11-deoxycorticosterone, which has significant mineralocorticoid activity.

30. **a. 17α hydroxypregnenolone concentration after ACTH stimulation**

Ref: Yen & Jaffe's 8th/ed p 87; Speroff 8th/ed p 353

- This is most likely deficiency of 3β-hydroxysteroid dehydrogenase enzyme.
- These are membrane-bound enzymes localized to endoplasmic reticulum and mitochondria.
- These enzymes catalyse dehydrogenation of 3β-hydroxyl group to yield delta 4 ketone structure.

- They convert
  1. Pregnenolone into progesterone
  2. 17α-hydroxypregnenolone to 17α-hydroxyprogesterone
  3. Dehydroepiandrosterone to androstenedione
- Basal levels of D^5-3β-hydroxy steroids (pregnenolone, 17α-hydroxypreg-nenolone, DHEA and DHEAS) generally are elevated in affected individuals.
- An increased ratio of D^5/D^4 steroids is a better indication of a possible 3β-HSD deficiency.
- The most reliable diagnostic criterion is the serum 17α-hydroxypregnenolone concentration after ACTH stimulation.
- Proposed threshold values are based on observations in patients with documented mutations (neonates, ≥ 12,600 ng/dL; Tanner stage I children ≥ 5,490 ng/dL, children with premature pubarche, ≥ 9,790 ng/dL; adults ≥ 9,620 ng/dL).
- The pathway is as follows

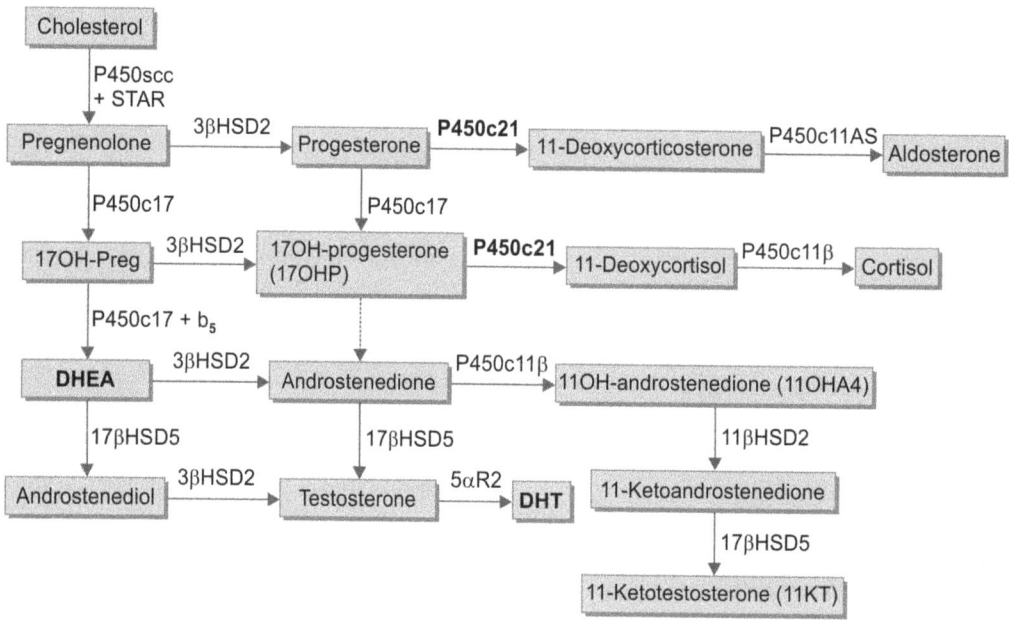

31. b. 4–5 weeks

Ref: Speroff 8th/ed p 355

- Dexamethasone is not metabolized by the placenta and crosses effectively into the fetal circulation.

Prenatal maternal treatment with dexamethasone (up to 1.5 mg daily in divided doses) can greatly decrease or prevent fetal female genital virilization.

- For maximum effectiveness, treatment should begin at 4 to 5 weeks of gestation, and not later than 9 weeks.
- Prenatal maternal treatment poses some potential risks for the fetus, such as postnatal failure to thrive and psychomotor developmental delay, and can have significant maternal side effects, including severe abdominal striae, hyperglycemia, hypertension, gastrointestinal symptoms, and emotional lability.

32. a. Delayed puberty

Ref: Speroff 8th/ed p 358

- Children with classical CAH are at increased risk for early puberty and short stature because high levels of sex steroids promote **premature epiphyseal closure**.
- In treated patients with classical CAH, adult height usually is lower than in reference populations, by an average of approximately 10 cm.
- Obesity is a common complication of glucocorticoid treatment. In obese children, the incidence of hypertension also increased.

33. b. Bedtime

Ref: Speroff 8th/ed p 358

When administered at bedtime in a dose ranging between 0.25 and 0.75 mg, ACTH is effectively suppressed for most of the following day.

Bedtime treatment effectively inhibits the peak of ACTH secretion, which occurs between 2:00 A.M. and 10:00 A.M.

34. d. Hydrocortisone treatment should be replaced by dexamethasone treatment in pregnancy as placenta can metabolize dexamethasone

Ref: Speroff 8th/ed p 359

It is otherwise.

Treatment with long-acting glucocorticoids should be discontinued **in favor of treatment with hydrocortisone**, which is metabolized by the placenta and thereby avoids the risk of suppressing the fetal hypothalamic-pituitary-adrenal axis.

Even when maternal androgen levels cannot be suppressed to normal, the high capacity of placental aromatase activity effectively protects the fetal female genitalia.

35. a. P450 Oxidoreductase (POR) deficiency

Ref: Yen & Jaffe's 8th/ed p 364

P450 Oxidoreductase (POR) Deficiency

- POR is a **flavoprotein** that is required for action of all microsomal P450 enzymes.
- POR deficiency is recently characterized cause of CAH, which affects the enzymatic activity of all microsomal P450 enzymes, including steroidogenic enzymes P450c17, P450c21, and P450aro.
- As many enzymes are involved, POR deficiency presents with a wide range of phenotypes.

36. b. Newly described steroidogenic enzyme as a cause of CAH

Ref: Yen & Jaffe's 8th/ed p 364, Speroff 8th/ed p 360

The classical forms of CAH all are caused by mutations in genes encoding steroidogenic enzymes, resulting in reduced or absent enzyme activity.

A newly described form of CAH results from a deficiency in the P450 oxidoreductase (POR) enzyme.

Although **not a steroidogenic enzyme** per se, POR nonetheless affects several steroidogenic pathways and now is recognized as a cause of both 46, XX disorders of sexual development (female virilization) and 46, XY disorders of sexual development (incomplete male virilization).

37. a. Liver

Ref: Yen & Jaffe's 8th/ed p 77, Speroff 8th/ed p 384

Aromatase Deficiency

- It is an endoplasmic reticulum enzyme.
- It is also designated as P450arom and CYP19A1.
- The aromatase protein is encoded by a single large gene, CYP19A1 located on chromosome 15 (15p21.1).
- It catalyzes the conversion of 19-carbon androgens (androstenedione, testosterone, 16a-hydroxy DHEA) to aromatic 18-carbon estrogens (estrone, estradiol, and estriol, respectively).
- The enzyme is active in the gonads, the placenta, the brain, and in adipose; tissue-specific regulation is controlled, in part, by alternative tissue-specific promoters.
- Aromatase deficiency is a rare autosomal recessive disorder caused by mutations in the CYP19A1 gene.
- As a consequence, fetal androgens are not converted to estrogens in the placenta, resulting in female fetal virilization (due to the accumulation of fetal androgens), low maternal serum estrogen levels, and maternal hirsutism.

38. c. Catalyzes conversion of 21 carbon to 18 carbon compound

Ref: Yen & Jaffe's 8th/ed p 77

Aromatase catalyzes three sequential hydroxylations of a C19 substrate by using three molecules of NADPH and three molecules of molecular oxygen to produce one molecule of C18 steroid with a phenolic A ring.

The first hydroxylation yields a C19 hydroxyl derivative, which is converted in a second hydroxylation to yield C19 aldehyde.

39. a. Clitoromegaly

Ref: Speroff 8th/ed p 362

The possible or probable extent of fetal virilization relates to **the time** of exposure to maternal androgens.

Time of exposure	Effect
Exposure during early pregnancy	Labioscrotal fusion Clitoromegaly
Exposure after 12 weeks of gestation	Clitoral hypertrophy only

40. d. All

Ref: Speroff 8th/ed p 362

Maternal Gestational Hyperandrogenism

It is cause of fetal virilization and may result from maternal ingestion of androgens or drugs having androgenic actions, or from excess maternal androgen production.

Luteomas and theca-lutein cysts are the most common causes.

Virilizing ovarian or adrenal tumors are rarely encountered during pregnancy.

41. b. High risk of female child becoming virilized

Ref: Speroff 8th/ed p 364

Theca-Lutein Cysts

- Ovaries containing theca-lutein cysts can become quite enlarged, reaching 10-15 cm in diameter.

- Histologically, the ovarian cortex usually exhibits focal hyalinization.
- Approximately **30%** of pregnant women with clinically apparent theca-lutein cysts become hirsute or virilize.
- In most of those who exhibit virilization, serum concentrations of testosterone and androstenedione are elevated; cord serum testosterone levels also may be elevated in their infants, but no cases of virilized female infants have been reported.

42. **c. Affected patients often have cardiac anomalies**

Ref: Yen & Jaffe's 8th/ed p 207

Mayer-Rokitansky-Kuster-Hauser Syndrome (MRKH)

- It is the congenital aplasia or severe hypoplasia of adult derivatives of Müllerian duct, including fallopian tubes, uterus, cervix, and upper vagina.
- Incidence: 1 in 4500 women.
- Subclassified into two types
- Type I: isolated Müllerian hypoplasia
- Type II: also known as Müllerian Renal Cervico-thoracic Somite (MURCS association), involving renal, skeletal, and hearing defects, as well as occasional cardiac and digital anomalies.
- More recently, a third distinct entity, MRKH association with hyperandrogenism, has been reported and association with four different defects in WNT4 gene have been confirmed.
- Typically, the ovaries are entirely normal, although one or both also may be undescended, hypoplastic, or associated with an inguinal hernia.
- Affected patients often also have urologic anomalies (unilateral renal agenesis, ectopic or horseshoe kidney, and duplication of the collecting systems) and skeletal malformations (e.g., hemiverterbrae and scoliosis, or the Klippel-Feil syndrome, which includes a short neck, low hairline, limited range of motion, and neurologic symptoms, resulting from one or more fused vertebrae).

43. **b. Swyer syndrome**

Ref: Yen & Jaffe's 8th/ed p 412

Swyer Syndrome

- Complete gonadal dysgenesis.
- Individuals have intra-abdominal, bilateral, fibrous streaks which do not secrete AMH or testosterone.
- Phenotypically, pure XY gonadal dysgenesis individuals are unambiguously phenotypic females but usually internally possess hypoplastic Müllerian structures.
- Affected individuals generally present after the expected time of puberty with delayed sexual maturation, primary amenorrhea, normal pubic hair, and normal female internal and external genital anatomy.
- Evaluation reveals hypergonadotropic hypogonadism, prompting a karyotype that establishes the diagnosis.
- They are at increased risk of gonadoblastoma because dysgenetic gonads carrying Y chromosome have an increased risk for neoplastic changes.

44. **a. Steroid 5α reductase deficiency**

Ref: Cambridge. Infertility in the male. 4th/ed p 262

5α-reductase Deficiency

- Autosomal recessive disorder
- Karyotype: 46, XY
- Defective conversion of testosterone to DHT leading to impaired virilization during embryogenesis
- Severe perineal hypospadias

The **distinguishing feature** of the disorder is that affected individuals virilize, to varying degrees, at the time of puberty.

Hormonal profile:
- Mild elevation in testosterone
- Decreased to absent levels of DHT
- Normal LH and FSH levels

Because of the failure to convert testosterone to DHT, DHT-sensitive organs do not develop normally. Patients present with a spectrum of ambiguous genitalia, abnormal prostate development, and abnormal virilization at puberty.

- These men usually have sperm production adequate to initiate a pregnancy, but, because of their genital-urinary anatomic defects, intrauterine insemination may be necessary.

45. **c. 17α-hydroxylase deficiency**

Ref: Speroff 8th/ed p 369

17α-Hydroxylase Deficiency

- The CYP17A1 gene encodes an enzyme having both 17α-hydroxylase and 17,20-lyase activities, which are required for synthesis of cortisol, androgens and estrogens.
- The compensatory increase in ACTH stimulation that accompanies decreased cortisol synthesis stimulates increased production of 11-deoxysteroids (via 21-hydroxylase), including corticosterone and the mineralocorticoids 11-deoxycorticosterone and 18-hydroxy-deoxycorticosterone.

- Females with 17α-hydroxylase deficiency typically present with delayed puberty, primary amenorrhea, and hypergonadotropic hypogonadism; most are hypertensive (due to hypernatremia and hypervolemia) and some also have hypokalemia.
- Affected males have female external genitalia, a blind vagina, and intra-abdominal testes; most raised as girls, with underlying disorder recognized only later during evaluation for delayed puberty.

46. **c. Congenital lipoid adrenal hyperplasia**

    Ref: Speroff 8th/ed p 371

- Congenital lipoid adrenal hyperplasia is the rarest and most severe form of CAH.
- Autosomal recessive disorder.
- Mutations in the gene encoding the steroidogenic acute regulatory (StAR) protein.

Congenital Lipoid Adrenal Hyperplasia

- Characterized by a deficiency of all adrenal and gonadal steroid hormones, increased ACTH secretion, and marked adrenal hyperplasia associated with progressive accumulation of cholesterol esters.
- StAR facilitates **transport of cholesterol** from the outer to the inner mitochondrial membrane, the rate-limiting step in steroidogenesis.
- It is expressed in the adrenal cortex and gonads, but not in the placenta.
- All steroidogenic pathways are affected, resulting in a **global deficiency of steroid hormones** that reflects both the intrinsic defect in steroidogenesis and the progressive cellular damage that results from the accumulation of cholesterol.
- Serum cortisol and aldosterone concentrations are very low, ACTH and plasma renin activity levels are very high, sex steroid concentrations are low and serum gonadotropin levels are elevated, even in young children.
- Present very soon after birth or in early infancy with symptoms of severe adrenal insufficiency (vomiting, diarrhea, volume depletion, hyponatremia, hyperkalemia).
- Male infants usually have female external genitalia due to the severe androgen deficiency.
- **Females are normally developed** at birth and even may undergo spontaneous puberty, possibly because the prepubertal ovary, unlike the adrenals and testes, is relatively dormant and thus may escape cellular damage from cholesterol accumulation.

47. **a. Steroidogenic acute regulatory (StAR) protein**

    Ref: Speroff 8th/ed p 371

48. **a. Congenital lipoid adrenal hyperplasia**

    Ref: Speroff 8th/ed p 371

49. **d. Mutations of StAR gene**

    Ref: Speroff 8th/ed p 371

Congenital lipoid adrenal hyperplasia caused by mutations of the StAR gene, located on chromosome 8p11.2, are the only inherited disorder of steroidogenesis not caused by a defect in one of the steroidogenic enzymes.

50. **d. Ovarian granulosa cell**

    Ref: Speroff 8th/ed p 40

In the adrenal gland pathway to cortisol, very little 17,20-lyase activity is expressed.

In the ovarian theca cells, the testicular Leydig cells, and the adrenal reticularis, both 17-hydroxylase and 17,20-lyase activities are expressed, directing the steroidogenic pathway via dehydroepiandrosterone (DHEA).

Granulosa cells lack 17-hydroxylase enzyme.

In the corpus luteum, the principal pathway is via progesterone.

51. **b. 17β-hydroxysteroid dehydrogenase**

    Ref: Speroff 8th/ed p 41

- The 17β-hydroxysteroid dehydrogenase and 5α-reductase reactions are mediated by non-P450 enzymes.
- The 17β-hydroxysteroid dehydrogenase is bound to the endoplasmic reticulum and the 5α-reductase to the nuclear membrane.
- The 17β-hydroxysteroid dehydrogenase enzymes convert
    - Estrone to estradiol
    - Androstenedione to testosterone
    - DHEA to androstenediol, and vice versa.

Eight different isozymes have been cloned and characterized.

The cell-specific production of each of these isoforms is a method for regulating the local concentration of estrogens and androgens.

52. **a. Complete androgen insensitivity syndrome**

    Ref: Cambridge Infertility in Male. 4th/ed p 258

- The AR gene is located on the X chromosome **(Xq12).**
- Complete AIS follows an **X-linked recessive** pattern of inheritance.

Androgen Insensitivity Syndrome

- The three main clinical phenotypes resulting from androgen insensitivity are defined as complete, partial, and minimal androgen insensitivity (CAIS, PAIS, and MAIS).
- Kennedy syndrome, also known as X-linked spinal and bulbar muscular atrophy (SBMA), is a form of androgen insensitivity associated with aging, which results in reduced fertility.
- These diseases also include Reifenstein syndrome, testicular feminization (male pseudohermaphroditism), Lub syndrome, and Rosewater syndrome.
- Androgen resistance can be present in men who are undervirilized or infertile.

53. c. AIS always follows Mendelian inheritance pattern

Ref: Speroff 8th/ed p 373

- 40% of patients with complete AIS have no family history of the disorder, presumably representing de novo mutations.

Inheritance in AIS

- Complete AIS can result from a wide variety of inactivating mutations in the AR gene, including major gene deletions, premature stop codons, splicing abnormalities, and missense mutations that result in amino acid substitutions in the androgen receptor.
- The AR gene is located on the X chromosome (Xq12) and complete AIS therefore follows an X-linked recessive pattern of inheritance.
- One in three phenotypic sisters of an affected individual and one in six female offspring of a normal sister will have XY karyotype.

54. a. Complete androgen insensitivity syndrome

Ref: Cambridge Infertility in Male. 4th/ed p 258

- The diagnosis of complete AIS should be suspected in girls with inguinal hernias or labial masses, and in women with primary amenorrhea.
- In the adolescent or adult, diagnosis usually is not difficult.
- The CAIS individuals are 46, XY pseudohermaphrodites (genotypic males) displaying an unambiguously female appearance.
- Female external genitalia develop because, despite high circulating testosterone levels, the tissues are resistant to androgen action. Thus DHT-dependent masculinization of the external genital primordia is absent.
- Patients with CAIS have underdeveloped labia, a blind-ending vagina, and paucity of axillary or pubic hair.
- Because the labial or abdominal testes continue to produce AMH, the uterus, ovaries, and fallopian tubes are absent.
- CAIS occurs in about 2–5/100 000 births, and these patients are sterile.
- So, in summary most patients with complete AIS present with primary amenorrhea, normal breast development, absent or scant pubic and axillary hair, a short vagina, and an absent cervix and uterus; a serum testosterone in the normal male range and a 46, XY karyotype establish the diagnosis.

55. c. Gonadectomy is indicated soon after diagnosis due to significant risk of germ cell tumors in AIS

Ref: Speroff 8th/ed p 374

- Gonadectomy is indicated **soon after diagnosis** of Swyer syndrome due the significant risk for development of germ cell tumors in occult testicular elements (20–30%).

In patients with complete AIS, gonadectomy generally is best delayed until after puberty is completed (approximately age 16–18) because pubertal development generally proceeds more smoothly in response to endogenous hormone production, and because the overall risk for tumor development is quite low (5–10%), particularly before puberty.

56. b. Partial androgen insensitivity syndrome

Ref: Speroff 8th/ed p 374

Reifenstein syndrome

57. b. Incomplete AIS

Ref: Speroff 8th/ed p 374

Reifenstein Syndrome

- Individuals having a predominantly male phenotype who are **undervirilized**.
- Chief clinical presentation: infertile man with a bifid scrotum and perineoscrotal hypospadias.
- However, the appearance of the external genitalia can vary widely, from a microphallus with a normal penile urethra to complete failure of scrotal fusion.
- The internal genitalia are male but not completely developed; Müllerian structures are absent.
- The testes can be:
  - Cryptorchid
  - Small
  - Exhibit **maturation arrest**

- Men with Reifenstein syndrome have normal axillary and pubic hair but, typically, little or no chest or facial hair.
- They have a male body habitus but usually develop gynecomastia at the time of puberty.
- Gender identity corresponds with the sex of rearing and sexual dysfunction is common in those raised as males.

58. a. LH receptor defects

Ref: Speroff 8th/ed p 376

- Leydig cell hypoplasia, describing the absence of mature Leydig cells in the testes, is a rare autosomal recessive 46,XY disorder of sexual development caused by inactivating mutations in the LH/hCG receptor.
- The phenotype of patients with Leydig cell hypoplasia otherwise generally correlates with the level of residual LH/hCG receptor activity, ranging from completely female external genital development to nearly normal male genitalia.
- Those having no significant testosterone production appear female at birth and present at puberty with primary amenorrhea and sexual infantilism, lacking both pubic hair development (due to the lack of testosterone) and breast development (due to the absence of aromatizable substrate)
- The serum LH concentration is elevated and testosterone levels are abnormally low.

59. b. Uterine hernia syndrome

Ref: Speroff 8th/ed p 377; Infertility in the male. Cambridge. 4th/ed p 264

Hernia Uterine Inguinale Syndrome

- Rare autosomal recessive disorder.
- Results from failure of Müllerian duct regression, due to mutations in the genes encoding AMH or its receptor.
- Affected patients appear as normal males having an inguinal hernia containing relatively well-differentiated müllerian duct structures, usually including a uterus and fallopian tubes.
- They have normal male internal and external genitalia and, usually, cryptorchid testes.

60. d. Short stature

Ref: Yen & Jaffe's 8th/ed p 411

- The sine qua non of turner syndrome is short stature.
- Approximately 95% of individuals with TS have short stature.
- Haploinsufficiency for the short stature homeobox-containing (SHOX) gene, located in the pseudoautosomal region of the X chromosome, contributes to the short stature and skeletal abnormalities associated with TS.

Common skeletal features include:
- Cubitus valgus
- Shortened fourth metacarpals
- Short neck
- High arched palate
- Madelung deformity
- Scoliosis (may develop during the adolescent years)

61. d. All

Ref: National Organisation of Rare Disorders. Melissa L. 2019

Synonyms of Turner Syndrome

- 45, X syndrome
- Bonnevie-Ullrich syndrome
- Monosomy X
- Ullrich-Turner syndrome

62. d. Sporadic

Ref: National Organization for Rare Disorders. Melissa L. 2019

In females with Turner syndrome, all or a portion of one of the second sex chromosome is missing.

The reason that this occurs is unknown and is believed to result from a random event.

In some cases, the chromosomal abnormality appears to arise spontaneously (de novo) due to an error in the division of a parent's reproductive cells, either in the sperm or oocyte.

This results in the genetic error being contained in all cells of the body.

63. a. Noonan syndrome

Ref: Yen & Jaffe's 8th/ed p 439

Other names for Noonan syndrome:
- Male Turner syndrome
- Female pseudo-Turner syndrome
- Turner phenotype with normal chromosomes karyotype

Noonan Syndrome

- Clinical features of Noonan syndrome include short stature, hypertelorism, short webbed neck, mental retardation, bleeding disorders, and right-sided cardiac anomalies.
- The estimated incidence ranges from 1:1000 to 1:2500 live births.
- Though inherited in an **autosomal-dominant** manner, 60% of cases are sporadic.
- **Cryptorchidism** is common in affected males.
- Reproductive function tends to be normal in women.
- Post-pubertal men tend to have elevated LH and FSH concentrations and declining AMH and inhibin B concentrations suggesting that Sertoli and/or germ cell function progressively deteriorates, resulting in impaired spermatogenesis and subfertility.

Differences between Noonan and Turner syndrome:
1. Noonan syndrome affects both males and females
2. Normal karyotype in Noonan syndrome.

64. a. Small X-ring chromosome

Ref: Yen & Jaffe's 8th/ed p 436, American journal of medical genetics, 1992

Patients with Turner syndrome typically have normal intelligence. The rare patient having a **small X-ring chromosome** may have severe mental retardation, because the ring chromosome does not undergo X-inactivation.

Mental retardation is typical for girls with ring X chromosomes lacking the XIST gene (the gene responsible for X inactivation) because one copy of certain genes is not activated.

65. c. 45, XO/45, XY

Ref: Yen & Jaffe's 8th/ed p 436

- Girls with TS and evidence of virilization or presence of a marker chromosome should be thoroughly evaluated for presence of Y chromosomal material. If Y chromosomal sequences are present, the risk for development of gonadoblastoma is estimated to be 7% to 10%.
- Such gonadoblastomas may secrete testosterone or estrogens and become calcified, but rarely become malignant.
- For patients with 45, X/46, XY karyotypes, prophylactic gonadectomy needs to be considered.

Turner Syndrome

- Turner syndrome (TS) is due to deletions or structural rearrangements of the X chromosome.
- The reported incidence of liveborn females - 1:2000 to 1:5000.
- Initially, the process of ovarian differentiation proceeds normally in fetuses with TS.
- During the 4th week of gestation, the primitive germ cells begin to migrate from their extra-gonadal site of origin to the genital ridge.
- Premature degeneration of ovarian follicles begins by 18 weeks of gestation. Ovarian follicles are replaced by abundant connective tissue (streak gonad). This accelerated prenatal and postnatal follicular atresia is generally associated with ovarian failure.
- Majority of girls with TS do not spontaneously enter puberty.
- 25% to 30% of girls show partial pubertal development at the appropriate time, and 2% to 5% may have spontaneous menses.
- Spontaneous pubertal development is more common among girls with mosaic karyotypes.

66. b. 48, XXY

Ref: Infertility in the male, Cambridge, 4th/ed p 251

Klinefelter Syndrome

- Klinefelter syndrome occcuring in approximately 1 in 500 to 1 in 1000 live births, is most common cause of **classic hypergonadotropic hypogonadism**.
- It is underlying genetic anomaly in 10% of nonobstructive azoospermic men.
- The most common karyotype associated with the disorder is 47, XXY, but additional X chromosomes (e.g., 48, XXXY) and mosaics (e.g., 46, XY/47, XXY) also have been described.
- Klinefelter syndrome results from **nondisjunction of the sex chromosomes** of either parent during meiosis; mosaics likely result from mitotic nondisjunction.

67. a. Caput epididymidis

Ref: Infertility in the male, Cambridge, 4th/ed p 262

- The caput epididymidis, made up of the efferent ductules, is always present and will be full and firm, as it is distended with fluid from the testis.
- The corpus and cauda are occasionally found as well.
- The vasa are absent bilaterally to palpation.
- Since the seminal vesicles are typically absent or atrophic, although occasionally large and cystic, the ejaculate consists only of prostatic fluid and is thin, watery, of low volume (0.6 mL), and low pH (6.5).

68. b. Nervous system

Ref: Infertility in the male, Cambridge, 4th/ed p 263

- The most life-threatening and morbid clinical component of CF is the **obstructive pulmonary disease** resulting from thickened, tenacious respiratory secretions that begin a cycle of repetitive infections in the small airways and alveoli.
- For similar biochemical reasons, the pancreatic exocrine system may fail. This is a less morbid issue because of the availability of oral pancreatic enzyme replacement.
- Spermatogenesis is intrinsically normal.

69. d. All

Ref: Infertility in the male, Cambridge, 4th/ed p 264

Syndromes that adversely affect extratesticular ductal system, thus leading to male infertility:
- CBAVD
- Persistent Müllerian duct syndrome
- Failure of mesonephric duct differentiation
- Prune belly syndrome
- Young syndrome

70. **c. C**

Ref: Endocrine society guidelines on CAH. J Clin Endocrinol Metab 103: 4043–4088, 2018

- The US Food and Drug Administration classifies Dexamethasone as a **category C drug** whose safety in pregnancy is not established.

According to the US Food and Drug Administration, "Animal reproduction studies have shown an adverse effect on the fetus and there are no adequate and well-controlled studies in humans, but potential benefits may warrant use of the drug in pregnant women despite potential risks".

Consistent with animal data that Dexamethasone can cause cleft palate, the National Birth Defects Prevention Study reviewed 1769 infants with cleft lip with/ without cleft palate born to women who received glucocorticoids during the first trimester, finding statistically increased risks of orofacial clefts compared with 4143 controls.

A recent case report cited the first known instance of an orofacial cleft in a girl affected with CAH treated prenatally with Dexamethasone.

Acute encephalopathy was reported in two infants who had received prenatal Dexamethasone.

CHAPTER 7

Endocrinology of Pubertal Development

Multiple Choice Questions

1. A girl 11 years of age, presents in your clinic along with her mother with complain that she is feeling growth in size of breast buds. As her physician what will be the correct order of pubertal events which you will explain her to decrease her anxiety?
   a. Thelarche > Pubarche > Menarche
   b. Menarche > Pubarche > Thelarche
   c. Thelarche > Menarche > Pubarche
   d. Pubarche > Thelarche > Menarche

2. How many times Hypothalamo-pituitary-gonadal axis gets activated in total, ultimately getting activated for the final time at adolescence?
   a. Once   b. Twice
   c. Thrice   d. Four times

3. During embryogenesis, the olfactory placode is the place of origin of GnRH neurons. They migrate to their final destination in:
   a. Medial basal hypothalamus
   b. Lateral basal hypothalamus
   c. Supraoptic nucleus
   d. Paraventricular nucleus

4. Development of portal venous system is completed by how many weeks?
   a. 9-10 weeks
   b. 19-20 weeks
   c. 25-26 weeks
   d. 32-33 weeks

5. Puberty is result of activation of hypothalamo-pituitary-gonadal axis. When is this axis gets activated for the first time?
   a. In early pregnancy   b. In late pregnancy
   c. Infancy   d. Adolescence

6. In response to pulsatile GnRH, pituitary secretes FSH and LH into fetal circulation by the end of:
   a. 22 weeks   b. 12 weeks
   c. 32 weeks   d. Only postpartum

7. Juvenile pause refers to interval between:
   a. Infancy and puberty
   b. Birth and puberty
   c. Birth and infancy
   d. Adolescence

8. Gonadostat theory forms the basis of juvenile pause. Most likely postulated hypothesis for gonadostat theory:
   a. Central inhibition of pulsatile secretion
   b. Heightened sensitivity to negative feedback effect of sex steroids
   c. Both of the above
   d. None of the above

9. All of the following holds true for puberty, *except*:
   a. Early stages of puberty are associated with nocturnal rise of LH
   b. GnRH pulse generator activity is abolished during juvenile pause phase
   c. Central inhibition of pulsatile secretion of GnRH is the most likely explanation for juvenile pause
   b. Minipuberty is associated with rise of FSH more in girls and LH more in boys

10. Final maturation of HPG axis is characterised by:
    a. Development of estrogen positive feedback, culminating in ovulation
    b. Onset of menses
    c. Attainment of final adult height
    d. None of the above

11. All of the following are associated with inhibition of onset of puberty, *except*:
    a. GABA   b. Neuropeptide Y
    c. Ghrelin   d. Leptin

12. Functional antagonist of leptin, inhibiting release of GnRH:
    a. Ghrelin   b. Neuropeptide Y
    c. GABA   d. Glutamate

13. All are associated with earlier onset of puberty, *except*:
    a. Suppressed leptin levels
    b. Elevated IGF-1 levels
    c. Insulin resistance
    d. High animal protein intake

14. As per Frisch hypothesis, what is the percentage of fat in body necessary for initiation of puberty?
    a. 27%
    b. 7%
    c. 37%
    d. 17%

15. Neurons in the arcuate nucleus functioning as a "pubertal clock," or as a growth-tracking "somatometer," which are critical component of the neurobiologic mechanism that regulates the activity of the hypothalamic pulse generator?
    a. Kisspeptins
    b. Neuropeptins
    c. Angiopeptins
    d. Lipopectins

16. True about kisspeptins, all *except*:
    a. Kisspeptin neurons are located in preoptic and infundibular are of hypothalamus
    b. Activating mutations in KISS1R leads to hypogonadotropic hypogonadism
    c. Kisspeptin neurons are upstream regulatory neurons of GnRH neurons
    d. Continuous kisspeptin infusion downregulates GPR54, suppressing both LH pulse amplitude and frequency

17. Recombinant leptin has role in all of the following conditions, *except*:
    a. Precocious puberty
    b. Hypogonadotropic hypogonadism
    c. Delayed puberty
    d. None of the above

18. All of the following all true for adrenarche, *except*:
    a. Activation of zona reticularis of adrenal cortex
    b. Recognized clinically as pubarche
    c. Adrenarche is dependent of the maturation of the hypothalamic-pituitary-gonadal axis
    d. Starts around the age of 6 years

19. Biochemical indicators of adrenarche in girls:
    a. Serum DHEAS
    b. Serum testosterone
    c. Androstenedione
    d. 5 DHT

20. 1st sign of puberty in males:
    a. Prostatic growth
    b. Penile growth
    c. Testicular growth
    d. Deepening of voice

21. False statement for premature thelarche:
    a. Associated with marked acceleration of skeletal age
    b. Breast development before the age of 8 years
    c. Follow up needed to differentiate from CPP
    d. May occur in association with EDCs

22. Gold standard treatment for idiopathic central precocious puberty:
    a. Short acting GnRH agonists
    b. Long acting GnRH agonists
    c. GnRH antagonists
    d. Glucocorticoids

23. All holds true for treatment of precocious puberty with GnRH agonists, *except*:
    a. Reproductive potential is found to be decreased in girls who received treatment with GnRH agonists
    b. Most effective when treatment started before the age of 6 years
    c. Increase in final adult height up to 10 cm can be seen
    d. Gonadal function is promptly restored after cessation of treatment

24. Which of the following is not the cause of peripheral precocious puberty?
    a. Juvenile granulosa cell tumors
    b. McCune-Albright syndrome
    c. Primary hypothyroidism
    d. Congenital adrenal hyperplasia

25. A 7-year-old girl presenting in OPD with her mother with complain of breast development. On examination, breast Tanner stage 2, evidence of hyperpigmented spots with jagged borders all over-body. On X-ray of non-dominant wrist-bone age accelerated to chronological age. Long bone X-ray showed dysplastic areas. Lab investigations: FSH, LH levels within normal range, E2 elevated. Which of the following is not true for above condition?
    a. Above condition is an example of cause of central precocious puberty
    b. Activating mutations in GNAS1 gene
    c. More common in girls
    d. May be associated with other endocrinopathies

26. **Peak IGF-1 levels are seen in which phase of human life?**
    a. Infancy
    b. Puberty
    c. Reproductive age
    d. Menopause

27. **Zona reticularis exhibits a unique enzymatic profile with following hormones showing high activity, *except*:**
    a. 3 β hydroxysteroid dehydrogenase
    b. 17 α hydroxylase
    c. 17, 20 lyase
    d. Steroid sulfotransferase

28. **A 9-year-old girl presents to you in your OPD along with her mother with complaints of increase in size of breast buds with no other complain. She is overweight. What will you explain mother and girl regarding this situation?**
    a. Age of onset of puberty has been declining and she should not panic over onset of thelarche at this age
    b. Higher weight and body fat mass are associated with an increased likelihood of early menarche
    c. Early pubertal development is associated with slightly decreased adult height and an increased risk for obesity, compared to a late menarche
    d. All of the above

29. **Priya, 11-year-old girl presents in your clinic with development of breast buds and pubic hair but tells you that she has not attained menarche yet. Which hormone will not be detectable in her until she gets menstrual cycles?**
    a. Inhibin A
    b. Inhibin B
    c. Estradiol
    d. Testosterone

30. **All of the following conditions merit thorough evaluation when girl presents with precocious puberty, *except*:**
    a. 6 year old girl presenting with Pubarche
    b. 7 year old girl presenting with both Thelarche and Pubarche
    c. 7 year old girl presenting with isolated thelarche
    d. 7 year old girl presenting with both Thelarche and advanced bone age

31. **A 6-year-old girl presenting in your clinic along with her mother with complaint of breast budding and spotting per vaginum. Lab investigations showed elevated serum estradiol levels with low both basal and GnRH stimulated gonadotropin concentrations. What is the most common cause of above condition?**
    a. Functional ovarian follicular cysts
    b. McCune -Albright syndrome
    c. Granulosa cell tumors
    d. Iatrogenic

32. **A 7-year-old presents with her aunt with thelarche and pubarche in your clinic. She does not give any history of spotting per vaginum. Aunt tells that her height is same as her peers. What is the next line of evaluation?**
    a. GnRH stimulation test
    b. Bone age assessment
    c. Ultrasonography pelvis
    d. MRI brain

33. **The same girl as mentioned above, bone age shows advanced bone age than chronological age. What is now next step in evaluation?**
    a. GnRH stimulation test
    b. Head MRI
    c. Ultrasonography pelvis
    d. ACTH stimulation test

34. **A 14-year-old girl presents in your clinic with her mother. Girl tells her height is less than her peers and she feels bad about it. On history taking she tells she has not attained menarche yet. On examination you see, breast is prepubertal and very sparse pubic hair. Her chest appear shield like and she has slight webbing of neck. You order karyotyping for child and it comes out as 45XO. After all investigations you plan to put her on hormone replacement therapy as treatment for delayed puberty. You start her with transdermal estrogen. When should you start progesterone?**
    a. Once menses have begun
    b. Once breast grows Tanner stage 4
    c. Along with estrogen
    d. After 12 months of estrogen therapy

35. **A 14-year-old girl presents in your clinic with her mother with complaints of lack of breast development and non-attainment of menarche. What will be your next line of management?**
    a. FSH, LH, E2
    b. Karyotyping
    c. Head MRI
    d. Bone age

36. **Same bone age girl comes out to be delayed, what will be your next line of evaluation?**
    a. FSH, LH, E2
    b. Karyotyping
    c. Head MRI
    d. DHEAS

37. A 9-year-old girl visits your clinic with her mother. Mother complains that her girl's height is not at par with her peers, so she is worried regarding short stature of her child. On examination, you see, breast pre pubertal and no pubic hairs. What is your next line of evaluation?
    a. Karyotype
    b. Bone age
    c. Head MRI
    d. Serum IGF-1

38. The Bayley-Pinneau can be used to determine a predicted adult height. What are the parameters on which Bayley- Pinneau tables are based?
    a. Current height and bone age
    b. Current height only
    c. Bone age only
    d. Current weight

39. Which of the following causes of precocious puberty associated with delayed bone age?
    a. Hypothalamic hamartoma
    b. Primary hypothyroidism
    c. Endocrine disruptive chemicals
    d. McCune-Albright syndrome

Answer with Explanations

1. **a. Thelarche > Pubarche > Menarche**

   Ref: Yen & Jaffe's 8th/ed p 394

   - In general, the first sign of puberty in most adolescent girls is an acceleration of growth, followed by breast budding (thelarche), the appearance of pubic hair (pubarche), and finally, the onset of menses (menarche).
   - Although the physical sequelae of gonadarche and adrenarche generally occur concomitantly a discordance of the two processes may also occur in normal development.

   - Puberty consists of a series of events that vary in timing, sequence, and pace.
   - Puberty in humans is defined as the period of first becoming capable of reproducing, and is marked by maturation of the genital organs, development of secondary sex characteristics, acceleration in linear growth velocity, changes in affect and, in the female, the occurrence of menarche.
   - In humans, the transition into puberty is driven by two physiological processes: gonadarche and adrenarche.
   - Gonadarche comprises growth and maturation of the gonads and is associated with increased secretion of sex steroids and with the initiation of folliculogenesis and ovulation in the female and spermatogenesis in the male. Gonadarche leads to thelarche and menarche in girls and testicular enlargement in boys.

2. **c. Thrice**

   Ref: Kamini A Rao 2nd/ed p 122

   - HPG axis gets activated for the first time early in intrauterine life when anterior pituitary starts secreting FSH and LH into fetal circulation by the end of 12 weeks.
   - HPG axis gets activated for the second time in infancy and rise in gonadotropins soon after birth is due to reactivation of HPG axis rather than the escape of HPG axis from negative feedback effect only. It is more of a function of development of the HPG axis than its mere escape.
   - With onset of puberty, the HPG axis reawakens for the third time which is the final time for activation, and GnRH neurons begin secretion in pulsatile form.

3. **a. Medial basal hypothalamus**

   Ref: Kamini A Rao 2nd/ed p 121

   - During embryogenesis, the olfactory placode is the place of origin of GnRH neurons from where they migrate to arcuate nucleus located in medial basal hypothalamus between 6 and 9 weeks of pregnancy.
   - The axon of the GnRH neurons setup contacts with the capillaries of the hypophyseal portal venous system in the median eminence.
   - The hypothalamus-gonadal axis starts functioning in utero during early fetal development.

4. **b. 19–20 weeks**

   Ref: Speroff 8nd/ed p 392

   - The hypothalamic-pituitary-gonadal axis becomes functional even before birth.

   Neurons that synthesize GnRH originate in **olfactory placode** and migrate to the hypothalamus between 6 and 9 weeks. By 10 weeks, the hypothalamus contains significant amount of GnRH.

   Development of portal venous system starts at 6–10 weeks of gestation and is completed by 19–20 weeks.

5. **a. In early pregnancy**

   Ref: Kamini A Rao 2nd/ed p 121; Speroff 8th/ed p 392

   In response to pulsatile GnRH secretion, anterior pituitary starts secreting FSH and LH into fetal circulation by the end of 12 weeks, reaching peak at 20-24 weeks, gradually falling over last 10 weeks of pregnancy, probably due to a developed sensitivity to the negative feedback effects of high circulating estrogen and progesterone concentrations derived from the placenta. Thus, HPG axis is active in early intrauterine life.

6. **b. 12 weeks**

   Ref: Kamini A Rao 2nd/ed p 121

7. **a. Infancy and puberty**

   Ref: Kamini A Rao 2nd/ed p 122

   Juvenile pause is the interval between infancy and puberty when HPG axis lies dormant.

8. **a. Central inhibition of pulsatile secretion**

   Ref: Speroff 8th/ed p 393

   Juvenile pause is the interval between infancy and puberty, when hypothalamic-pituitary-gonadal axis lies dormant.

The typical "diphasic" pattern of gonadotropin secretion from infancy to puberty results primarily from changing levels of central inhibition of pulsatile GnRH secretion, and to a lesser extent, from a high sensitivity to low levels of gonadal steroid feedback.

9. b. GnRH pulse generator activity is abolished during juvenile pause phase

Ref: Speroff 8th/ed p 393

After birth, steroid levels fall precipitously due to the loss of maternal and placental hormones, allowing the newborn's hypothalamic-pituitary-gonadal axis to escape their suppressive effects.

The characteristic pulsatile pattern of hypothalamic GnRH secretion emerges, and serum gonadotropin concentrations rise again promptly, with a striking sex difference.

FSH rises to a greater extent in females	LH to a greater extent in males

During juvenile pause, although the GnRH pulse generator is active, the frequency and amplitude of pulsatile GnRH secretion generally are irregular and very low.

Low amplitude pulses of gonadotropin secretion can be detected in prepubertal children as young as 5 years of age, primarily during sleep. So, HPG axis lies dormant, activity of GnRH pulse generator is not abolished.

10. a. Development of estrogen positive feedback culminating in ovulation

Ref: Speroff 8th/ed p 406

- The **hallmark** of the maturation of the hypothalamic-pituitary-ovarian axis and of the completion of puberty is the development of **estrogen positive feedback**, which stimulates the midcycle LH surge and ovulation.

Menarche occurs in late puberty, after a year-long rise in daily estrogen production, probably when estradiol and inhibin B levels become sufficient to exert significant negative feedback on gonadotropin secretion, resulting in cyclic estrogen production.

Cycle length and menstrual characteristics vary until the positive feedback relationship between estradiol and gonadotropin secretion matures and ovulation becomes established, often a year or more after menarche.

11. d. Leptin

Ref: Yen & Jaffe's 8th/ed p 264

- Leptin is key regulator of satiety and body mass index.
- Its levels are thought to reflect the amount of energy stores and nutritional state.
- It coordinates body mass status with reproductive function.

Leptin

- A 146-amino acid protein produced primarily by **adipocytes**.
- Leptin **decreases food intake** and body weight via its hypothalamic receptor.
- How Leptin acts as a permissive factor in reproduction?

Pulsatile hypothalamic GnRH secretion does not occur unless leptin levels reach a threshold value. Such a mechanism may ensure that energy stores are sufficient to support a pregnancy.

12. a. Ghrelin

Ref: Yen & Jaffe's 8th/ed p 408

- Ghrelin and leptin appear to act as **reciprocal regulators of energy homeostasis** exerting opposing influences on the hypothalamic-pituitary-gonadal axis.

Ghrelin

- It is a small peptide, secreted predominantly by the **stomach**, which circulates in two forms. The active form is acetylated and promotes GH secretion.
- Circulating ghrelin concentrations are higher during fasting and decrease after food intake.
- Ghrelin concentrations peak during the first 2 years of life and decrease during puberty.
- The ghrelin receptor, GH secretagogue receptor-1a (GHSR-1a) is expressed in human hypothalamus, pituitary, testis, and ovaries.
- **Resistin** and **adiponectin** are two recently described hormones secreted by adipocytes, which appear to provide metabolic and nutritional status information.

13. a. Suppressed leptin levels

Ref: Kamini A Rao 2nd/ed p 125

- Puberty is associated with elevated leptin levels.
- Leptin is produced by adipocytes and it might act as a somatic stimulus for the onset of puberty.
- Leptin-deficient mice and rats fail to enter puberty, and treatment with leptin induces the onset of puberty.

Gamma-Aminobutyric Acid (GABA)

- Inhibitory neurotransmitter.
- Produced by specialized neurons in the hypothalamus.
- Release of GABA into the median eminence decreases as pulsatile GnRH secretion increases at the onset of puberty.

Neuropeptide Y (NPY)

- Hypothalamic peptide involved in the control of food intake behavior and reproductive function in adults.
- NPY, like GABA, is an important component of the **"neurobiologic brake"** that restrains the GnRH pulse generator in prepubertal primates.

Glutamate

- Excitatory neurotransmitter.
- Produced in the hypothalamus.
- Stimulates GnRH release via N-methyl-D-aspartate (NMDA) receptors.

14. d. 17%

Ref: Kamini A Rao 2nd/ed p 125

- The leptin-ghrelin story has restored credibility to the critical weight hypothesis originally proposed by Rose Frisch in the 1970s.
- The **critical weight hypothesis** states that the onset and regularity of menstrual function necessitate maintaining weight above a critical level, and, therefore, above a critical amount of body fat.

As per Frisch hypothesis, percentage of fat in body necessary for initiation of puberty is **17 percent**. The brain tracks the somatic cues and thus is thought of as the **somatometer**.

Recombinant human leptin administration to women with hypothalamic amenorrhea secondary to exercise or weight loss is associated with an increase in the levels of gonadotropins, free thyroxine, and insulin-like growth factor, with a resumption of ovarian activity.

15. a. Kisspeptins

Ref: Yen & Jaffe's 8th/ed p 13

- It is believed to be requisite for normal GnRH secretion, serving as a **"gatekeeper" of puberty** and helping to mediate the effects of sex steroids and metabolic cues on GnRH secretion.

The Kisspeptin System

- The importance of the kisspeptin system in reproduction was initially revealed by members of two consanguineous families with KISS1R mutations leading to pubertal failure and normosmic hypogonadotropic hypogonadism.
- Inactivating KISS1 mutations leading to pubertal failure and normosmic hypogonadotropic hypogonadism have also been described in four sisters.
- Mouse models with targeted knockouts of KISS1 and KISS1R exhibit hypogonadotropic hypogonadism with impaired sexual maturation, reduced gonadal size, failure of estrous cyclicity (females), impaired spermatogenesis (males), and infertility.
- The kisspeptin receptor is expressed by a majority of GnRH neurons; kisspeptin can directly depolarize GnRH neurons; and kisspeptin stimulation of gonadotropin secretion is completely blocked by GnRH antagonists.
- However, kisspeptin may also work indirectly, as kisspeptin increases GABAergic and glutamatergic postsynaptic currents onto GnRH neurons in the presence (but not absence) of estrogen in the mouse model.
- Kisspeptin does not stimulate LH secretion in KISS1R knockout mice, suggesting that kisspeptin acts exclusively through its cognate receptor.

16. b. Activating mutation in KISS1R leads to hypogonadotropic hypogonadism

Ref: Kamini A Rao 2nd/ed p 124

- Isolated idiopathic hypogonadotropic hypogonadism may be related to "loss of function" mutations in KISS1R.
- Activating mutations in KISS1R leads to central precocious puberty.

Kisspeptins are neuropeptides (encoded by the KISS1 gene) that signal via the G-protein coupled receptor, GPR54 (encoded by the KISS1R gene). Several members of a large consanguineous family with hypogonadotropic hypogonadism and delayed puberty were found to harbor homozygous inactivating mutations for GPR54.

Neurons expressing KISS1 are located exclusively in the **arcuate nucleus**, where GnRH neurons also express GPR54. Hypothalamic kisspeptin secretion is distinctly pulsatile and highly correlated with that of GnRH. Taken together, these observations indicate that hypothalamic kisspeptin-GPR54 signaling is a key component of the neurobiologic mechanism that triggers the onset of puberty. They further suggest that kisspeptin neurons may provide the fuel for the hypothalamic GnRH pulse generator.

17. **a. Precocious puberty**

    Ref: "Effects of recombinant leptin therapy in a child with congenital leptin deficiency" N Engl J Med 1999 Sep 16;341(12):879-84

Recombinant leptin can have role in hypogonadotropic hypogonadism and delayed puberty in patients with congenital leptin deficiency.

18. **c. Adrenaline is dependent of the maturation of the hypothalamic-pituitary-gonadal axis**

    Ref: Speroff 8th/ed p 397

- Although adrenarche is independent of the maturation of the hypothalamic-pituitary-gonadal axis, the two often are temporally related.

Adrenarche

- Term used to describe the increase in adrenal androgen production that begins at approximately **6 years** of age in both boys and girls.
- The increase in adrenal androgen production results from a change in the adrenal response to adrenocorticotropic hormone (ACTH) stimulation, characterized by a shift towards:
    - Increased production of D^5-3b-hydroxysteroid intermediates (17a-hydroxypregnenolone; dehydroepiandrostendione, DHEA)
    - Decreased production of D^4-ketosteroids (17a-hydroxyprogesterone, 17-OHP; androstendione)
    - No change in cortisol secretion
- Consequently, an **increase in serum DHEA-sulfate (DHEA-S)** levels heralds the onset of adrenarche.

19. **a. Serum DHEAS**

    Ref: Speroff 8th/ed p 398

- The best indicator of adrenarche is a serum DHEA-S concentration greater than **40 mg/dL**, which is higher than that normally seen in children 1-5 years of age (5-35 mg/dL).

Adrenal androgens derive from the **zona reticularis**, the innermost layer of the adrenal cortex, which begins to form at approximately 3 years of age and becomes well defined coincident with the increase in DHEA-S production at adrenarche.

20. **c. Testicular growth**

    Ref: Kamini A Rao 2nd/ed p127

- 1st sign of puberty in males is growth and **enlargement of testes** occurring around 11.5 years.

Rising testosterone levels lead to deepening of voice and increase bulk in muscle mass.

Testosterone is converted to DHT by 5a-reductase which leads to growth of penis and scrotum, enlargement of prostate and pubic hair. DHT leads to growth of facial hair.

21. **a. Associated with marked acceleration of skeletal age**

    Ref: Kamini A Rao 2nd/ed p128

- **Exaggerated thelarche:** Premature thelarche with increased growth velocity and/or advanced bone age.

Premature Thelarche

- Defined as isolated breast development in girls before the age of **8 years** without:
    - Any other signs of early puberty.
    - Marked acceleration of skeletal age.
- In girls, premature thelarche usually is a **benign condition** considered a variant of normal puberty.
- The evaluation of premature thelarche, like that of premature adrenarche, should focus on determining whether breast development is an isolated phenomenon or associated with other signs of precocious puberty; here again, the **most important initial test is an evaluation of bone age.**
- In children with Tanner stage 2 breast development and normal bone age, precocious puberty is unlikely and expectant management is appropriate, with re-evaluation at 6 months and periodically thereafter.
- Follow-up is needed to differentiate it from central precocious puberty.
- Premature thelarche is benign and may occur due to exposure to endocrine disruptive chemicals.

22. **b. Long acting GnRH agonists**

    Ref: Abnormal female puberty. Appelbaum p 29

Long-term GnRH Agonist Therapy

- GnRH agonists, such as the monthly or quarterly leuprolide acetate depot IM injection or yearly histrelin subdermal implantation, will introduce a constant, non-pulsatile GnRH milieu, effectively desensitizing and decreasing gonadotropin release.
- These formulations have not been directly compared to each other in randomized trials, but appear to have a similar effect in suppressing the axis.
- Response is judged on subsequent physical examination, during which signs of puberty should be noted to have stopped progressing and then to regress over the first 6 months of treatment.
- Growth velocity should return to a typical prepubertal rate. Gonadotropin and estradiol levels should

decrease to prepubertal levels within a month following treatment.
- Patients who do not have very advanced bone ages prior to treatment tend to have better results with respect to gaining back their height potential.
- Discontinuation of therapy should be based on
  - Patient's age
  - Growth velocity
  - Bone age
  - Height prediction
  - Psychosocial readiness
- Treatment with GnRH agonists appears to have **no significant long-term effects** on the pituitary-gonadal axis.
- Bone density may decrease during prolonged therapy, but is regained after treatment, therefore monitoring of bone density is not required.

23. **a. Reproductive potential is found to be decreased in girls who received GnRH agonists**
    Ref: Abnormal female puberty. Appelbaum p 29; Speroff 8th/ed p 417

Long-acting GnRH Agonists

1. Have proven both safe and effective for the treatment of idiopathic gonadotropin-dependent precocious puberty.
2. In girls under 6 years of age with idiopathic gonadotropin-dependent precocious puberty, treatment with a GnRH agonist can be expected to add 9-10 cm to adult height.
3. In older children already past their peak with slowing growth velocity, treatment can be expected to slow it further, to delay epiphyseal fusion, and to yield slow but steady increases in predicted adult height.
4. In girls between 6 and 8 years of age, GnRH agonist treatment typically results in a gain of 4-7 cm in height, less if bone age is significantly advanced.
5. Treatment with GnRH agonists does not appear to have any significant long-term adverse effects on function of the hypothalamic-pituitary-gonadal axis.
6. It **can be continued until the epiphyses are fused** or until the pubertal and chronological ages are appropriately matched.
7. **Prompt reactivation** of the pituitary-gonadal axis and pubertal development, in a pattern similar to that in normal adolescents, generally follows the discontinuation of treatment.

24. **c. Primary hypothyroidism**
    Ref: Yen & Jaffe's 8th/ed p 418

Primary Hypothyroidism and Precocious Puberty

- Girls with primary hypothyroidism can, on rare occasions, present with breast development or isolated vaginal bleeding.
- On ultrasound, enlarged **multicystic ovaries** may be noted.
- Additional features may include **delayed bone age**, ascites, and pleural and pericardial effusions.
- This is the only etiology for precocious puberty associated with delayed bone age. (Remember otherwise precocious puberty is associated with advanced bone age.)
- Thyroid hormone replacement therapy is associated with regression and resolution of the cysts; surgical treatment is not indicated.
- The mechanism underlying the ovarian stimulation is unclear. One possibility is that the excessively elevated TSH concentrations cross-react with the FSHR to promote estrogen secretion.

25. **a. Above condition is an example of cause of central precocious puberty**
    Ref: Speroff 8th/ed p 412; Yen & Jaffe's 8th/ed p 416

- McCune-Albright syndrome is a rare disorder characterized classically by:
  - Precocious puberty
  - Café-au-lait skin pigmentation
  - Polyostotic fibrous dysplasia of bone

McCune-Albright Syndrome

- It is caused by a **somatic mutation** of the alpha subunit of the G-protein (encoded by the GNAS1 gene), which results in a mosaic distribution of cells bearing **constitutively active** adenylate cyclase.
- The mutation results in continuous stimulation of endocrine function and, in addition to precocious puberty, also can cause gigantism, Cushing syndrome, adrenal hyperplasia, and thyrotoxicosis, in varying combinations.
- Early and repeated exposure to elevated sex steroid levels can result in **accelerated growth**, **advanced bone age**, and reduced adult height; it also may induce early maturation of the hypothalamic-pituitary-gonadal axis, resulting in secondary **gonadotropin-dependent** precocious puberty.
- McCune-Albright syndrome is more common in **girls** than in boys. The diagnosis merits consideration in girls presenting with recurrent functional ovarian follicular cysts and episodic menses.

Endocrinology of Pubertal Development

26. **b. Puberty**

Ref: Speroff 8th/ed p 401

IGF-I and Growth and Development

- It is synthesized and secreted by the **liver** in response to GH stimulation
- Circulates in serum bound to high affinity IGF binding proteins (IGFBPs).
- The genes encoding IGF-I, IGF-II, and insulin all belong to the same family.
- IGF-I receptor concentrations are controlled by GH, thyroxine, and other growth factors such as fibroblast growth factor and platelet-derived growth factor.
- The family of IGFBPs includes six proteins having greater affinities for IGF-I than the IGF-I receptor.
- IGFBP-3 is the most abundant in serum and has the highest affinity for IGF-I, but generally is saturated. Although present in lower concentrations, IGFBP-1 is unsaturated and therefore has greater impact on the levels of free IGF-I.
- The serum IGFBP-1 concentration is regulated by insulin, increasing during fasting when insulin levels are low, and decreasing after feeding or administration of insulin.
- IGF-I levels are decreased in diseases associated with malnutrition such as inflammatory bowel disease and in hypothyroidism.
- IGF-I augments the effects of FSH and LH in the ovary, the effect of ACTH on adrenal steroidogenesis, and the thyroid response to TSH.
- IGF-I levels rise 7-fold from very low concentrations at birth to **peak values at puberty**, fall rapidly by approximately 50% by age 20, then decline slowly with advancing age.

27. **a. 3β-hydroxysteroid dehydrogenase**

Ref: Speroff 8th/ed p 398

The unique enzymatic profile of Zona reticularis:
1. The activity of 3b-hydroxysteroid dehydrogenase/D^5-D^4 isomerase (3b-HSD), which catalyzes the oxidation and isomerization of D^5-3b-hydroxysteroid precursors into D^4-ketosteroids, is low.
2. The activities of P450c17, including both 17a-hydroxylase (catalyzing the conversion of pregnenolone to 17a-hydroxpregnenolone) and 17,20 lyase (catalyzing the conversion of 17a-hydroxpregnenolone to DHEA), are high, as is steroid sulfotransferase activity.

28. **d. All of the above**

Ref: Abnormal female puberty. Appelbaum p 135; Speroff 8th/ed p 403

The Timing of Puberty

- In females timing when puberty starts is the result of a combination of genetic and environmental factors.
- In the last 200 years, there has been a trend towards earlier puberty, a result of better overall health and nutrition in women in industrialized countries. However, in the past 30 years, girls have begun entering puberty and experiencing menarche at even younger ages.
- As this phenomenon has occurred in parallel with the increased rates of childhood and adolescent obesity, it has been hypothesized that the earlier onset of puberty and menarche in girls is associated with overnutrition and adiposity.
- Historically, the trend to an earlier onset of sexual development has been attributed to improved nutrition and less stressful living conditions.
- Indeed, higher weight and body fat mass are associated with an increased likelihood of early menarche. Importantly, early pubertal development is associated with slightly decreased adult height and an increased risk for obesity, compared to a late menarche.

29. **a. Inhibin A**

Ref: Speroff 8th/ed p 394

Inhibin in Puberty

- Inhibin B levels, which are low or undetectable in prepubertal girls, increase sharply in mid-puberty, then decline in its later stages, first reflecting increasing ovarian stimulation, then the onset of the menstrual cycle and the appearance of a luteal phase, when levels are low.
- Inhibin A concentrations, undetectable or very low through early puberty, increase gradually thereafter but reach adult levels only after menarche, consistent with the corpus luteum being the primary source.
- Menarche occurs in late puberty, after a year-long rise in daily estrogen production, probably when estradiol and inhibin B levels become sufficient to exert significant negative feedback on gonadotropin secretion, resulting in cyclic estrogen production.
- Cycle length and menstrual characteristics vary until the positive feedback relationship between estradiol and gonadotropin secretion matures and ovulation becomes established, often a year or more after menarche.

30. **c. 7 years old girl presenting with isolated thelarche**

Ref: Speroff 8th/ed p 410

Factors associated with an increased risk for intracranial pathology that clearly warrant complete evaluation and imaging
- Onset of puberty before age 6
- Rapid pubertal progression
- Associated symptoms of headache, seizures, or focal neurologic deficits

Indications for Evaluation of Precocious Puberty

- All girls under the age of 6 who have either breast or pubic hair development and girls under age 8 having both breast and pubic hair development merit a thorough evaluation to determine the cause.
- Girls under 8 years of age having only early breast development (premature thelarche) or pubic hair growth (premature adrenarche or pubarche) warrant a careful history and physical examination and, at a minimum, an evaluation of bone age and close follow-up to determine their linear growth rate in efforts to identify those who may be at risk for decreased growth potential.
- Between the ages of 6 and 8 years, clinicians must make individual judgments regarding the extent of evaluation, based on the results of the initial evaluation and, inevitably, on the level of anxiety in the patient and her parents.

31. a. Functional ovarian follicular cysts

Ref: Abnormal female puberty. Appelbaum p 13;
Speroff 8th/ed p 411

- This patient has precocious puberty as evidenced by the presence of thelarche prior to the age of 8 years. In this patient, 6 year old, estradiol is elevated but gonadotropins are suppressed. This goes in favour of peripheral, or gonadotropin-independent, precocious puberty.
- The most common cause of gonadotropin independent precocious puberty (GIPP) is autonomously functioning **ovarian follicular cysts**.
- GIPP should be strongly considered in the differential diagnosis where thelarche is the predominant or initial sign of pubertal development (as opposed to pubarche).
- It is important to distinguish benign premature thelarche from PP; girls with benign premature thelarche do not have growth acceleration or an advanced bone age.
- If a diagnosis of precocious puberty is made in context of an autonomously functioning ovarian cyst, the patient should be evaluated for possible McCune-Albright syndrome (MAS).
- Gonadotropin-independent precocious puberty can result from excess sex steroids secretion from the gonads or adrenals or from exposure to exogenous estrogens.

32. b. Bone age assessment

Ref: Speroff 8th/ed p 413

First line of management in girl comes with either thelarche or pubarche before the age of 8 years is bone age assessment.

The single most important and useful test is an **X-ray wrist joint of the nondominant hand** for bone age.

Those who warrant further endocrine assessment:
- Children with advanced bone age
- Those having normal bone age accompanied by both breast and pubic hair development
- Normal bone age with evidence of accelerated growth and breast or pubic hair development.

33. a. GnRH stimulation test

Ref: Speroff 8th/ed p 415

The GnRH Stimulation Test

- Basal and GnRH-stimulated serum gonadotropin levels differentiate gonadotropin-dependent from gonadotropin-independent precocious puberty, which then guides further evaluation.
- Serum gonadotropin concentrations should be measured using ultra-sensitive assays having low detection limits for pediatric patients (approximately 0.1 IU/L).
- The GnRH stimulation test is performed by obtaining blood samples before and 30–40 minutes after a single dose of GnRH (100 mg), administered intravenously.
- Synthetic GnRH is not available, so a GnRH agonist can be used instead, obtaining blood samples before and 60 minutes after a single dose of leuprolide acetate (20 mg/kg) is administered subcutaneously.
- The stimulated serum LH concentration is the most useful diagnostic parameter, a stimulated LH value of **3.3–5.0 IU/L** defines the upper limit of normal for prepubertal children (Tanner stage 1, T1) with most assays.
- Both basal and stimulated serum LH concentrations have high specificity and positive predictive value for diagnosis of gonadotropin-dependent precocious puberty.

34. **a. Once menses have begun**
    Ref: Abnormal female puberty. Appelbaum p 81; Speroff 8th/ed p 423

- Oral or transdermal estrogen therapy can be used, beginning at doses well below those used for adults (e.g., 0.25-0.5 mg oral micronized estradiol or its equivalent), increasing gradually at intervals of 3-6 months according to response (Tanner stage, bone age), with the goal of completing sexual maturation over a period of 2-3 years.
- Progestin should not be added to the treatment regimen **until there is substantial breast development** and full contour breast growth has plateaued, because premature progestin treatment can adversely affect breast growth or contours. In general, progestin therapy can safely begin **once menses have begun**, or after 12-24 months of estrogen treatment.

35. **d. Bone age**
    Ref: Kamini A Rao 2nd/ed p 132; Speroff 8th/ed p 422

Evaluation of Delayed Puberty

- First step in evaluation of delayed puberty is assessment of bone age by X-ray wrist joint of non-dominant hand.
- A measurement of bone age should be obtained for comparison with chronological age and for assessment of the potential for future growth.
- Patients with **constitutional delay** of puberty typically exhibit a **bone age between 12 and 13.5 years**, which generally does not progress further without the exposure to gonadal steroids that is required for epiphyseal closure.
- A karyotype should be obtained in all girls with hypergonadotropic hypogonadism to detect chromosomal abnormalities, except when a history of previous chemotherapy or gonadal radiation provides an obvious explanation.
- The most common disorder of this type is gonadal dysgenesis, with Turner syndrome (45, X) being the prototype. In addition to other structural X chromosome abnormalities (e.g., deletions, rings and isochromosomes), karyotype will identify those harboring a Y chromosome (e.g., 46,XY, Swyer syndrome), in whom gonadectomy will be indicated due to the significant risk for malignant transformation in occult testicular elements (20-30%).

- A head MRI should be obtained in patients with hypogonadotropic hypogonadism and those with neurologic signs or symptoms. In addition to detecting mass lesions, imaging can reveal the presence or absence of the olfactory bulbs and tracts (absent in Kallmann syndromes).

36. **a. FSH, LH, E2**
    Ref: Kamini A Rao 2nd/ed p 132; Speroff 8th/ed p 422

- Now after bone age assessment, next step comes laboratory evaluation.
- The laboratory evaluation of girls with delayed puberty is aimed first at differentiating primary (hypergonadotropic) from secondary (hypogonadotropic) hypogonadism, which typically can be accomplished by measuring the serum FSH, LH, and estradiol concentrations.
- By mid-adolescence, gonadotropin levels, particularly FSH, are grossly elevated in girls with primary gonadal failure.
- In patients with hypogonadism, low basal gonadotropin levels are consistent with the diagnosis of constitutional delay of puberty, but also with congenital GnRH deficiency or pituitary gonadotropin deficiency.
- Ultra-sensitive immuno-fluorometric assays for FSH and LH may help to distinguish the low but detectable concentrations typically observed in those with constitutional delay from the undetectable levels in patients with congenital GnRH deficiency.

37. **b. Bone age**
    Ref: Kamini A Rao 2nd/ed p 134

The basic and essential laboratory test in the evaluation of perceived abnormal growth is a left hand/wrist X-ray for bone age.

The Bayley-Pinneau tables along with Greulich-Pyle Atlas can aid to predict the adult height.

38. **a. Current height and bone age**
    Ref: Speroff 8th/ed p 424

The Bayley-Pinneau tables can be used to determine a predicted adult height, based on current height and bone age.

39. **b. Primary hypothyroidism**
    Ref: Yen & Jaffe's 8th/ed p 418

Primary hypothyroidism is the only etiology for precocious puberty associated with delayed bone age.

CHAPTER 8

Endocrinology of Amenorrhea

Multiple Choice Questions

1. Which of the following patients should be evaluated for amenorrhea?
   a. No menses by age 14 in the absence of growth or development of secondary sexual characteristics
   b. No menses by age 16 regardless of the presence of normal growth and development of secondary sexual characteristics
   c. No menses for an interval of time equivalent to a total of at least three previous cycles, or 6 months
   d. All

2. Cryptomenorrhea can result from all *except*:
   a. Imperforate hymen
   b. Mullerian aplasia
   c. Transverse vaginal septum
   d. Cervical atresia

3. A 16-year-old girl presents to OPD with complain of primary amenorrhea. Secondary sexual characters are well developed. On per speculum examination, vagina is patent and cervix can be seen. What will be your likely possibility?
   a. Mullerian agenesis
   b. Androgen insensitivity syndrome
   c. Cervical stenosis
   d. Asherman syndrome

4. Most common overall cause of amenorrhea lie at the level of:
   a. Ovary
   b. Hypothalamo-pituitary
   c. Outflow tract
   d. Uterus

5. Methods for assessing the level of ovarian estrogen production:
   a. Amount and character of cervical mucus
   b. Progestin challenge test
   c. Measurement of endometrial thickness by transvaginal ultrasonography
   d. All

6. The progestin challenge test will be considered negative after:
   a. 7 days
   b. 14 days
   c. 21 days
   d. 28 days

7. Which of the following not suggests ovarian failure?
   a. FSH 6 IU/L, E2 50 pg/mL
   b. FSH 7 IU/L, E2 100 pg/mL
   c. FSH 17 IU/L, E2 40 pg/mL
   d. FSH 12 IU/L, E2 80 pg/mL

8. A 16-year-old girl presented to OPD with complaint of primary amenorrhea. She does not complain of any significant physical, nutritional, or emotional stress. Progestin challenge test negative. Ultrasound shows presence of uterus. Hormone profile: TSH-2.3 mIU/L, Prolactin 20 ng/dL, FSH 3 IU/L, E2 30 pg/dL. What should be the next investigation?
   a. Skull X-ray
   b. Karyotyping
   c. Head MRI
   d. USG abdomen

9. A 26-year-old woman presented to OPD with complaint of secondary amenorrhea. She does not complain of any significant physical, nutritional, or emotional stress. Progestin challenge test negative. Ultrasound shows thin endometrium and small ovaries. Hormone profile: TSH-2.3 mIU/L, Prolactin 20 ng/dL, FSH 25 IU/L, E2 20 pg/dL. All of the following are we justified doing, *except*:
   a. Karyotyping
   b. Anti CYP21 antibodies
   c. FMR 1 premutation testing
   d. MRI head

10. Least risk of ending up with premature ovarian failure:
    a. Numerical and structural chromosomal abnormalities
    b. Hypothyroidism
    c. Fragile X premutations
    d. Autoimmune disease

11. **Which of the following statements is not true regarding premature ovarian failure?**
    a. In all patients with premature ovarian failure, a karyotype must be obtained
    b. Karyotype showing Y chromosome runs 30% risk of malignant transformation of gonads
    c. Many patients with Y chromosome, do not exhibit any sign of excess androgen production
    d. Women with short stature with ovarian failure merit karyotype

12. **Which of the following is not true regarding Fragile X syndrome?**
    a. POF associated with premutations may reflect FMR1 mRNA loss-of-function toxicity
    b. Most common inherited cause of mental retardation and autism
    c. Results from abnormal expansion of an unstable trinucleotide (CGG) repeat sequence in the *FMR1* gene
    d. Women with POF should be offered testing for FMR1 premutations

13. **Which of the following is not true regarding autoimmune ovarian failure?**
    a. Addison's disease has the strongest association with POF
    b. The prevalence of other autoimmune diseases is higher among women with POF
    c. The presence of thyroid autoantibodies prove autoimmune ovarian failure
    d. Women with POF should be tested for anti-adrenal antibodies and for anti-thyroid antibodies

14. **A 30-year-old woman presents with secondary amenorrhea. She gives history of puerperal retention of products of conception and secondary hemorrhage for which curettage was done. She breastfed her child for 6 months. Her menses did not resume post delivery. Progesterone challenge test negative. Hormonal assays are within normal range. Which of the following is not true regarding this condition?**
    a. Amenorrhea traumatica, most common cause is curettage done for postpartum hemorrhage
    b. Most women with intrauterine adhesions present with dysmenorrhea, hypomenorrhea, infertility, or recurrent pregnancy loss, rather than amenorrhea
    c. Saline infusion sonography is definitive test for diagnosis
    d. Operative hysteroscopy is the primary method for treatment of intrauterine adhesions

15. **Which of the following leads to Asherman's syndrome?**
    a. Uterine artery embolization
    b. Tuberculosis
    c. Schistosomiasis
    d. All

16. **Which of the following is incorrect regarding Asherman's syndrome?**
    a. Very severe adhesions can be seen following post-partum curettage or postpartum hypogonadism
    b. Hematometra occur inevitably
    c. Can present as recurrent pregnancy loss or infertility
    d. Pregnancy is frequently complicated by placenta accreta

17. **Most common causes of primary amenorrhea:**
    a. Gonadal dysgenesis
    b. Mullerian agenesis
    c. Androgen insensitivity syndrome
    d. Swyer syndrome

18. **Which of the following does not go in favor of transverse vaginal septum?**
    a. No visible cervix
    b. No obvious vaginal orifice
    c. No distention of bulge with Valsalva maneuver
    d. Palpable hematocolpos

19. **Which of the following does not hold true for müllerian agenesis?**
    a. Second most common cause of primary amenorrhea
    b. Normal, symmetrical breast and pubic hair development
    c. Laparoscopy is necessary for diagnosis of Müllerian agenesis
    d. May present with cryptomenorrhea

20. **A 15-year-old girl presents with primary amenorrhea. She has well developed tanner stage 4 secondary sexual characteristics. Ultrasound reveals absence of uterus. Karyotype is 46,XX. Which of the following statement does not hold correct for the present situation?**
    a. Ovaries can be entirely normal, undescended, hypoplastic, or associated with an inguinal hernia
    b. Urologic anomalies are seen in 40% cases
    c. Skeletal malformations can be seen in 10–15% of patients
    d. May result from inactivating mutation in the gene encoding AMH or its receptor

21. A 18-year-old girl presents in OPD with primary amenorrhea. She has well developed breasts but scanty pubic hair. Ultrasound reveals absence of uterus. She has a younger sister 16 years old who has not attained menarche yet. Karyotyping reveals 46, XY. Which of the following statement is incorrect regarding this situation?
    a. Third most common cause of primary amenorrhea
    b. Gonads show evidence of spermatogenesis
    c. Half of patients with complete AIS have an inguinal hernia
    d. Other family members such as a sister or maternal aunt are often affected

22. Which of the following points help to distinguish above patient from that of primary amenorrhea due to MRKH syndrome?
    a. Serum testosterone and serum LH concentration
    b. Karyotyping
    c. Asymmetrical secondary sexual development
    d. All

23. In which of the following is the only exception to the rule that gonads with a Y chromosome should be removed as soon as a diagnosis is made?
    a. Complete AIS   b. Partial AIS
    c. Minimal AIS   d. Swyer syndrome

24. Which of the following is incorrect regarding Turner syndrome and karyotyping?
    a. Risk for developing gonadoblastoma is less than 5%
    b. 5% of women with Turner syndrome have a karyotype containing all or part of a Y chromosome
    c. Further analysis with FISH will identify another 5% having occult Y chromosome material
    d. FISH analysis is most clearly indicated for those exhibiting any evidence of virilization or having a chromosomal fragment of uncertain origin

25. A 18-year-old girl presenting with complain of secondary amenorrhea and short stature. On examination, she has stage 3 breast and pubic hair development. She gives history of onset of menarche at the age of 16 years. On ultrasonography, she has small sized uterus and small ovaries. Her FSH is 20 IU/L, Estradiol value 20 pg/mL. Karyotype comes out to be 45, X/46, XX. Which of the following is not true regarding counselling this patient?
    a. Mosaic 46, XX cell line (e.g. 45, X/46, XX), the gonad may contain functional ovarian cortical tissue
    b. Gonadectomy is indicated being at high risk of gonadoblastoma
    c. Approximately 5% complete puberty and begin menstruation
    d. Approximately one-third has cardiovascular anomalies

26. A 18-year-old girl present with primary amenorrhea. Breast development corresponds to tanner stage On ultrasonography, uterus and cervix seen but gonad appeared streak. Karyotype revealed 46, XY. Which of the following statement is incorrect regarding this?
    a. Exhibit normal growth and intellectual development
    b. No comorbid specific medical problems
    c. Gonadectomy can be delayed till pubertal development is fully achieved
    d. Pregnancy can be achieved with in vitro fertilization using donor oocytes

27. Women with gonadal dysgenesis can present with secondary amenorrhea. The abnormal karyotype most commonly associated with this:
    a. Mosaics (45, X/46, XX)
    b. Deletions of short or long arm of X chromosome
    c. 47, XXX
    d. 45, X

28. Functional ovarian failure resulting from disorder of follicular development with hypergonadotropic hypogonadism is known as:
    a. Swyer syndrome
    b. Sheehan syndrome
    c. Simmond syndrome
    d. Savage syndrome

29. Resistant ovary syndrome leading to hypergonadotropic hypogonadism can result from all of the following *except:*
    a. Pituitary failure
    b. Disorders of intraovarian regulation
    c. Steroidogenic enzyme defects
    d. Inactivating mutations in β-subunit of LH or FSH

30. Which is not correct about pituitary adenomas causing amenorrhea?
    a. The large majority of pituitary adenomas are functional prolactin-secreting lactotroph adenomas
    b. Pituitary adenomas are true neoplasms and mostly malignant
    c. The large majority are monoclonal
    d. Activating mutations in the *GNAS1* gene

31. Pituitary adenoma. False statement:
    a. Nonfunctioning adenomas do not have functional consequences
    b. MRI is the best method for imaging the pituitary gland
    c. The classical complaint is bitemporal hemianopsia
    d. Prolactin deficiency has no known symptoms other than failed lactation after delivery

32. Prevalence of premature ovarian insufficiency:
    a. 0.1%
    b. 1%
    c. 10%
    d. 5%

33. Which of the following is incorrect regarding gonadotroph adenomas?
    a. The large majority of gonadotroph adenomas are functional
    b. Account for 80-90% of all nonfunctional pituitary adenomas
    c. FSH-secreting adenomas may cause anovulation and spontaneous ovarian hyperstimulation
    d. Hyperprolactinemia can be seen in gonadotroph adenomas

34. A 30-year-old woman presents with secondary amenorrhea since her last childbirth. Pregnancy test is negative. She gives history of severe PPH in last pregnancy for which she received 5 units of blood transfusion. She was not able to breastfeed her child as milk formation was not enough. Which of the following statements is not correct for this situation?
    a. Acute infarction and ischemic necrosis of posterior pituitary gland
    b. Most common cause is hypovolemic hypotension from postpartum hemorrhage
    c. Failed lactation after delivery is the classical presenting symptom
    d. Skull X ray shows partially or completely empty sella

35. Which of the following is incorrect regarding amenorrheic exerciser?
    a. Shows bone loss like seen in postmenopausal women
    b. Requires hormone replacement therapy
    c. Not at risk of stress fracture
    d. Menses resume on decreases excercise

36. The critical level of body fat required for the onset and regularity of menstrual function corresponds to:
    a. 17% for menarche, and at 22% for regular menstruation
    b. 27% for menarche, and at 22% for regular menstruation
    c. 17% for menarche, and at 27% for regular menstruation
    d. 22% for menarche, and at 17% for regular menstruation

37. Which is not true for Kallmann's syndrome?
    a. Congenital GnRH deficiency is associated with anosmia or hyposmia
    b. Always X-linked inheritance
    c. Cleft lip/palate, urogenital tract anomalies, or syndactaly may be associated
    d. Associated with hypoplastic or absent olfactory sulci

38. Perimenopausal transition is associated with:
    a. High FSH, high LH
    b. Low FSH, high LH
    c. High FSH, normal LH
    d. Normal FSH, normal LH

39. Which of the following statements is false?
    a. Third most common cause of primary amenorrhea is AIS
    b. Approximately 30% patients with Y chromosome will develop signs of virilization
    c. Gonadal dysgenesis associated with normal karyotype and neurosensory deafness is Perrault syndrome
    d. 30% women with hyperprolactinemia have galactorrhea

40. Which of the following statements is true?
    a. Midcycle LH surge is approximately 3 times baseline level
    b. Galactosemia is associated with hypogonadotropic hypogonadism
    c. Women with gonadal dysgenesis present only with primary amenorrhea
    d. Mullerian agenesis is most common cause of primary amenorrhea

41. Which of the following situation is not associated with hypogonadotropic state?
    a. Anorexia nervosa
    b. Large pituitary tumors
    c. Ovarian failure
    d. Negative progesterone challenge test

42. Which of the following statements is incorrect regarding coned-down lateral view of sella turcica?
    a. Can detect craniopharyngioma
    b. Can detect microadenomas reliably
    c. Suprasellar tumors can be missed
    d. When combined with a prolactin assay can determine when to obtain MRI

43. Most distinguishing feature of Kallmann's syndrome:
    a. Short stature
    b. Tall stature
    c. Anosmia
    d. Syndactaly

44. Which of the following is incorrect statement regarding congenital GnRH deficiency?
    a. Presence of adrenarche can help distinguish congenital GnRH deficiency from constitutional delay as cause of delayed puberty
    b. More common in females than in males
    c. Gonads respond normally to exogenous gonadotropin stimulation
    d. When congenital GnRH deficiency is associated with hyposmia, it is known as Kallmann's syndrome

Answer with Explanations

1. **d. All**

   Ref: Speroff 8th/ed p 436

   Following patients need evaluation for amenorrhea:
   - No menses by age 14 in the absence of growth or development of secondary sexual characteristics
   - No menses by age 16 regardless of the presence of normal growth and development of secondary sexual characteristics
   - No menses for an interval of time equivalent to a total of at least three previous cycles, or 6 months.

2. **b. Mullerian aplasia**

   Ref: Speroff 8th/ed p 438

   Obstructed menstrual flow is known as cryptomenorrhea. Causes can be:
   - Imperforate hymen
   - Transverse vaginal septum
   - Cervical atresia.

3. **c. Cervical stenosis**

   Ref: Speroff 8th/ed p 440

   In those with primary or secondary amenorrhea having a patent vagina and visible cervix, the likelihood of a genital outflow tract abnormality is very small. The only possibilities:
   - Cervical stenosis
   - Intrauterine adhesions (Asherman's syndrome)
   - Endometrial damage from surgical trauma or infection

4. **a. Ovary**

   Ref: Speroff 8th/ed p 441; Kamini A Rao 2nd/ed p 138

   > - Gonadal agenesis and dysgenesis leading to primary ovarian failure alone accounts for 40% cases of amenorrhea

   Abnormalities of ovarian function are the **most common** overall cause of amenorrhea and include a wide variety of disorders ranging from simple chronic anovulation, as in women with PCOS, obesity, thyroid disorders and hyperprolactinemia, to complete ovarian failure relating to chromosomal abnormalities or other genetic disorders such as Fragile X (FMR1) premutations and galactosemia, autoimmune disease, radiation or chemotherapy.

5. **d. All**

   Ref: Speroff 8th/ed p 442

   Methods for assessing the level of ovarian estrogen production include:
   - Measurement of the serum estradiol concentration
   - The "bioassays" based on clinical observations of:
     - The amount and character of cervical mucus
     - The results of a "progestin challenge test"
     - Measurement of endometrial thickness by transvaginal ultrasonography

6. **b. 14 days**

   Ref: Kamini A Rao 2nd/ed p 140

Progestin Challenge Test

- Based on the premise that progestin treatment will induce menses only in those having normal circulating estrogen concentrations.
- A pure progestational agent must be used because endogenous estrogen status cannot be inferred from the response to an OCP that contains both estrogen and progestin.
- The more potent synthetic progestins such as medroxyprogesterone acetate are a better choice than oral micronized progesterone, which must be administered in relatively high doses (e.g. 300 mg daily) to achieve a response.
- A positive test—bleeding within 2-14 days after completion of progestin treatment—implies normal estrogen production and ovarian function, and a negative test—no withdrawal menses—suggests hypogonadism.
- Scant withdrawal bleeding or spotting suggests marginal levels of endogenous estrogen production.
- However, the overall correlation between withdrawal bleeding and estrogen status is far from perfect; both false positive (withdrawal bleeding despite generally low levels of estrogen production) and false negative results (absent bleeding despite significant estrogen production) are relatively common.
- Up to 40-50% of women whose amenorrhea relates to stress, exercise, weight loss, hyperprolactinemia, or ovarian failure, in whom estrogen levels generally are low, exhibit withdrawal bleeding.
- Up to 20% of amenorrheic women with significant estrogen production have no withdrawal bleeding, in

some because the endometrium is decidualized by high circulating androgen levels.

7. **a. FSH 6 IU/L, E2 50 pg/mL**

    Ref: The Boston IVF Handbook of infertility. 3rd/ed p 21

- The normal feedback relationship between ovarian estrogen production and pituitary gonadotropin secretion dictates that low estrogen levels should cause a **compensatory increase in FSH** release to stimulate ovarian follicular development and estrogen secretion, just as they do during the early follicular phase of the normal cycle.
- When estrogen production is abnormally low, a low serum FSH concentration (<5 IU/L) indicates that inadequate or ineffective gonadotropin secretion is the cause and that even basic central feedback mechanisms in the HPO axis are not functioning.
- When estrogen levels are clearly low, a serum FSH level in the low normal range (5-10 IU/L) has the same interpretation and clinical implication, for two reasons.
    - First, because the FSH level should be high when estrogen production is grossly low, even a "normal" value is, in fact, abnormally low in that clinical context.
    - Second, although the measured level of immunoreactive FSH may be normal, the level of biologically active FSH clearly is not.

Interpretation of cycle Day 3 hormone levels

FSH levels (miu/mL)	Estradiol levels (pg/mL)	Ovarian reserve
>10	<70	Reduced
>10	>70	Reduced
2–10	>70	Reduced
2–10	<70	Normal

8. **c. Head MRI**

    Ref: Speroff 8th/ed p 451

- When there is no clear explanation for hypogonadotropic hypogonadism (e.g. significant physical, nutritional, or emotional stress) or for hyperprolactinemia (e.g. medications), further evaluation with imaging is indicated to exclude tumors and to help distinguish between pituitary and hypothalamic causes.
- The **method of choice is MRI** (with gadolinium contrast) because it is more sensitive and accurate than other imaging techniques for detection of abnormalities within and near the sella turcica.
- MRI can demonstrate the nearby optic chiasm and can detect blood, allowing hemorrhage and vascular abnormalities to be distinguished from other sellar mass lesions.
- Most sellar masses are pituitary adenomas, which account for 10% of all intracranial neoplasms.
- In the absence of any demonstrable mass lesion in the sellar region or relevant history suggesting another specific cause for pituitary damage, there is no need to perform any additional specific pituitary function tests.

Flowchart below explains the same.

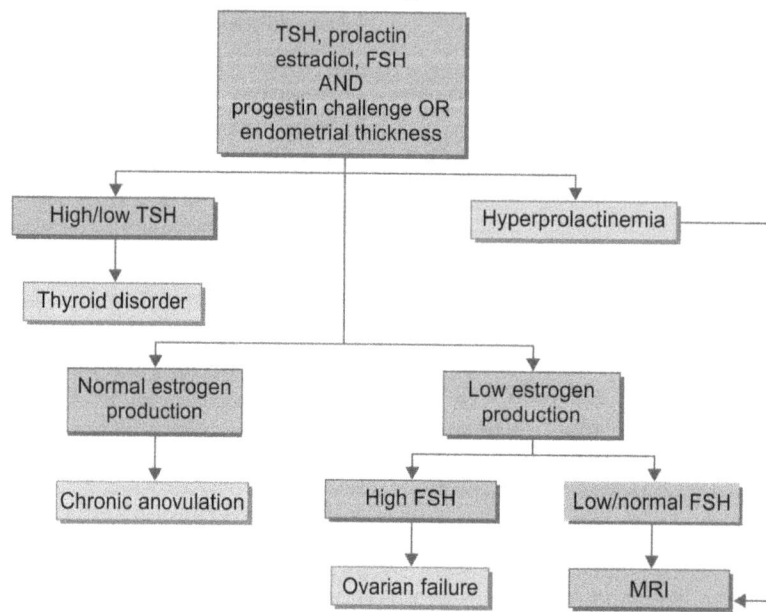

9. d. MRI head

Ref: Speroff 8th/ed p 464

This is a case of premature ovarian failure. Following investigations should be done in case of ovarian failure:

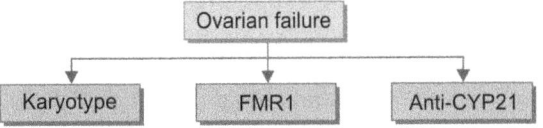

10. b. Hypothyroidism

Ref: Speroff 8th/ed p 449

Numerical and structural chromosomal abnormalities like translocations, deletions and mosaicism runs high risk of premature ovarian failure.

Convincing evidence has demonstrated an association between premature ovarian failure (POF) and fragile X "premutations".

Ovarian failure sometimes may be the consequence of **autoimmune disease**.

11. a. In all patients with premature ovarian failure a karyotype must be obtained

Ref: Speroff 8th/ed p 449

Premature Ovarian Failure

- When evaluation reveals low estrogen production and consistently high serum FSH, the diagnosis of ovarian failure is established.
- In all patients under the age 30 with premature ovarian failure, a karyotype must be obtained to exclude chromosomal translocations, deletions and mosaicism.
- A karyotype showing Y chromosome runs **30% risk of malignant transformation** in occult testicular elements, hence gonadectomy is indicated.
- Signs of virilization cannot reliably identify subset of women at risk because many having a Y chromosome exhibit no signs of excess androgen production.
- **Karyotype after age 30 is unnecessary** because most tumors in patients with a Y chromosome arise before age 20, and virtually all before age of 30. (So, not all patients with premature ovarian failure require karyotyping)
- After age 30, women with short stature or a family history of early menopause still merit a karyotype to exclude X chromosome deletions and translocations.

12. a. POF associated with permutations may reflect FMR1 mRNA loss of functional toxicity

Ref: Frontiers in Gynecological Endocrinology. Andrea R Genazzani. Vol 3 p 23; Speroff 8th/ed p 465

Fragile X Syndrome

- Most common inherited cause of mental retardation and autism.
- Results from abnormal expansion of an unstable trinucleotide (CGG) repeat sequence in the *FMR1* (Fragile X Mental Retardation) gene, located on the long arm of the X chromosome (Xq27.3).
- The gene normally contains about 30 CGG repeats, but in those with Fragile X syndrome, the number exceeds 200.
- Convincing evidence has demonstrated an association between premature ovarian failure (POF) and fragile X "premutations," characterized by 55–200 CGG repeats.
- Whereas the full mutation silences the FMR1 gene, resulting in little or no production of the corresponding mRNA or gene product (fragile X mental retardation protein, FMRP), the POF associated with premutations may reflect FMR1 mRNA **gain-of-function toxicity**.
- Women with premutations often exhibit endocrine evidence of early ovarian aging and up to one-third have an early menopause.

Prevalence of premutations	
Familial POF	14%
Sporadic cases of POF	1%–7%

Women with POF therefore should be offered testing for FMR1 premutations.

13. c. The presence of thyroid auto-antibodies prove autoimmune ovarian failure

Ref: Speroff 8th/ed p 450

POF and Autoimmune Oophoritis

- Ovarian failure sometimes may be the consequence of autoimmune disease.
- Addison's disease (autoimmune adrenocortical insufficiency) has the strongest association with POF.
- The prevalence of other autoimmune diseases (e.g. thyroid autoimmunity, Type I diabetes, and myasthenia gravis) is higher among women with POF than in the general population.
- Autoimmune ovarian failure generally occurs as part of a specific autoimmune polyendocrine syndrome (APS) that includes adrenal insufficiency.
- Women with POF should be tested for anti-adrenal antibodies (most easily demonstrated against the 21-hydroxylase enzyme, CYP21), and for anti-thyroid antibodies (anti-thyroid peroxidase and anti-thyroglobulain antibodies).

- The presence of anti-adrenal antibodies strongly implies autoimmune oophoritis as the cause of POF and identifies women who should be carefully evaluated and followed to exclude adrenal insufficiency.
- Patients with positive anti-adrenal antibodies should be further evaluated to exclude asymptomatic adrenal insufficiency, by measuring the morning (6:00-9:00 AM) serum cortisol level.
- The presence of thyroid autoantibodies does not prove autoimmune ovarian failure but identifies women at risk for developing autoimmune thyroid disorders.

14. c. Saline infusion test is definitive test for diagnosis

Ref: Speroff 8th/ed p 459

This is suggestive of Asherman's Syndrome
- Also known as "amenorrhoea traumatica,"
- Results from intrauterine adhesions that obstruct or obliterate the uterine cavity, as a consequence of trauma.
- Risk for developing intrauterine adhesions is increased by inflammation, as may result from endometritis or retained products of conception, and when the endometrium is relatively thin and inactive, as it is during the postpartum period. Consequently, most cases arise in close temporal proximity to a pregnancy and are associated with surgical trauma, primarily curettage.
- Most women with intrauterine adhesions present with dysmenorrhea, hypomenorrhea, infertility, or recurrent pregnancy loss, rather than amenorrhea.
- Sonohysterography or hysterosalpingography (HSG) provide more specific information regarding the location and extent of adhesions that partially or completely obliterate or obstruct the endometrial cavity or the cervical canal, and **hysteroscopy is definitive**.
- Operative hysteroscopy is the primary method for treatment of intrauterine adhesions that may be lysed by scissors, electrodissection, or with a laser; most prefer sharp dissection, which may have less risk for causing further injury.

15. d. All

Ref: Kamini A Rao 2nd/ed p 140

Asherman syndrome might result from:
- Cesarean section
- Abdominal or hysteroscopic myomectomy or metroplasy
- Uterine artery embolization
- Elective endometrial ablation
- Tuberculosis
- Schistosomiasis

16. b. Hematometra occur inevitably

Ref: Speroff 8th/ed p 459

Adhesions in Asherman's syndrome may partially or completely obliterate the endometrial cavity, the internal cervical os, the cervical canal. But surprisingly, despite stenosis or atresia of internal os, hematometra does not inevitably occur.

Very severe adhesions have been noted following postpartum curettage and postpartum hypogonadism, e.g. in Sheehan's syndrome.

17. a. Gonadal dysgenesis

Ref: Kamini A Rao 2nd/ed p 138

Gonadal agenesis and dysgenesis lead to 40% cases of primary amenorrhea.

18. b. No obvious vaginal orifice

Ref: Speroff 8th/ed p 454

Transverse vaginal septum can be differentiated from imperforate hymen by following points:

Distinguishing parameter	Transverse vaginal septum	Imperforate hymen
Vaginal orifice	Normal	Not well appreciable
Vaginal length	Shortened vagina of varying length	Not well appreciable
Bulge	Thick	Thin, often bulging
Valsalva maneuver	No distention at introitus	Distention at introitus
Color of membrane	Pink	Blue

19. c. Laparoscopy is necessary for diagnosis of Müllerian agenesis

Ref: Speroff 8th/ed p 456

- Laparoscopy usually is not necessary for diagnosis of müllerian agenesis.

Ultrasonography may help to define the size and symmetry of any pelvic reproductive organs, but MRI is more accurate and is indicated when doubt remains.

20. d. May result from inactivating mutation in the gene encoding AMH or its receptor

Ref: Speroff 8th/ed p 455; Kamini A Rao 2nd/ed p 141

Mayer-Rokitansky-Küster-Hauser Syndrome

- The failure of müllerian development is second most common cause of primary amenorrhea next only to gonadal dysgenesis in prevalence.
- The cause is unknown. Although usually sporadic, some cases of müllerian agenesis are associated with chromosomal translocations or occur in familial aggregates, suggesting a genetic basis for the disorder.

- Müllerian agenesis might be attributed to an **activating mutation** in the gene encoding AMH or its receptor, causing excess AMH activity.
- Inactivating mutations in these genes causing persistence of müllerian structures in otherwise normally virilized males have been described.
- The prevalence of a mutation in the galactose-1-phosphate uridyl transferase (GALT) gene (different from that associated with classical galactosemia) is increased in daughters with müllerian agenesis and their mothers.
- The observation suggests that errors in fetal or maternal galactose metabolism resulting in increased intrauterine galactose exposure may have adverse effects on müllerian development.
- Patients typically present in late adolescence or as young adults, well after menarche was expected, with primary amenorrhea as their only complaint.
- They exhibit normal, symmetrical breast and pubic hair development, no visible vagina, and have no symptoms or signs of crytomenorrhea because the rudimentary uteri contain no functional endometrium.
- In approximately 10%, functional islands of endometrium may result in a hematometra and symptoms of cyclic pain.

21. b. Gonads show evidence of spermatogenesis
Ref: Speroff 8th/ed p 457; Yen & Jaffe's 8th/ed p 366

- The testes may be intra-abdominal, but often are partially descended; more than half of patients with complete AIS have an inguinal hernia.
- The testes frequently are palpable in the inguinal canals, most commonly at the level of the external inguinal ring. They generally resemble any cryptorchid testes but may be nodular.
- After puberty, the testes contain immature seminiferous tubules lined by immature germ cells and Sertoli cells, with no evidence of spermatogenesis.

22. d. All
Ref: Yen & Jaffe's 8th/ed p 237, 366

Points to distinguish AIS from MRKH Syndrome:
- They exhibit asymmetrical secondary sexual development (breast development with absent or scant pubic hair). The breasts may become relatively large and have subtle abnormalities; lacking the actions of progesterone, they have little glandular tissue, small nipples and pale areolae.
- Serum estradiol levels are in range of 50 pg/mL, comparable to early follicular-phase levels.
- A serum testosterone concentration is normal or modestly elevated above the range observed in normal males and well above the normal range for females. Serum LH levels also are elevated, reflecting androgen insensitivity at the hypothalamic-pituitary level.
- A karyotype (46, XY) firmly establishes the diagnosis.

23. a. Complete AIS
Ref: Yen & Jaffe's 8th/ed p 375; Speroff 8th/ed p 458

- Complete AIS is the only exception to the rule of immediate gonadectomy in presence of Y chromosome.

DSD conditions are accompanied by variable risk of germ cell tumor, which should be taken into consideration on long-term management of these patients.

Higher risk of gonadal tumors has been shown in gonadal dysgenesis positive for the presence of TSPY (testis-specific protein Y) encoded on Y chromosome, and for partial androgen insensitivity syndromes with intraabdominal gonads.

Lower risks are observed in ovotesticular DSD and complete androgen insensitivity syndrome.

Whereas gonadectomy is recommended at time of diagnosis in other intersex states such as XY gonadal dysgenesis (Swyer syndrome), it is better delayed in those with AIS, for two reasons.

i. The smooth pubertal development that results from endogenous hormone production is difficult to achieve with exogenous hormone treatment.
ii. Gonadal tumors develop less often in patients with AIS and rarely before puberty (5-10%).

Therefore, gonadectomy and hormone therapy (physiologic estrogen treatment) generally are best postponed until after pubertal development is complete, by approximately age 16-18.

In patients with the incomplete form of AIS, surgery should not be postponed because prompt gonadectomy will prevent further unwanted virilization.

24. a. Risk of developing gonadoblastoma is less than 5%
Ref: Yen & Jaffe's 8th/ed p 354; Speroff 8th/ed p 461

Karyotyping in Turner Syndrome

- A karyotype is definitive, and specifically indicated, in part because it may reveal a cell line containing a Y chromosome otherwise not suspected or identified (e.g. 45, X/46, XY)
- Approximately 5% of women with Turner syndrome have a karyotype containing all or part of a Y chromosome.

- Further analysis with fluorescence in situ hybridization (FISH) will identify another 5% having occult Y chromosome material.
- Whereas it is important to identify a Y chromosome because affected individuals are at significant increased risk for developing gonadoblastoma (20-30%), that risk appears lower (5-10%) in women with Turner syndrome and limited to those having detectable Y chromosome on their karyotype.
- FISH analysis is most clearly indicated for those exhibiting any evidence of virilization or having a chromosomal fragment of uncertain origin.

25. **b. Gonadectomy is indicated being at high risk of gonadoblastoma**

    Ref: Yen & Jaffe's 8th/ed p 436; Speroff 8th/ed p 461

- Mosaicism in women with Turner syndrome has important clinical implications besides those relating to a cell line containing a Y chromosome.
- In those with a mosaic 46, XX cell line (e.g. 45, X/46, XX), the gonad may contain functional ovarian cortical tissue, resulting in some degree of sexual development, or even menses and the possibility of pregnancy.
- Depending on the degree of gonadal dysgenesis, up to 30% undergo some degree of spontaneous puberty and approximately 5% complete puberty and begin menstruation.
- It is estimated that 2% to 5% of patients have potential for spontaneous pregnancy.
- Approximately one-third has cardiovascular anomalies, including a bicuspid aortic valve, coarctation of the aorta, mitral valve prolapse, and aortic aneurysm.
- Renal anomalies also are common and include horseshoe kidney, unilateral renal agenesis or pelvic kidney, rotational abnormalities, and partial or complete duplication of the collecting system(s).
- Autoimmune disorders are common in Turner syndrome and include thyroiditis, type 1 diabetes, autoimmune hepatitis and thrombocytopenia, and celiac disease.
- Hearing loss also is common.

26. **c. Gonadectomy can be delayed till pubertal development is fully achieved**

    Ref: Yen & Jaffe's 8th/ed p 362; Speroff 8th/ed p 463

- Gonadoblastoma is a premalignant germ cell tumor, unique to intersex states like Swyer syndrome, and may contain or give rise to other highly malignant tumors, including dysgerminoma, endodermal sinus tumor, embryonal and choriocarcinomas.

This patient represents most likely **Swyer Syndrome**.
- Gonadectomy is indicated soon after diagnosis due the significant risk for malignant transformation in occult testicular elements (20-30%).
- The risk of gonadoblastoma formation in XY gonadal dysgenesis patients increases with age and has been estimated to be as high as 30% by 30 years of age.

27. **a. Mosaics (45, X/46, XX)**

    Ref: Speroff 8th/ed p 463

A wide variety of numerical and structural chromosomal abnormalities may be identified in women presenting with ovarian failure.

A review of karyotypes obtained in women with secondary amenorrhea revealed the spectrum of possibilities and demonstrates the importance of a karyotype in women with POF.

Half of the observed abnormalities were numerical, involving X chromosome mosaicism (including 45,X, 46,XX, and 47,XXX cell lines) or Y chromosome mosaicism (including 46,XY, 47,XYY, and 47,XXY cell lines); the remainder included an assortment of X chromosome translocations, deletions and other structural abnormalities, and even some with a pure 46,XY karyotype.

28. **d. Savage syndrome**

    Ref: Speroff 8th/ed p 470

- Savage syndrome is functional ovarian failure resulting from disorder of follicular development.

Whereas accelerated follicular depletion is the underlying mechanism for the most common causes of POF, a variety of rare genetic disorders causing impaired or abnormal follicular development may result in a functional ovarian failure.

Patients present with amenorrhea and hypergonadotropic hypogonadism and are resistant to high doses of exogenous gonadotropins, although their ovaries contain numerous follicles. Disorder is called as "resistant ovary syndrome" or "Savage syndrome".

Examples include:
- Disorders of intraovarian regulation
- Steroidogenic enzyme defects
- Abnormalities in gonadotropins and their receptors.

29. **a. Pituitary failure**

    Ref: Speroff 8th/ed p 471

Pituitary failure will lead to hypogonadotropic hypogonadism.

30. **b. Pituitary adenoma are true neoplasms and mostly malignant**

    Ref: Speroff 8th/ed p 478

Pituitary Adenomas

- True neoplasms but almost always are benign.
- The large majority are monoclonal.
- Activating mutations in the GNAS1 gene are identified in approximately 40% of GH-secreting somatotroph adenomas.

31. a. Nonfunctioning adenomas do not have functional consequences

Ref: Speroff 8th/ed p 474

If large enough, even nonfunctioning adenomas can have functional consequences, by compressing the pituitary stalk and interfering with the delivery of hypothalamic releasing or inhibiting factors, or by compressing surrounding cells known as 'The Stalk Effect'.

32. b. 1%

Ref: Frontiers in Gynecological Endocrinology. Andrea R Genazzani. Vol 3 p 53

- Incidence of POI is likely to rise as cure rates for cancers in childhood and young women continue to improve.

Premature ovarian insufficiency has been estimated to affect about:
- 1% of women younger than 40
- 0.1% of women under 30
- 0.01% of women under age 20.

POF generally results in secondary amenorrhea at some time after puberty is completed, but also may occur at any time before menarche and is distinguished from gonadal dysgenesis on the basis of ovarian morphology and histology; instead of streak gonads, the ovaries more closely resemble those of postmenopausal women.

33. a. The large majority of gonadotroph adenomas are functional

Ref: Speroff 8th/ed p 476

FSH Secreting Adenomas

- FSH-secreting adenomas may cause anovulation and spontaneous ovarian hyperstimulation, resulting in amenorrhea, multiple large ovarian cysts, and high serum FSH and estradiol levels.
- In prepubertal girls, they may cause breast development and vaginal bleeding. However, most patients with gonadotroph adenomas have normal or low serum gonadotropin concentrations because the **tumors are nonfunctional** and disrupt menstrual function only indirectly, via compression of the pituitary stalk or surrounding cells. They may inhibit gonadotropin secretion by interrupting the delivery of hypothalamic GnRH or by compressing normal gonadotrophs.
- Alternatively, they may cause hyperprolactinemia by interfering with the inhibitory actions of dopamine on lactotrophs, resulting in a secondary suppression of hypothalamic GnRH secretion and amenorrhea.
- Gonadotroph adenomas also may secrete large amounts of the a-subunit common to all of the pituitary glycoprotein hormones (having no intrinsic biological activity).
- In the presence of low or normal gonadotropin levels, an elevated level of free a-subunit also suggests a nonfunctioning gonadotroph adenoma.

34. a. Acute infarction and ischemic necrosis of posterior pituitary gland

Ref: Speroff 8th/ed p 483

Sheehan's Syndrome

- Acute infarction and ischemic necrosis of the pituitary gland resulting from postpartum hemorrhage and hypovolemic hypotension is known as Sheehan's syndrome. Anterior pituitary is most commonly involved.
- One of the most common causes of hypopituitarism in underdeveloped or developing countries.
- Failed lactation after delivery is the classical presenting symptom.
- The rest of the clinical picture varies with the severity of the pituitary insult, ranging from severe hypopituitarism soon after delivery, manifesting as lethargy, anorexia, and weight loss, to secondary amenorrhea, loss of sexual hair, and less severe symptoms of fatigue that emerge weeks and months later.
- Deficiencies in GH, prolactin, and gonadotropins are most common, although the majority also exhibit ACTH and TSH deficiencies.
- A partially or completely empty sella is a common later finding.

35. c. Not at risk of stress fracture

Ref: Reproductive endocrinology for MRCOG and beyond. Chapter 7 p 80

Amenorrheic excercisers usually have hypoestrogenic state.

Measurement of bone mineral density is indicated in amenorrheic women who are estrogen deficient.

Measurement are made in the lumbar spine and femoral neck.

The vertebral bone is more sensitive to estrogen deficiency and vertebral fractures tend to occur in a younger age group than fractures at the femoral neck.

Those who are not candidate for ovulation induction should receive HRT:
- Gonadal failure
- Hypothalamic amenorrhea
- Postgonadectomy patients

36. a. 17% for menarche and at 22% for regular menstruation

Ref: Speroff 8th/ed p 490; Reproductive Endocrinology for MRCOG and beyond. Chapter 7 p 83

Weight Related Amenorrhea

- A regular menstrual cycle is unlikely to occur if BMI is less than 19 kg/m^2.
- Fat appears to be critical to a normally functioning hypothalamic-pituitary-gonadal axis.
- The critical weight hypothesis holds that the onset and regularity of menstrual function require that weight remains above a critical threshold level, with a corresponding critical level of body fat, which is estimated at 17% for menarche, and at 22% for regular menstruation.
- This level enables extra ovarian aromatization of androgens to estrogen.
- To cause amenorrhea, the loss must be 10-15% of the women's normal weight for height.

37. b. Always X-linked inheritance

Ref: Yen & Jaffe's 8th/ed p 441

Kallmann's Syndrome

- When congenital GnRH deficiency is associated with anosmia or hyposmia (an absent or grossly impaired sense of smell), the disorder is known as Kallmann's syndrome.
- The classical X-linked form of the disorder is caused by a variety of genetic mutations in the *KAL* gene (located on the short arm of the X chromosome, Xp22.3) encoding anosmin-1, a neural adhesion molecule that promotes migration of GnRH neurons, and olfactory neurons, from the olfactory placode into the hypothalamus during embryonic development.
- Kallmann's syndrome also can be inherited in an autosomal dominant or recessive fashion.
- At puberty, both males and females with Kallmann's syndrome usually present with delayed growth and sexual development.
- The presence of pubic hair, reflecting a normal adrenarche, helps to distinguish them from those with a constitutional delay of puberty in whom adrenarche typically also is delayed.
- However, the most distinguishing feature of Kallmann's syndrome is the inability to perceive odors, such as coffee or perfume.
- Patients with the disorder also may have a family history of delayed puberty and other abnormalities, including cleft lip/palate, urogenital tract anomalies, or syndactaly.

38. c. High FSH, normal LH

Ref: Disorders of Menstruation. Marshburn & Hurst. Chapter 4 p 47

- During perimenopausal period it is normal for FSH levels to begin to rise even before bleeding has ceased. This is true whether the perimenopausal period is premature at age 25-35 or at the usual time.
- This increase in FSH is associated with a decrease in inhibin production by less competent ovarian follicles. Period of elevated levels of FSH can be followed by a pregnancy.
- The value of measuring both FSH and LH is again emphasized because this special perimenopausal condition is associated with a high FSH but a normal LH.

39. b. Approximately 30% patients with Y chromosome will develop signs of virilization

Ref: Speroff 8th/ed p 461

- Approximately 30% patients with Y chromosome **will not** develop signs of virilization. Therefore, even the normal appearing adult woman with elevated gonadotropin levels must be karyotyped.
- Third most common cause of primary amenorrhea is AIS after gonadal dysgenesis and mullerian agenesis.
- Gonadal dysgenesis associated with normal karyotype and neurosensory deafness is Perrault syndrome. Auditory evaluation should be considered in all 46, XX gonadal dysgenesis cases.
- 30% women with hyperprolactinemia have galactorrhea and 30% of women with galactorrhea have normal menses.

40. a. Midcycle LH surge is approximately 3 times baseline levels

Ref: Speroff 8th/ed p 470

- Mullerian agenesis is **second** most common cause of primary amenorrhea first being gonadal dysgenesis.

Midcycle LH surge is approximately 3 times baseline level. Therefore, if patient does not bleed 2 weeks after blood sample was obtained, a high level can be safely interpreted as abnormal.

Galactosemia is associated with hypergonadotropic hypogonadism. It is an autosomal recessive disorder of galactose metabolism caused by deficiency of enzyme galactose-1-phosphate uridyl transferase. It is a rare cause of premature ovarian failure. Affected women have fewer primordial follicles, due to cumulative toxicity of galactose metabolites on germ cell migration and survival.

Women with gonadal dysgenesis can also present with secondary amenorrhea.

41. c. Ovarian failure
Ref: Disorders of Menstruation. Marshburn & Hurst. Chapter 8 p 129

Ovarian failure is associated with hypergonadotropic hypogonadism.

42. b. Can detect microadenomas reliably
Ref: Disorders of Menstruation. Marshburn & Hurst. Chapter 8 p 130

X-ray coned-down lateral view of sella turcica does not offer enough information to focus in on potential diagnosis.

- This can detect presence of a large tumor, although rare suprasellar extension or small microadenomas might escape this method.
- It can detect craniopharyngioma
- When combined with a prolactin assay can determine when to obtain MRI.

43. c. Anosmia
Ref: Yen & Jaffe's 8th/ed p 441; Speroff 8th/ed p 493

When congenital GnRH deficiency is associated with anosmia or hyposmia, it is known as Kallmann's syndrome. Anosmia is most characteristic feature of syndrome.

44. b. More common in females than in males
Ref: Yen & Jaffe's 8th/ed p 441; Speroff 8th/ed p 492

Congenital GnRH deficiency is more common in males than in females with ratio of 5:1.

Most common form of inheritance is X-linked form of disorder with genetic mutation in KAL gene.

CHAPTER 9

Chronic Anovulation and Polycystic Ovary Syndrome

Multiple Choice Questions

1. Conditions associated with chronic anovulation:
   a. PCOS
   b. Obesity
   c. Hepatic disease
   d. All

2. Obesity is associated with chronic anovulation because:
   a. Increased peripheral aromatization
   b. Decreased SHBG
   c. Insulin resistance leading to hyperandrogenism
   d. All

3. How many percent of patients with chronic anovulation associated with polycystic ovaries do not have elevated LH levels?
   a. 20–40
   b. 10–20
   c. <10
   d. Elevated LH levels is the rule

4. Which of the following statement is not true?
   a. LH stimulation of androgen production in thecal cells is enhanced by IGF-1
   b. Insulin increases SHBG production by liver
   c. Androgens in low concentration promote aromatase enzyme activity
   d. Inhibin promotes LH stimulation of thecal androgen synthesis

5. Most common metabolic abnormality observed in women with PCOS:
   a. Dyslipidemia
   b. Hyperglycemia
   c. Hypertension
   d. Hyperuricemia

6. What does not hold correct regarding PCOS?
   a. Increased estrogen is due to peripheral aromatization
   b. Lipid profile in androgenized women with polycystic ovaries is similar to male pattern
   c. Characterized by fluctuating hormone levels
   d. There is a direct relationship between plasma insulin levels and blood pressure

7. PCOS is associated with high IGF-1 secretion. Which of the following is incorrect regarding PCOS?
   a. IGF-1 is produced in granulosa cells
   b. IGF-1 production is enhanced by estradiol and growth hormone
   c. Chronic anovulation is associated with endometrial and breast cancer
   d. IGF-1 receptors have structural similarity to insulin receptors

8. Which is not correct regarding hyperthecosis?
   a. Chronic anovulation
   b. High LH levels
   c. Patches of luteinized theca-like cells scattered throughout ovarian stroma
   d. Insulin resistance

9. BMI below which insulin resistance is not detected:
   a. < 27 kg/m^2
   b. <32 kg/m^2
   c. <30 kg/m^2
   d. <35 kg/m^2

10. Not component of HAIRAN syndrome:
    a. Hyperandrogenism
    b. Hypertension
    c. Insulin resistance
    d. Acanthosis nigricans

11. Not true about Acanthosis nigricans:
    a. Associated with insulin resistance
    b. Histological characteristics of acanthosis nigricans are hyperkeratosis and papillomatosis
    c. Acanthosis nigricans is an absolute marker for hyperandrogenism
    d. Gray brown velvety discoloration of skin

12. Hyperinsulinemia leads to all except:
    a. Decreased SHBG
    b. Increased IGFBP-1
    c. Increased free androgen
    d. Increased IGF-1

13. Ratio of fasting glucose to fasting insulin defining hyperinsulinemia:
    a. <4.5
    b. <4
    c. <5.5
    d. <6

14. Which statement is incorrect?
    a. Hyperthyroidism can lead to chronic anovulation
    b. Hypothyroidism can lead to hyperprolactinemia
    c. Chronic stress may lead to anovulation
    d. Polycystic ovary is result of a specific central defect

15. Following statement is incorrect regarding PCOS:
    a. The thick sclerotic capsule acts as mechanical barrier to ovulation
    b. Follicles in polycystic ovary are surrounded by hyperplastic theca cells
    c. Theca cells are often luteinized in response to high LH levels
    d. Polycystic ovary is end result of chronic anovulation

16. Leprechaunism all true *except*:
    a. Mutation in insulin receptor gene
    b. Severe insulin resistance
    c. Increased number of insulin receptors
    d. Polycystic ovaries

17. Which of the following is false?
    a. Hyperandrogenism induces hyperinsulinemia
    b. Evaluation of androgens in not necessary in patient with anovulation without features of hyperandrogenism
    c. Documentation of anovulation is unnecessary in view of menstrual irregularity with periods of amenorrhea
    d. SHBG is reduced with hyperinsulinemia

18. PCOS is characterized by chronic anovulation and is associated with high risk of endometrial cancer. Which statement is incorrect regarding this?
    a. Decision to perform endometrial biopsy is based on duration of exposure to unopposed estrogen
    b. Decision to perform endometrial biopsy is based on the age of patient
    c. Chronic anovulation is associated with 3 fold increased risk of carcinoma endometrium
    d. Progesterone supplementation for at least 12 days is warranted to combat risk of hyperestrogenic state

19. Activin is member of TGF-b superfamily. What is not correct about activin?
    a. Exists in two forms
    b. In early follicular phase, it enhances action of FSH
    c. Suppresses thecal androgen synthesis
    d. Prevents premature luteinization

20. Hormonal profile in women with PCOS show all *except*:
    a. High FSH
    b. High LH
    c. Low normal FSH
    d. High LH:FSH ratios

21. PCOS is associated with:
    a. Abnormal LH secretory dynamics
    b. Predominance of basic LH isoforms with greater bioactivity
    c. GnRH pulse generator less sensitive to the feedback inhibition of sex steroids
    d. All

22. Overall prevalence of insulin resistance in women with PCOS:
    a. 50–75%   b. 25–50%
    c. 10–20%   d. >75%

23. Overall prevalence of PCOS in women with insulin resistance:
    a. 15%   b. 25%
    c. 50%   d. 75%

24. The primary mechanisms driving increased ovarian androgen production in PCOS include:
    a. Increased LH stimulation resulting from abnormal LH secretory dynamics
    b. Increased LH bioactivity
    c. Hyperinsulinemia due to insulin resistance
    d. All

25. The primary mechanisms driving increased adrenal androgen production in PCOS include:
    a. Chronic estrogen stimulation due to anovulation could decrease adrenal 3b-HSD activity
    b. Increased pituitary ACTH secretion or increased sensitivity to ACTH
    c. Intrinsic upregulation of P450c17 17,20 lyase activity
    d. All

26. Least common clinical manifestation of hyperandrogenism:
    a. Androgenic alopecia   b. Hirsutism
    c. Acne   d. Clitoromegaly

27. Hirsutism is the growth of terminal hairs on the face or body in a male pattern affecting up to 70% of women with PCOS. What is false about the method used for assessing the severity of hirsutism?
    a. The modified Ferriman-Gallwey score is the most common method for grading the extent of hirsutism
    b. A score from 0-4 in each area is given
    c. The modified Ferriman-Gallwey score is most practical way to assess the severity of hirsutism
    d. 9 androgen-sensitive areas are taken

28. Most common cause of anovulation with normo-gonadotropic normogonadism:
    a. PCOS
    b. Hyperprolactinemia
    c. Pregnancy
    d. OCPs

29. The Rotterdam, 2003 criteria for PCOS include all *except*:
    a. Oligo/anovulation
    b. Clinical or biochemical signs of hyperandrogenism
    c. Raised AMH
    d. Polycystic ovaries

30. Polycystic ovaries can be seen in:
    a. Hyperprolactinemia
    b. Normal women
    c. Oral contraceptive users
    d. All

31. Which of the following women nonclassical CAH must be excluded?
    a. Early onset of hirsutism (pre-or peri-menarcheal)
    b. Family history of CAH
    c. High risk ethnic group
    d. All

32. Severe insulin resistance syndrome includes all *except*:
    a. PCOS
    b. HAIR-AN syndrome
    c. Leprechaunism
    d. Ovarian hyperthecosis

33. A follicular phase morning serum 17-OHP concentration less than.... ng/dL rules out nonclassical CAH:
    a. 500
    b. 800
    c. 200
    d. 1500

34. Which of the following is not true regarding Barker hypothesis?
    a. Macrosomia at birth
    b. High risk of type II diabetes
    c. Premature pubarche
    d. Childhood obesity

35. Most common reproductive endocrinopathy of women:
    a. Congenital adrenal hyperplasia
    b. PCOS
    c. Hyperprolactinemia
    d. Cushing syndrome

36. Which of the following is not true regarding familial occurrence of PCOS?
    a. Prevalence of insulin resistance is greater in relatives of PCOS patients
    b. First degree male relatives show high circulating DHEA-S levels
    c. PCOS does not carry familial risk
    d. Early onset baldness may be seen in first degree male relatives

37. Which of the following conditions is associated with polycystic ovaries?
    a. Congenital adrenal hyperplasia
    b. Female to male transsexuals
    c. Women recovering from hypogonadotropic hypogonadism
    d. All

38. Which is not true regarding insulin resistance seen in PCOS?
    a. First degree relative show insulin resistance
    b. Fasting hyperglycemia but postprandial hypoglycemia
    c. Metformin can be given as insulin sensitizer
    d. Thiazolidinediones are not given in patients with liver diseases

39. Which of the following is rare severe side effect of metformin therapy?
    a. Renal failure
    b. Liver failure
    c. Lactic acidosis
    d. Agranulocytopenia

40. The reason because of which first generation thiazolidinediones were withdrawn?
    a. Renal failure
    b. Liver toxicity
    c. Neurotoxicity
    d. Lactic acidosis

41. Which of the following is WHO group 2 cause of anovulation?
    a. PCOS
    b. Hypothalamic causes
    c. Pituitary causes
    d. Hyperprolactinemia

42. Why female fetus is not affected by high androgen levels in women with PCOS during pregnancy?
    a. Increased circulating levels of SHBG
    b. Metabolic capacity of placental aromatase enzyme
    c. Reduced biologically available fraction of testosterone
    d. All

43. Anti-Mullerian hormone is a member of TGF-beta superfamily. Which of the following is incorrect regarding AMH?
    a. It inhibits recruitment of primordial follicles
    b. Increases follicle sensitivity to gonadotropin stimulation
    c. Inhibits action of FSH induced aromatase production
    d. Increased levels are seen in PCOS

44. Leading cause of dyslipidemia among reproductive age women:
    a. CAH   b. Cushing syndrome
    c. PCOS   d. Type II diabetes

45. Cardinal feature for diagnosis of PCOS as per Androgen Excess PCOS Society criteria:
    a. Hyperandrogenism   b. Oligoanovulation
    c. Polycystic ovaries d. All should be present

46. Which PCOS phenotype is associated with least metabolic risk?
    a. PCOS-A   b. PCOS-B
    c. PCOS-C   d. PCOS-D

47. Which of the following phenotypes of PCOS is associated with lower body mass index and lesser degrees of hyperinsulinemia and hyperandrogenism?
    a. PCOS-A   b. PCOS-B
    c. PCOS-C   d. PCOS-D

48. Which of the following area is not scored by Ferriman-Gallwey Score?
    a. Lower legs   b. Arms
    c. Thighs   d. Chin

49. Irregular menstrual cycles. Which of the following is incorrect for them?
    a. Normal in first year postmenarche
    b. > 1 to < 3 year post menarche, cycles are considered irregular if they come >35 days interval
    c. >3 years postmenarche to perimenopause cycles coming at interval less than 21 days are considered irregular
    d. < 8 cycles per year are considered abnormal

50. Which of the following is least accurate method to assess total or free testosterone in PCOS?
    a. Liquid chromatography
    b. Mass spectrometry and extraction
    c. Chromatography immunoassays
    d. ELISA

51. Ludwig visual score is used for is used to score:
    a. Hirsutism   b. Acne
    c. Clitoromegaly d. Alopecia

52. Which of the following is incorrect regarding newer recommendations for ultrasound in PCOS?
    a. In transabdominal ultrasound reporting is best focused on ovarian volume with a threshold of ≥ 12 mL
    b. Ultrasound should not be used for the diagnosis of PCOS in those with a gynaecological age of < 8 years
    c. Follicle number per ovary >20 is considered polycystic
    d. Volume >10 mL is abnormal

53. Value of AMH used as cut off as a single test to diagnose PCOS:
    a. 3.4 ng/dL   b. 4.4 ng/dL
    c. 5.4 ng/dL   d. None of the above

54. OGTT is recommended in PCOS women with:
    a. BMI >25 Kg/m^2
    b. Asians with BMI >23 Kg/m^2
    c. History of impaired glucose tolerance tests
    d. All of the above

55. Not true about COCP usage in PCOS:
    a. The 35 microgram ethinyl estradiol plus cyproterone acetate preparations is considered first line in PCOS
    b. The COCP alone should be recommended in adult women with PCOS for management of hyperandrogenism
    c. The COCP alone should be recommended in adult women with PCOS for management of irregular menstrual cycles
    d. PCOS specific risk factors such as high BMI, hyperlipidemia and hypertension need to be considered.

56. Indications to add antiandrogens in women with PCOS:
    a. To treat hirsutism when 6 months or more of COCPs have failed
    b. Androgen related alopecia
    c. Resistant hirsutism
    d. All of above

57. First line pharmacological agent used for ovulation induction in PCOS:
    a. Clomiphene
    b. Letrozole
    c. Gonadotropins
    d. LOD

58. As per PCOS 2018 guidelines, which of the following is incorrect for Laparoscopic ovarian drilling?
    a. Second line therapy for women with PCOS, who are clomiphene citrate resistant
    b. Runs risk for periadnexal adhesions
    c. Should never be used as first line therapy
    d. Associated with risk of low ovarian reserves

59. Conception should be avoided for how many months post-bariatric surgery?
    a. 12
    b. 18
    c. 24
    d. 36

60. Which is the preferred protocol for ovarian stimulation for IVF/ICSI in PCOS women?
    a. Antagonist protocol
    b. Long agonist protocol
    c. Microflare protocol
    d. Short protocol

61. Following are used to decrease risk of OHSS in PCOS women, *except:*
    a. Starting stimulation with lower doses of gonadotropins
    b. hCG trigger
    c. Cycle segmentation
    d. Antagonist protocol

62. Which is least effective method to reduce risk of OHSS in women with PCOS?
    a. IVM
    b. Agonist trigger
    c. Albumin therapy
    d. Calcium gluconate

Answer with Explanations

1. **d. All**
   Ref: Speroff 8th/ed p 498

   Conditions causing chronic anovulation are associated with sustained high levels of estrogen negative feedback preventing any significant increase in FSH levels:
   - Increased production
   - Decreased clearance
   - Decreased metabolism

   Conditions associated with chronic anovulation:
   - PCOS
   - Obesity
   - Hepatic disease
   - Thyroid disease
   - Estrogen producing tumors

2. **d. All**
   Ref: Speroff 8th/ed p 500

   Obesity predisposes to chronic anovulation in at least three distinct ways:
   A. Increased peripheral aromatization of androgens, resulting in chronically elevated estrogen concentrations.
   B. Decreased levels of hepatic SHBG production, resulting in increased circulating concentrations of free estradiol and testosterone.
   C. Insulin resistance, leading to a compensatory increase in insulin levels that stimulates androgen production in the ovarian stroma, resulting in high local androgen concentrations that impair follicular development.

3. **a. 20-40%**
   Ref: Speroff 8th/ed p 503

   20-40% of patients with persistent anovulation associated with polycystic ovaries do not have elevated LH levels with reversal of LH:FSH ratio.

   Polycystic ovary may be associated with extragonadal sources of androgens or with ovarian androgen-producing tumors.

4. **b. Insulin increases SHBG production by liver**
   Ref: Speroff 8th/ed p 518

   Explaining each option one by one:
   - Insulin, IGF-1 and androgens inhibit SHBG production by liver. There is **inverse relationship** between body weight and SHBG secretion.
   - The right concentration of androgens in granulosa cells promote aromatase activity and inhibin production.
   - Inhibin promotes LH stimulation of thecal androgen synthesis.
   - LH stimulation of thecal androgen production is further enhanced by autocrine activity of IGF-1.

5. **a. Dyslipidemia**
   Ref: Speroff 8th/ed p 517; Cambridge Polycystic ovarian syndrome 2nd/ed p 88

   - Dyslipidemia is the most common metabolic abnormality observed in women with PCOS.
   - Dyslipidemia is more pronounced among obese subjects. It seems to affect women at younger age, increasing risk for atherosclerosis.
   - Women with menstrual irregularities are likely to be those exhibiting more pronounced dyslipidemia.

   Applying the National Cholesterol Education Program guidelines, nearly 70% have at least one borderline or elevated lipid level.

   Insulin resistance and hyperinsulinemia are associated with:
   - Decreased HDL cholesterol
   - Elevated triglyceride levels

   Hyperinsulinemia is usually not associated with elevated LDL concentrations, but can be seen in PCOS as a result from hyperandrogenism.

6. **c. Characterized by fluctuating hormone levels**
   Ref: Speroff 8th/ed p 517
   - Persistent anovulation is associated with **steady state** of gonadotropins and sex steroids, unlike normal menstrual cycle.
   - The ovary does not secrete increased amounts of estrogen, and estradiol levels are equivalent to early follicular phase. The increased total estrogen is due to peripheral conversion of increased amounts of androstenedione to estrone.
   - There exists a direct relationship between plasma insulin levels and blood pressure.

7. **a. IGF-1 is produced in granulosa cells**
   Ref: Speroff 8th/ed p 548
   - Chronic anovulation is associated with:
     - 3 fold increased risk of endometrial cancer
     - 3-4 fold increased risk of breast cancer appearing in postmenopausal years.

IGF-1 is produced in theca cells in response to gonadotropin stimulation, and this response is enhanced by estradiol and growth hormone.

Impressive correlation between the degree of hyperinsulinemia and hyperandrogenism: At high insulin concentrations, insulin binds to IGF-1 receptors which are similar to insulin receptors.

8. **b. High LH levels**

    Ref: Cambridge Polycystic Ovarian Syndrome 2nd/ed p 46; Yen & Jaffe's 8th/ed p 549

Hyperthecosis

- Refers to patches of luteinized theca-like cells scattered throughout the ovarian stroma.
- Characterized by same histologic findings as seen in polycystic ovaries.
- More intense androgenization as a result of greater androgen production.
- **Lower LH levels** due to high testosterone levels blocking estrogen action at hypothalamic-pituitary level.
- Greater degree of insulin resistance.

9. **a. < 27 kg/m^2**

    Ref: Speroff 8th/ed p 520

- The only known therapy for PCOS is **weight loss**.
- Both hyperinsulinemia and hyperandrogenism can be reduced with weight loss which is more than 5% of initial weight.
- Insulin resistance is not detected with a BMI less than 27 kg/m^2.

10. **b. Hypertension**

    Ref: Kamini A Rao 2nd/ed p 161

HAIRAN Syndrome:
- **H**yper**A**ndrogenism
- **I**nsulin **R**esistance
- **A**canthosis **N**igricans

11. **c. Acanthosis nigricans is an absolute marker for hyperandrogenism**

    Ref: Cambridge Polycystic ovarian syndrome 2nd/ed p 102

Points to be remembered for acanthosis nigricans:
- Gray brown velvety discoloration of skin.
- Histological characteristics of acanthosis nigricans are hyperkeratosis and papillomatosis.
- Cutaneous marker of insulin resistance.
- Because acanthosis nigricans can be present in normal women, its presence is not an absolute marker for hyperandrogenism.

12. **b. Increased IGFBP-1**

    Ref: Cambridge Polycystic ovarian syndrome 2nd/ed p 239

Hyperinsulinemia leads to decreased hepatic production of SHBG thus increasing serum free testosterone and decreased IGFBP-1 thus increasing IGF-1 levels.

13. **a. <4.5**

    Ref: Speroff 8th/ed p 516

- A baseline 2-hour OGTT is recommended for all women with PCOS, as
    - Up to 35% exhibit impaired glucose tolerance
    - Up to 10% have diabetes mellitus.

Ratio of fasting glucose to fasting insulin **less than 4.5** defines hyperinsulinemia. It is not certain what levels of insulin in fasting state or in response to an oral glucose tolerance test are correlated with clinical outcome.

The standard OGTT is the mainstay of methods for diagnosis of impaired glucose tolerance and diabetes mellitus and can be used to assess insulin sensitivity, when indicated.

Although techniques vary, all involve measures of plasma glucose and insulin at intervals over 2 to 4 hours after a 75-g or 100-g oral glucose load.

14. **d. Polycystic ovary is result of a specific central defect**

    Ref: Yen & Jaffe's 8th/ed p 523

Polycystic ovary is the result of a functional derangement, not a specific central or local defect. Any condition causing chronic anovulation can lead to polycystic ovaries.

Both hyperthyroidism and hypothyroidism can cause persistent anovulation by altering not only metabolic clearance but also the peripheral conversion rates among the various steroids.

15. **a. The thick sclerotic capsule acts as mechanical barrier to ovulation**

    Ref: Speroff 8th/ed p 501

The polycystic ovary is enlarged and has smooth pearly white capsule. It **was erroneously believed** for so many years that thick sclerotic capsule acted as a mechanical barrier to ovulation.

Follicles in polycystic ovary are surrounded by hyperplastic theca cells, often luteinized in response to the high LH levels.

16. **c. Increased number of insulin receptors**

    Ref: Speroff 8th/ed p 520

Leprechaunism is a rare syndrome in young girls characterized by **mutation in the insulin receptor gene** and is associated with:
- Severe insulin resistance
- Polycystic ovaries
- Hyperandrogenism
- Acanthosis nigricans

Chronic Anovulation and Polycystic Ovary Syndrome

17. a. Hyperandrogenism induces hyperinsulinemia
Ref: Yen & Jaffe's 8th/ed p 525
- It is hyperinsulinemia which leads to hyperandrogenism, not vice versa.
- Administration of insulin to women with polycystic ovaries increases circulating androgen levels.
- After normalization of androgens with GnRH agonist treatment, the hyperinsulinemic response to glucose tolerance testing remains abnormal in obese women with polycystic ovaries showing its hyperinsulinemia which leads to hyperandrogenism and not otherwise.

18. b. Decision to perform endometrial biospy is based on the age of patient
Ref: Speroff 8th/ed p 524
- The decision on whether to perform an endometrial biopsy **should not be based on the patient's age**, but on the duration of potential exposure to unopposed estrogen stimulation.
- Chronic anovulation, obesity, and hyperinsulinemia all are associated with risk for developing endometrial cancer.
- The mechanism relates to constant, unrelenting estrogen stimulation of the endometrium, predisposing to abnormal patterns of growth.
- Endometrial hyperplasia, and even endometrial cancer can be encountered in young anovulatory women.
- Overall, the risk for developing endometrial cancer may be increased by as much as 3-fold.
- Consequently, for those with long-standing anovulation, endometrial sampling to exclude endometrial hyperplasia is a prudent precaution.

19. a. Exists in two forms
Ref: Speroff 8th/ed p 213
Points to be remembered regarding activin:
- Member of TGF-β superfamily
- Exists in **3 forms**
- In early follicular phase, activin produced by granulosa in immature follicles
    - Enhances action of FSH leading to increased aromatase activity and FSH and LH receptor formation
    - Suppresses thecal androgen synthesis
- In late follicular phase, in mature granulosa, it **prevents premature luteinization** and progesterone production.

20. a. High FSH
Ref: Speroff 8th/ed p 503
Women with PCOS generally exhibit:
- Increased serum LH concentrations
- Low-normal FSH levels
- Increased LH:FSH ratios

The increase in serum LH levels results from abnormal LH secretory dynamics, characterized by an increase in LH pulse frequency, and to a lesser extent, also in pulse amplitude.

The decrease in FSH levels results from:
- Increase in GnRH pulse frequency
- Negative feedback effects of chronically elevated estrone concentrations (derived from peripheral aromatization of increased androstenedione)
- Modestly increased levels of inhibin B (derived from small follicles).

21. d. All
Ref: Speroff 8th/ed p 503
LH pulse frequency in women with PCOS does not exhibit the normal cyclic variation seen in ovulatory women and is relatively constant, at approximately one pulse per hour. The pattern presumably reflects a similar increase in hypothalamic GnRH pulse frequency, which favors secretion of LH more than FSH.

GnRH pulse generator also is **less sensitive** to the feedback inhibition of sex steroids. Treatment with an estrogen-progestin contraceptive slows LH pulse frequency in women with PCOS, but to a lesser extent than in normal women suggesting decreased sensitivity of GnRH pulse generator.

22. a. 50-75%
Ref: Speroff 8th/ed p 504; Cambridge Polycystic ovarian syndrome 2nd/ed p 239
A few points need to be remembered regarding PCOS and insulin resistance:
- The overall prevalence of insulin resistance ranges between 50% and 75%.
- Up to 35% of women with PCOS exhibit impaired glucose tolerance.
- 7-10% meet criteria for type 2 diabetes mellitus.
- Among all women with insulin resistance, the prevalence of PCOS is 15%.

23. a. 15%
Ref: Speroff 8th/ed p 504
Among all women with insulin resistance, the prevalence of PCOS is 15%.

24. d. All
Ref: Speroff 8th/ed p 505
The primary mechanisms driving increased ovarian androgen production in PCOS:
- Increased LH stimulation resulting from abnormal LH secretory dynamics
- Increased LH bioactivity
- Hyperinsulinemia due to insulin resistance potentiates the action of LH

- Increased volume of theca cells in an expanded ovarian stroma
- Increased sensitivity to LH stimulation due to over-expression of LH receptor in theca and interstitial (stromal) cells

25. d. All

Ref: Speroff 8th/ed p 507

Potential mechanisms for the increase in adrenal androgen production:
- Chronic estrogen stimulation due to anovulation could **decrease adrenal 3b-HSD activity**
- Increased pituitary **ACTH** secretion or increased sensitivity to ACTH
- Intrinsic upregulation of P450c17 **17,20 lyase** activity

26. a. Androgenic alopecia

Ref: Kamini A Rao 2nd/ed p 159

- Clinical evidence of hyperandrogenism includes hirsutism, acne, and androgenic alopecia, all of which relate to the effect of androgens on the pilosebaceous unit.
- Hirsutism is the most obvious clinical indicator of androgen excess and is an important feature of PCOS.
- Androgenic alopecia is an uncommon, feature of PCOS; less than 5% of women with PCOS complain of hair loss. Typically, the hair loss is **limited to the crown** and does not involve the frontal hair line.

27. c. The modified Ferriman-Gallwey score is most practical way to assess the severity of hirsutism

Ref: Speroff 8th/ed p 542

Points to be remembered for the modified Ferriman-Gallwey score:
- Most common method for grading the extent of hirsutism
- A score from 0 to 4 is assigned in each of **9 androgen-sensitive areas** including the upper lip, chin, chest, upper and lower abdomen, upper arm, thighs, and the upper and lower back
- The threshold value that defines hirsutism is not firmly established, but generally has ranged between 6 and 8
- Mild hirsutism: Scores less than 8
- Moderate hirsutism: 8–15
- Severe hirsutism: greater than 15
- The modified Ferriman-Gallwey score is the accepted standard for assessing the severity of hirsutism in clinical investigations
- However, in clinical practice, the **easiest and most practical** way is to determine the method and frequency of hair removal (e.g., shaving, plucking, waxing), which also provides a clinically relevant measure for assessing the response to treatment.

28. a. PCOS

Ref: Kamini A Rao 2nd/ed p 160

Most common cause of anovulation with normogonadotropic normogonadism is PCOS.

29. c. Raised AMH

Ref: Yen & Jaffe's 8th/ed p 520

The European Society for Human Reproduction and Embryology (ESHRE) and the American Society for Reproductive Medicine (ASRM), convened in Rotterdam, The Netherlands, in 2003, concluded that diagnosis of PCOS should be based on at least **two of three** major criteria, include:
1. Oligo/anovulation
2. Clinical or biochemical signs of hyperandrogenism
3. Polycystic ovaries (as identified by ultrasonography), also excluding other androgen excess disorders.

30. d. All

Ref: Speroff 8th/ed p 515

The prevalence of polycystic ovaries is quite high among women with androgen excess (>80%). However, polycystic ovaries can be seen in:
- Normal women (8% to 25%)
- Oral contraceptive users (14%)
- Normal pubertal development
- Hypothalamic amenorrhea
- Hyperprolactinemia

31. d. All

Ref: Speroff 8th/ed p 519

Nonclassical CAH should be excluded in all women with hyperandrogenism, but following group of women specifically need exclusion:
- Those having an early onset of hirsutism (pre- or peri-menarcheal, including girls with premature adrenarche)
- Family history of the disorder
- High-risk ethnic groups (Hispanic, Mediterranean, Slavic, Ashkenazi Jewish, or Yupic Eskimo heritage)

32. a. PCOS

Ref: Speroff 8th/ed p 520

Severe insulin resistance syndromes:

Type A insulin resistance syndrome
- Defects in the insulin receptor
- Affects primarily lean women

Type B syndrome
- Autoimmune disorder affecting the insulin receptor

Type C syndrome—hyperandrogenic-insulin resistant-acanthosis nigricans (HAIR-AN) syndrome
- Variant of type A-Absence of insulin receptor defects
- Characterized by marked acanthosis nigricans, hyperandrogenism, obesity

Other rare disorders involving severe insulin resistance:
- *Leprechaunism*: Insulin receptor mutations
- *Rabson*: Mendenhall syndrome
- Variety of lipodystropic syndromes

33. c. 200
Ref: Yen & Jaffe's 8th/ed p 601

The ACTH stimulation test is performed by obtaining blood samples before and 60 minutes after administering cosyntropin (synthetic ACTH 1–24; 0.25 mg).

A follicular phase morning serum 17-OHP concentration less than 200 ng/dL rules out nonclassical CAH.

Values >800 ng/dL establishes diagnosis.

Values between 200 ng/dL and 800 ng/dL require ACTH stimulation test.

34. a. Macrosomia at birth
Ref: Cambridge Polycystic ovarian syndrome 2nd/ed p 239; Kamini A Rao 2nd/ed p 481

The Barker hypothesis—Fetal origin of adult disease
- Intrauterine malnutrition predisposes to insulin resistance, imprinting future metabolic derangements in affected foetuses.
- IUGR alters development of adipose tissue during fetal life.
- Increased risk of type 2 diabetes, dyslipidemia, and hypertension in adults.
- Low birthweight and rapid childhood weight gain predict abnormalities of glucose tolerance.
- A prenatal origin of hyperandrogenism can be associated with development later in life of premature pubarche and hyperinsulinism in girls, and functional ovarian hyperandrogenism and disorders of glucose tolerance in adult women.

35. b. PCOS
Ref: Yen & Jaffe's 8th/ed p 520

It is estimated that prevalence of PCOS is 4% to 12% of women in their reproductive years of life, which designates this disorder as **the most common reproductive endocrinopathy** of women.

36. c. PCOS does not carry familial risk
Ref: Yen & Jaffe's 8th/ed p 525

First degree relatives of PCOS women are at significant risk for having PCOS, the finding support a genetic basis for hyperandrogenism.

37. d. All
Ref: Yen & Jaffe's 8th/ed p 521

All of the following can be associated with polycystic ovaries:
- PCOS
- Congenital adrenal hyperplasia
- Female to male transsexuals
- Women recovering from hypogonadotropic hypogonadism

38. b. Fasting hyperglycemia but postprandial hypoglycemia
Ref: Yen & Jaffe's 8th/ed p 525, Polycystic ovary syndrome, Cambridge. 2nd/ed p 65

Insulin resistance is associated with postprandial hyperglycemia.

Fasting blood glucose levels may be normal.

39. c. Lactic acidosis
Ref: Yen & Jaffe's 8th/ed p 553; Polycystic ovary syndrome, Cambridge. 2nd/ed p 73

- Rare side effect of metformin therapy is **lactic acidosis**. It may occur in individuals with systemic and debilitating diseases.
- Precautionary temporal withdrawal of metformin therapy is advised in patients undergoing radiological procedures involving iodinated contrast materials and surgery.
- Metformin should not be prescribed to patients with renal, hepatic or major cardiovascular diseases or hypoxia because these patients have a predisposition to elevated lactate levels.
- FDA recommends that prior to initiating treatment with metformin, the patient's serum creatinine concentration should be measured and demonstrated to be less than 1.4 mg/dL.

40. b. Liver toxicity
Ref: Yen & Jaffe's 8th/ed p 553; Polycystic ovary syndrome, Cambridge. 2nd/ed p 74

- Liver toxicity was associated with first generation drugs of thiazolidinediones group.
- However, both rosiglitazone and pioglitazone have been virtually devoid of liver effects.
- Thiazolidinediones should not be initiated in patients with evidence of liver disease.

41. a. PCOS
Ref: Kamini A Rao 2nd/ed p 479

Anovulatory disorders account for about 30-40% of female infertility, with PCOS accounting for 80-90% of WHO group 2, normogonadotropic normoestrogenic anovulation (hypothalamic-pituitary-ovarian dysfunction)

42. d. All
Ref: Kamini A Rao 2nd/ed p 479; Yen & Jaffe's 8th/ed p 270

High maternal serum testosterone levels do not confer clinical consequence in female fetus due to following reasons:
- Increased circulating levels of SHBG
- Metabolic capacity of placental aromatase enzyme
- Reduced biologically available fraction of testosterone

43. b. Increases follicle sensitivity to gonadotropin stimulation

Ref: Kamini A Rao 2nd/ed p 486; Yen & Jaffe's 8th/ed p 534

Anti-Mullerian hormone is a member of TGF-beta superfamily. AMH has following roles:
- It inhibits recruitment of primordial follicles into the pool of growing follicles to prevent early depletion.
- Decreases follicle sensitivity to gonadotropin stimulation to control large number of preantral and small antral follicles to reach preovulatory stage.
- Inhibits action of FSH induced aromatase production.

44. c. PCOS

Ref: Kamini A Rao 2nd/ed p 491

Dyslipidemia is the most common metabolic dysfunction in PCOS, and PCOS is the leading cause of dyslipidemia among reproductive age women.

45. a. Hyperandrogenism

Ref: Yen & Jaffe's 8th/ed p 521

The AE-PCOS Society criteria for diagnosis of PCOS considers hyperandrogenism as the cardinal feature of PCOS. AE-PCOS defines PCOS as
- Hyperandrogenism (clinical and/or biochemical) and
- Ovarian dysfunction (oligo-anovulation and/or polycystic ovaries),
- Excluding other androgen excess-related disorders.

46. d. PCOS-D

Ref: Yen & Jaffe's 8th/ed p 521; Kamini A Rao 2nd/ed p 481

NIH 2012 extension of ESHRE/ASRM 2003 included identification of specific phenotypes of PCOS

Parameter	Phenotype A	Phenotype B	Phenotype C	Phenotype D
Polycystic ovaries	+	–	+	+
Oligo-anovulation	+	+	–	+
Hyperandrogenism	+	+	+	–

Simple way to remember:
- **A**ll present: PCOS-**A**
- **C**ycles regular: PCOS **C**
- **B** mode normal: PCOS **B** (polycystic ovaries can be seen on ultrasound which we do on B mode)
- An**D**rogen normal: PCOS **D**

Women with PCOS-D appear least affected with respect to metabolic risk

47. c. PCOS-C

Ref: Yen & Jaffe's 8th/ed p 521; Kamini A Rao 2nd/ed p 481

Ovulatory PCOS (Phenotype C) patients have lower body mass index and lesser degrees of hyperinsulinemia and hyperandrogenism, thus lower risk of developing reproductive and metabolic abnormalities.

48. a. Lower legs

Ref: Yen & Jaffe's 8th/ed p 522; Speroff 8th/ed p 542

9 androgen-sensitive areas including the upper lip, chin, chest, upper and lower abdomen, upper arm, thighs, and the upper and lower back.

49. b. >1 to < 3 year postmenarche, cycles are considered irregular if they come >35 days interval

Ref: PCOS 2018 Evidence based guidelines

Irregular menstrual cycles are defined as:
- Normal in the **first year post menarche** as part of the pubertal transition
- 1 to < 3 years post menarche: < 21 or > 45 days
- 3 years postmenarche to perimenopause: < 21 or > 35 days or < 8 cycles per year
- 1 year postmenarche > 90 days for any one cycle
- Primary amenorrhea by age 15 or > 3 years post-thelarche
- When irregular menstrual cycles are present a diagnosis of PCOS should be considered and assessed according to the guidelines.

So, cycles are considered normal between 1-3 years postmenarche, if they are coming every 35 days. Cycles coming at interval of >45 days are considered abnormal.

50. d. ELISA

Ref: PCOS 2018 Evidence based guidelines

High quality assays such as liquid chromatography–mass spectrometry (LCMS)/mass spectrometry and extraction/chromatography immunoassays, should be used for the most accurate assessment of total or free testosterone in PCOS.

Direct free testosterone assays, such as radiometric or enzyme-linked assays, preferably should not be used in assessment of biochemical hyperandrogenism in PCOS, as they demonstrate poor sensitivity, accuracy and precision.

51. d. Alopecia

Ref: PCOS 2018 Evidence based guidelines

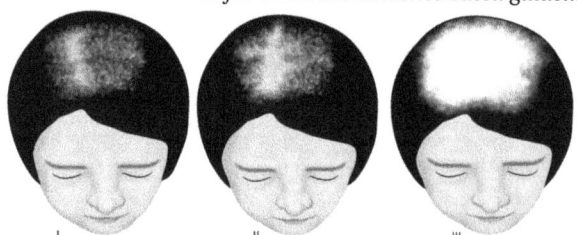

The **Ludwig scale** is a method of classifying female pattern baldness (androgenic alopecia), and ranges from stages I to III.
- *Stage I*: Thinning on the top of the head.
- *Stage II*: Scalp starts to show.

- *Stage III*: All of the hair at the crown of the head may be lost.

However, the scale is used merely for general categorization. Many women do not actually fit into the Ludwig stages.

52. a. In transabdominal ultrasound reporting is best focused on ovarian volume with a threshold of ≥12 mL

Ref: PCOS 2018 Evidence based guidelines

Salient features for ultrasonography in PCOS 2018 Evidence based guidelines

- Ultrasound should not be used for the diagnosis of PCOS in those with a gynaecological age of <8 years (<8 years after menarche), due to the high incidence of multi-follicular ovaries in this life stage.
- The transvaginal ultrasound approach is preferred in the diagnosis of PCOS, if sexually active and if acceptable to the individual being assessed.
- Using endovaginal ultrasound transducers with a frequency bandwidth that includes 8 MHz, the threshold for PCOM should be on either ovary, a follicle number per ovary of >20 and/or an ovarian volume ≥10 mL, ensuring no corpora lutea, cysts or dominant follicles are present.
- If using older technology, the threshold for PCOM could be an ovarian volume ≥10 mL on either ovary.
- In patients with irregular menstrual cycles and hyperandrogenism, an ovarian ultrasound is not necessary for PCOS diagnosis; however, ultrasound will identify the complete PCOS phenotype.
- In transabdominal ultrasound reporting is best focused on ovarian volume with a threshold of ≥10 mL, given the difficulty of reliably assessing follicle number with this approach.

So, volume threshold is same, whether done transabdominally or transvaginally i.e, 10 mL.

53. d. None of the above

Ref: PCOS 2018 Evidence based guidelines

Serum AMH levels should not yet be used as an alternative for the detection of PCOM or as a single test for the diagnosis of PCOS.

54. d. All of the above

Ref: PCOS 2018 Evidence based guidelines

An oral glucose tolerance test (OGTT), fasting plasma glucose or HbA1c should be performed to assess glycaemic status.

In high-risk women with PCOS an OGTT is recommended:

- BMI >25 kg/m^2 or in Asians >23 kg/m^2
- History of impaired fasting glucose, impaired glucose tolerance or gestational diabetes
- Family history of diabetes mellitus type 2 or hypertension
- High-risk ethnicity.

A 75-g OGTT should be offered in all women with PCOS preconception when planning pregnancy or seeking fertility treatment, given the high risk of hyperglycaemia and the associated comorbidities in pregnancy.

If not performed preconception, an OGTT should be offered at < 20 weeks gestation, and all women with PCOS should be offered the test at 24-28 weeks gestation.

55. a. The 35 microgram ethinyl estradiol plus cyproterone acetate preparations is considered first line in PCOS

Ref: PCOS 2018 Evidence based guidelines

- The 35 microgram ethinyloestradiol plus cyproterone acetate preparations **should not be considered** first line in PCOS as per general population guidelines, due to adverse effects including venous thromboembolic risks.

When prescribing COCPs in adults and adolescents with PCOS:

- Various COCP preparations have similar efficacy in treating hirsutism
- The lowest effective estrogen doses (such as 20-30 micrograms of ethinyloestradiol or equivalent), and natural estrogen preparations need consideration, balancing efficacy, metabolic risk profile, side effects, cost and availability
- The generally limited evidence on effects of COCPs in PCOS needs to be appreciated with practice informed by general population guidelines
- The relative and absolute contraindications and side effects of COCPs need to be considered and be the subject of individualised discussion
- PCOS specific risk factors such as high BMI, hyperlipidemia and hypertension need to be considered.

56. d. All of the above

Ref: PCOS 2018 Evidence based guidelines

- In PCOS, antiandrogens must be used with effective contraception, to avoid male foetal undervirilization.
- Variable availability and regulatory status of these agents is notable and for some agents, potential **liver toxicity** requires caution.

Indications to add antiandrogens in women with PCOS as per newer recommendations:

- In combination with the COCP, antiandrogens should only be considered in PCOS to treat **hirsutism**, after six months or more of COCP and cosmetic therapy have failed to adequately improve symptoms.
- In combination with the COCP, antiandrogens could be considered for the treatment of **androgen-related alopecia** in PCOS.

57. b. Letrozole
Ref: PCOS 2018 Evidence based guidelines

Letrozole should be considered **first line** pharmacological treatment for ovulation induction in women with PCOS with anovulatory infertility and no other infertility factors to improve ovulation, pregnancy and live birth rates.

Health professionals and women need to be aware that the risk of multiple pregnancy appears to be less with letrozole, compared to clomiphene citrate.

58. c. Should never be used as first line therapy
Ref: PCOS 2018 Evidence based guidelines

- Laparoscopic ovarian surgery could be second line therapy for women with PCOS, who are clomiphene citrate resistant, with anovulatory infertility and no other infertility factors.
- Laparoscopic ovarian surgery **could potentially be offered as first line treatment if laparoscopy is indicated for another reason** in women with PCOS with anovulatory infertility and no other infertility factors.
- Where laparoscopic ovarian surgery is to be recommended, the following need to be considered:
- Comparative cost
- Expertise required for use in ovulation induction
- Intra-operative and post-operative risks are higher in women who are overweight and obese
- There may be a small associated risk of lower ovarian reserve or loss of ovarian function
- Periadnexal adhesion formation may be an associated risk.

59. a. 12
Ref: PCOS 2018 Evidence based guidelines

- Bariatric surgery should be considered an experimental therapy in women with PCOS, or the purpose of having a healthy baby, with risk to benefit ratios currently too uncertain to advocate this as fertility therapy.
- If bariatric surgery is to be prescribed, the following need to be considered:
    - Comparative cost.
    - The need for a structured weight management program involving diet, physical activity and interventions to improve psychological, musculoskeletal and cardiovascular health to continue post-operatively.
    - Perinatal risks such as small for gestational age, premature delivery, possibly increased infant mortality.
    - Potential benefits such as reduced incidence of large for gestational age fetus and gestational diabetes.
    - Recommendations for pregnancy avoidance during periods of rapid weight loss and for at least 12 months after bariatric surgery with appropriate contraception.
    - If pregnancy occurs, the following need to be considered:
    - Awareness and preventative management of pre- and post-operative nutritional deficiencies is important, ideally in a specialist interdisciplinary care setting monitoring of fetal growth during pregnancy.

60. a. Antagonist protocol
Ref: PCOS 2018 Evidence based guidelines

A gonadotropin releasing hormone antagonist protocol is preferred in women with PCOS undergoing an IVF/ICSI cycle, over a gonadotropin releasing hormone agonist long protocol, to reduce:
- The duration of stimulation,
- Total gonadotropin dose
- Incidence of ovarian hyperstimulation syndrome (OHSS).

61. b. hCG trigger
Ref: PCOS 2018 Evidence based guidelines

About Trigger, following points should be taken care of:
- Human chorionic gonadotropins is best used at the lowest doses to trigger final oocyte maturation in women with PCOS undergoing an IVF/ICSI cycle to reduce the incidence of OHSS.
- Triggering final oocyte maturation with a gonadotropin-releasing hormone (GnRH) agonist and freezing all suitable embryos could be considered in women with PCOS having an IVF/ICSI cycle with a GnRH antagonist protocol and at an increased risk of developing OHSS or where fresh embryo transfer is not planned.

62. c. Albumin therapy
Ref: PCOS 2018 Evidence based guidelines

The term in vitro maturation (IVM) treatment cycle is applied to "the maturation in vitro of immature cumulus oocyte complexes collected from antral follicles" encompassing both stimulated and unstimulated cycles, but without the use of a human gonadotropin trigger.

Albumin therapy has Grade C evidence in prevention of OHSS.

CHAPTER 10

Endocrinology of Hyperprolactinemia

Multiple Choice Questions

1. Hyperprolactinemia can be associated with:
   a. Short luteal phase
   b. Oligomenorrhea
   c. Amenorrhea
   d. All of the above

2. Hyperprolactinemia can present as all *except*:
   a. Precocious puberty
   b. Delayed puberty
   c. Primary amenorrhea
   d. Secondary amenorrhea

3. Following conditions are associated with transient increase in prolactin levels, *except*:
   a. Sleep
   b. Hyperthyroidism
   c. Exercise
   d. Breast stimulation

4. The predominant form of prolactin which is most biologically active is:
   a. Monomer
   b. Dimmer
   c. Trimer
   d. Tetramer

5. Which of the following statement is incorrect regarding hyperprolactinemia?
   a. Generalized increase in hypothalamic dopaminergic neuronal activity is most common cause for anovulation
   b. Only about one-third of women with hyperprolactinemia exhibit galactorrhea
   c. Hyperthyroidism may be associated with hyperprolactinemia
   d. Renal insufficiency can be associated with hyperprolactinemia

6. Apart from pituitary, prolactin can be found in all of the following areas, *except*:
   a. Endometrium
   b. Hypothalamus
   c. Placenta
   d. Kidneys

7. Which of the following does not increase prolactin levels?
   a. Estrogen
   b. Progesterone
   c. Epidermal growth factor
   d. Thyrotropin releasing hormone

8. Which of the following statements regarding hyperprolactinemia is not true?
   a. Medication-induced hyperprolactinemia often cross 100 mcg/L
   b. Macroprolactinemia need not be treated
   c. Females have higher incidence of hyperprolactinemia
   d. Prolactin variants are due to proteolytic cleavage, alternative splicing or post-translational modifications

9. Men with hyperprolactinemia may present as all of the following *except*:
   a. Hypogonadism
   b. Impotence
   c. Increased libido
   d. Retrograde ejaculation

10. Which of the following is termed as WHO type 4 anovulation?
    a. Hyperprolactinemia
    b. PCOS
    c. Hypothalamic causes
    d. Pituitary causes

11. A gradual decrease in their regular intermenstrual interval, followed by increasing oligomenorrhea, and finally, amenorrhea is menstrual pattern suggestive of following *except*:
    a. Hyperprolactinemia
    b. PCOS
    c. Premature ovarian failure
    d. Physiological menopause

12. Which is not correct regarding hyperprolactinemia?
    a. Measurement of the serum prolactin and TSH concentrations are justified in all women with amenorrhea
    b. TRH leads to gradual depletion of hypothalamic dopamine, thus causing galactorrhea
    c. On thyroxine replacement in hypothyroidism, breast secretions show rapid response
    d. TRH causes constant stimulation of pituitary lactotropes

13. **Which is true about bromocriptine treatment?**
    a. A clinical response usually demonstrates a restoration of ovulation and menses prior to galactorrhea
    b. Macroadenoma does not respond to medical therapy
    c. Complete cessation of galactorrhea occur within days of start of therapy
    d. Galactorrhea remains suppressed even with discontinuation of therapy

14. **Most common pituitary adenoma:**
    a. Nonfunctional lactotroph adenoma
    b. Nonfunctional gonadotroph adenoma
    c. Functional gonadotroph adenoma
    d. Functional prolactin secreting lactotroph adenoma

15. **Pituitary adenomas may present as:**
    a. Visual impairment
    b. Nonspecific headaches
    c. Cerebrospinal fluid rhinorrhea
    d. All of the above

16. **Which of the following is not true regarding prolactinoma?**
    a. Polyclonal origin
    b. Accounts for 40% of all clinically recognized pituitary adenomas
    c. Microadenomas usually are associated with serum prolactin concentrations less than 200 ng/mL
    d. Dopamine agonists are the first treatment of choice irrespective of size

Newer Questions Based on Guidelines

17. **Which of the following holds false for diagnosis of hyperprolactinemia?**
    a. Dynamic testing of prolactin secretion is required due to pulsatile secretion of prolactin
    b. Prolactin level > 500 ng/mL is diagnostic of macroadenoma
    c. Assay-specific normal values are higher in women than in men and are generally < 25 ng/mL
    d. Risperidone and metoclopramide may cause prolactin elevations above 200 ng/mL

18. **When there is significant discrepancy between a very large pituitary tumor and mildly elevated prolactin level, what should be next step?**
    a. MRI should be planned
    b. Repeat serum prolactin levels next day
    c. Serial dilutions of sample
    d. Rule out macroprolactinemia

19. **Which of the following statements is false for drug induced hyperprolactinemia?**
    a. No treatment is necessary in the asymptomatic patient with medication-induced hyperprolactinemia
    b. In case of hypogonadal symptoms or low bone mass, estrogen or testosterone therapy should be considered
    c. In a symptomatic patient with suspected drug-induced hyperprolactinemia, discontinuation of the medication for 3 d, followed by remeasurement of serum prolactin is indicated
    d. Medication-induced hyperprolactinemia is rare cause of nontumoral hyperprolactinemia

20. **Which dopamine agonist is recommended as first line in treatment of hyperprolactinemia?**
    a. Cabergoline
    b. Bromocriptine
    c. Quinagolide
    d. All are equal efficacy

21. **In patients who begin dopamine agonist therapy, which of the following is correct regarding follow up?**
    a. Periodic prolactin measurement starting 1 month after therapy to guide treatment intensification to achieve normal prolactin level and reversal of hypogonadism
    b. Visual field examinations in patients with macroadenomas at risk of impinging the optic chiasm
    c. Assessment and management of comorbidities, e.g. sexsteroid-dependent bone loss, persistent galactorrhea
    d. All of the above

22. **Patients on dopamine agonist therapy, repeat MRI is indicated at the interval of three months in all of the following situations, *except:***
    a. Macroprolactinoma
    b. Microadenomas
    c. If prolactin levels continue to rise while patient is receiving dopaminergic agents
    d. If new symptoms, e.g. galactorrhea, visual disturbances, headaches, or other hormonal disorders, occur

23. **Recommended treatment option for asymptomatic woman harbouring macroprolactinoma:**
    a. Dopamine agonist therapy
    b. OCPs
    c. Surgery
    d. Follow-up

24. **Treatment options for hypogonadal premenopausal women with microadenomas who are not desirous of pregnancy?**
    a. Cabergoline
    b. Bromocriptine
    c. OCPs
    d. All of the above

25. **Which of the following is false for Dopamine agonist resistance?**
    a. Failure to achieve a normal prolactin level on maximally tolerated doses of dopamine agonist and a failure to achieve a 50% reduction in tumor size
    b. Failure to restore fertility in patients receiving standard doses of dopamine agonist
    c. Severe side effects of the agonists precluding their use
    d. Discordant responses with reduction in tumor size without normalization of prolactin levels and vice versa

26. **Not true about dopamine agonist resistance:**
    a. Microadenomas are less resistant to dopamine agonists than are macroadenomas
    b. Ten percent of patients with microadenomas are resistant
    c. Women are more likely than men to be dopamine agonist resistant
    d. High-dose cabergoline runs potential risk of cardiac valvular regurgitation

27. **Which of the following is not true about dopamine therapy in pregnancy?**
    a. Continuation of dopamine agonist therapy in microadenomas
    b. To continue dopaminergic therapy throughout the pregnancy in macroadenomas
    c. Both bromocriptine and cabergoline appears to be safe in pregnancy
    d. Surgery is considered as last option

28. **Which of the following drug given to treat hyperprolactinemia, not safe in pregnancy?**
    a. Cabergoline
    b. Quinagolide
    c. Bromocriptine
    d. All are considered unsafe

29. **Which of the following regarding hyperprolactinemia during pregnancy is not suggested by endocrine society?**
    a. Visual field assessment followed by MRI is indicated in pregnant women with prolactinomas who experience severe headaches
    b. Bromocriptine therapy is recommended in patients who experience symptomatic growth of a prolactinoma during pregnancy
    c. Serum prolactin measurements during pregnancy are recommended to monitor microadenomas
    d. Routine pituitary MRI during pregnancy in patients with microadenomas or intrasellar macroadenomas is not recommended unless there is clinical evidence for tumor growth

30. **Patients with macroadenoma who do not undergo surgery or irradiation before pregnancy, runs risk of symptomatic pituitary tumor enlargement by:**
    a. 30%
    b. 50%
    c. 90%
    d. Risk of tumor growth in pregnancy is very low

31. **Drug of choice for treatment of symptomatic hyperprolactinemia in pregnancy:**
    a. Cabergoline
    b. Bromocriptine
    c. Both are equally recommended
    d. Surgery is best option

Answer with Explanations

1. d. All of the above
Ref: Speroff 8th/ed p 497

Hyperprolactinemia stimulates increase in dopaminergic activity, intended to suppress prolactin secretion but also inhibiting GnRH neurons.

Spectrum of ovulatory dysfunction ranges from short luteal phase to hypogonadotropic hypogonadism, depending on the extent to which gonadotropin secretion is disturbed.

Normal prolactin	Mild hyperprolactinemia (20–50 ng/mL)	Moderate hyperprolactinemia (50–100 ng/mL)	Severe hyperprolactinemia (>100 ng/mL)
Normal ovulation	Short luteal phase	Anovulation or oligomenorrhea or amenorrhea	Frank hypogonadism

2. a. Precocious puberty
Ref: Speroff 8th/ed p 447

Hyperprolactinemia is among the most common causes of secondary amenorrhea and also may result in delayed puberty and primary amenorrhea when it arises before menarche.

3. b. Hyperthyroidism
Ref: Speroff 8th/ed p 447; Kamini A Rao 2nd/ed p 149

A serum prolactin concentration is justified in all women with amenorrhea.

A normal random measurement (<15–20 ng/mL in most clinical laboratories) excludes hyperprolactinemia.

Physiological Causes of Hyperprolactinemia
- Pregnancy
- Lactation
- Stress
- Nipple stimulation
- Sleep
- Coitus
- Exercise
- Meals

To avoid otherwise unnecessary and costly imaging, mildly elevated prolactin levels (20–40 ng/mL) are best repeated and confirmed before the diagnosis of hyperprolactinemia is made.

4. a. Monomer
Ref: Yen & Jaffe's 8th/ed p 59

- In about 10% of patients with hyperprolactinemia, macroprolactinemia can be diagnosed.
- Prolactin circulates in various forms that have varying bioactivity (manifested by galactorrhea) and immunoactivity (recognition by immunoassay).
- The predominant form (80–95%) is **monomeric** (molecular weight 23 kDa), which is **more biologically active** than larger glycosylated forms that may combine to form dimmers or trimers ("big prolactin," 50–60 kDa) and other even larger varieties (macroprolactin, >100 kDa), which result from the aggregation of smaller prolactin molecules bound together with immunoglobulins (mainly IgG).
- Adding **polyethylene glycol (PEG)** to the serum, the larger molecular weight forms precipitate and monomeric form is left behind.

5. c. Hyperthyroidism may be associated with hyperprolactinemia
Ref: Speroff 8th/ed p 445; Disorders of menstruation. Marshburn & Hurst. Chapter 4 p 47

Discussing all the options:
Hyperprolactinemia may result from hypothyroidism. Discussed in detail below.

- The mechanism by which hyperprolactinemia results in anovulation and amenorrhea: disruption of the normal hypothalamic GnRH pulse rhythm > ineffective or frankly low levels of gonadotropin secretion.
- Hyperprolactinemia > generalized increase in hypothalamic dopaminergic neuronal activity > inhibition of GnRH neurons.
- Only about **one-third** of women with hyperprolactinemia exhibit galactorrhea, probably because breast milk production requires estrogen and hyperprolactinemia often results in anovulation or a more severe secondary hypogonadotropic hypogonadism and low circulating estrogen levels.
- Renal insufficiency and macroprolactinemia may cause hyperprolactinemia, due to decreased clearance.

6. d. Kidneys
Ref: Speroff 8th/ed p 445; Kamini A Rao 2nd/ed p 148

Initially found to be secreted in a pulsatile manner from lactotrophs of anterior pituitary, prolactin has been isolated in:
- Hypothalamus
- Placenta
- Mammary glands
- Endometrium

7. **b. Progesterone**

   Ref: Kamini A Rao 2nd/ed p 148

   Factors increasing prolactin levels:
   - Estrogen
   - Antidopaminergics
   - Epidermal growth factor
   - Thyrotropin-releasing hormone

8. **a. Medication-induced hyperprolactinemia often cross 100 mcg/L**

   Ref: Kamini A Rao 2nd/ed p 149; Yen & Jaffe's 8th/ed p 65

   - Females have higher incidence of hyperprolactinemia as compared to males, with peak prevalence at 25–34 years.

   ## Medication-induced Hyperprolactinemia

   - Medications mostly associated with hyperprolactinemia: neuroleptics, antipsychotics, anticonvulsants, antihistaminics, opiates and antidepressants.
   - Antihypertensive drugs like Verapamil have been associated with sustained hyperprolactinemia. Verapamil blocks hypothalamic generation of dopamine.
   - Protease inhibitors are associated with galactorrhea.
   - Medications are **most common cause** of non-tumoral hyperprolactinemia
   - Most patients have prolactin levels between 25–100 ng/mL, except some atypical antipsychotics which are associated with higher levels of prolactin.
   - Hyperprolactinemia resolves **within 4 days** after discontinuation of offending agent.

   ## Macroprolactinemia

   - Majority of the prolactin exists as **23 kDa** molecule, variants occur due to proteolytic cleavage, alternative splicing or post-translational modifications
   - Big and big prolactin causes macroprolactinemia
   - Delayed renal clearance of macroprolactin causes a false elevation in prolactin levels
   - Macroprolactin is detected by polyethylene glycol precipitation of the serum
   - If it is confirmed to be the only cause of hyperprolactinemia, no further treatment is required.

9. **c. Increased libido**

   Ref: Kamini A Rao 2nd/ed p 150; Yen & Jaffe's 8th/ed p 64

   - Galactorrhea in men has been reported in 10–20% of cases.
   - Upto 25% of men presenting with erectile dysfunction are hyperprolactinemic.

   In human sperm, prolactin increases fructose utilization, glycolysis, and glucose oxidation.

   Men with hyperprolactinemia may present with:
   - Decreased libido
   - Impotence
   - Hypogonadism
   - Infertility
   - Oligospermia
   - Retrograde ejaculation
   - Gynecomastia

   Chronic hyperprolactinemia results in impotence and decreased libido in over 90% of cases.

10. **a. Hyperprolactinemia**

    Ref: Kamini A Rao 2nd/ed p 149

    Hyperprolactinemia has been also called as **WHO type 4 anovulation**, due to hypogonadism caused by high prolactin levels.

11. **b. PCOS**

    Ref: Speroff 8th/ed p 497

    A gradual decrease in their regular intermenstrual interval, followed by increasing oligomenorrhea, and finally, amenorrhea is the menstrual pattern often seen in women with hyperprolactinemia or premature ovarian failure.

12. **c. On thyroxine replacement in hypothyroidism, breast secretions show rapid response**

    Ref: Speroff 8th/ed p 445

    ## Hypothyroidism and Hyperprolactinemia

    - The likelihood of hyperprolactinemia increases with the duration of hypothyroidism
    - Galactorrhea is more common in young women with higher prolactin levels.
    - The mechanism involves
      - The gradual depletion of hypothalamic dopamine (the putative prolactin-inhibiting factor)
      - Constant stimulation of pituitary lactotropes by thyrotropin-releasing hormone (TRH), which may cause pituitary hypertrophy or hyperplasia and sometimes even enlargement or erosion of the sella turcica.
    - Although hormone levels rapidly normalize with appropriate treatment, the disappearance of breast secretions in those with galactorrhea is gradual and can take several months.

13. **a. A clinical response usually demonstrates a restoration of ovulation and menses prior to galactorrhea**

    Ref: Speroff 8th/ed p 447

    Complete cessation of galactorrhea occurs in an average time of 12.7 weeks.

    Loss of galactorrhea is slower and less certain response as compared to restoration of ovulation and menses.

14. **d. Functional prolactin secreting lactotroph adenoma**

    Ref: Speroff 8th/ed p 474

    - Pituitary adenomas are classified by cell type and size and may be functional (hormone-secreting) or nonfunctional.
    - Large majority of pituitary adenomas are **functional prolactin-secreting lactotroph adenomas** or non-functional adenomas, most of which derive from gonadotrophs.
    - Functional thyrotroph adenomas (secreting TSH and causing hyperthyroidism), somatotroph adenomas (secreting GH and causing acromegaly) and corticotroph adenomas (secreting ACTH and causing Cushing's disease) are rare.

15. **d. All of the above**

    Ref: Yen & Jaffe's 8th/ed p 71

Pituitary Tumors and Mass Effects

- Local mass effects may cause symptoms in patients with macroadenomas, depending upon size and extent of extrasellar extension.
- Visual field defects due to chiasmal compression depend upon the amount of suprasellar extension.
- Because of great variation in how these tumors grow superiorly with respect to location of chiasm, visual field defects can range from the classical, complete bitemporal hemianopsia to small, partial quadrantic defects, to scotomas.
- Decreased visual acuity develops with more severe compression of the chiasm and diplopia (blurred vision) results from lateral extension and compression of the oculomotor nerve.
- Other neurologic symptoms include nonspecific headaches (from expansion of the sella), cerebrospinal fluid rhinorrhea (from inferior extension of the tumor), and pituitary apoplexy (caused by sudden hemorrhage into the adenoma).

16. **a. Polyclonal origin**

    Ref: Yen & Jaffe's 8th/ed p 67; Speroff 8th/ed p 478

Prolactinomas

- Accounts for 40% of all clinically recognized pituitary adenomas.
- Most arise **de novo** as intrinsic disorders of pituitary due to single cell mutation with monoclonal cell proliferation.
- They also may occur as part of the MEN1 syndrome
- Approximately 10% of adenomas that secrete prolactin also secrete GH, leading some to recommend measuring the serum IGF-1 concentration, even in women with microadenomas.
- In women with lactotroph adenomas, serum prolactin concentrations generally correlate with the size of the adenoma.
- Microadenomas usually are associated with serum prolactin concentrations less than 200 ng/mL and macroadenomas with higher levels, but exceptions in either case are not uncommon.
- In some women with large lactotroph macroadenomas, prolactin levels are only modestly elevated because the tumor is largely cystic.
- Dopamine agonists are the first treatment of choice for women with functional prolactin-secreting lactotroph adenomas of all sizes.
- The failure of a tumor to shrink significantly in size despite a normalization of prolactin levels strongly suggests it is a nonfunctioning adenoma, rather than a functional lactotroph adenoma.
- Menses, ovulation, and fertility typically return when normal prolactin levels are restored.
- In those who cannot tolerate dopamine agonist treatment and therefore remain hyperprolactinemic and anovulatory, ovulation induction can be induced with exogenous gonadotropins.

17. **a. Dynamic testing of prolactin secretion is required due to pulsatile secretion of prolactin**

    Ref: Diagnosis and Treatment of Hyperprolactinemia: An Endocrine Society Clinical Practice Guideline 2011

    "To establish the diagnosis of hyperprolactinemia, we recommend a single measurement of serum prolactin; a level above the upper limit of normal confirms the diagnosis as long as the serum sample was obtained without excessive venipuncture stress"

    We recommend **against dynamic testing** of prolactin secretion for the diagnosis of hyperprolactinemia.

18. **c. Serial dilutions of sample**

    Ref: Diagnosis and Treatment of Hyperprolactinemia: An Endocrine Society Clinical Practice Guideline 2011

Hook Effect

- When there is a discrepancy between a very large pituitary tumor and a mildly elevated prolactin level, we recommend serial dilution of serum samples to eliminate an artifact that can occur with some immunoradiometric assays leading to a falsely low prolactin value—"hook effect"

- Hook effect is an assay artifact that may be observed when high serum prolactin concentrations saturate antibodies in the two-site immunoradiometric assay.
- The second (signaling) antibody binds directly to the excess prolactin remaining in the solution and, therefore, is less available to the prolactin already bound to the first (coupling) antibody. Therefore, artifactually low results are obtained.
- The guideline recommends that when prolactin values are not as high as expected, the assay should be repeated after a 1:100 serum sample dilution to overcome a potential hook effect.

19. **d. Medication-induced hyperprolactinemia is rare cause of nontumoral hyperprolactinemia**

    Ref: Diagnosis and Treatment of Hyperprolactinemia: An Endocrine Society Clinical Practice Guideline 2011

- Medication induced hyperprolactinemia is **most common** cause of nontumoral hyperprolactinemia.
- No treatment is necessary in the asymptomatic patient with medication-induced hyperprolactinemia.
- In case of **hypogonadal symptoms** or low bone mass, estrogen or testosterone therapy should be considered.
- In a symptomatic patient with suspected drug-induced hyperprolactinemia, discontinuation of the medication for **3 days**, followed by remeasurement of serum prolactin is indicated.

20. **a. Cabergoline**

    Ref: Diagnosis and Treatment of Hyperprolactinemia: An Endocrine Society Clinical Practice Guideline 2011

- Guidelines say that **cabergoline is preferred to other dopamine agonists** because it has higher efficacy in normalizing prolactin levels, as well as a higher frequency of pituitary tumor shrinkage.

It is unclear why cabergoline is more effective than bromocriptine, but the greater efficacy may be explained by the fact that:

- Cabergoline has a higher affinity for dopamine receptor binding sites.
- Because the incidence of unpleasant side effects is lower with cabergoline, drug compliance may be superior for this medication.
- No clinical trials have directly compared the mass-reducing effects of different dopamine agonists.
- Studies indicate that bromocriptine decreases pituitary tumor size by approximately 50% in two thirds of patients, compared with a 90% decrease with cabergoline.

21. **d. All of the above**

    Ref: Diagnosis and Treatment of Hyperprolactinemia: An Endocrine Society Clinical Practice Guideline 2011

In patients who begin dopamine agonist therapy, follow-up includes:

- Periodic prolactin measurement starting 1 month after therapy to guide treatment intensification to achieve normal prolactin level and reversal of hypogonadism.
- Repeat MRI in 1 year (or in 3 months in patients with macroprolactinoma, if prolactin levels continue to rise while patient is receiving dopaminergic agents, or if new symptoms, e.g. galactorrhea, visual disturbances, headaches, or other hormonal disorders, occur).
- Visual field examinations in patients with macroadenomas at risk of impinging the optic chiasm.
- Assessment and management of comorbidities, e.g. sex steroid-dependent bone loss, persistent galactorrhea in the face of normalized prolactin levels, and pituitary trophic hormone reserve.

22. **b. Microadenomas**

    Ref: Diagnosis and Treatment of Hyperprolactinemia: An Endocrine Society Clinical Practice Guideline 2011

Patient on dopamine agonist therapy with microadenomas, repeat MRI is indicated annually.

23. **d. Follow-up**

    Ref: Diagnosis and Treatment of Hyperprolactinemia: An Endocrine Society Clinical Practice Guideline 2011

Endocrine society guidelines suggest to not to treat asymptomatic women harbouring microprolactinomas with dopamine agonists as microadenomas rarely grow.

24. **d. All of the above**

    Ref: Diagnosis and Treatment of Hyperprolactinemia: An Endocrine Society Clinical Practice Guideline 2011

- Hypogonadal premenopausal women with microadenomas who are not desirous of pregnancy may be treated with oral contraceptives instead of dopamine agonist therapy.
- Women with microadenomas who are not desirous of pregnancy may be treated with a dopamine agonist or oral contraceptives.
- No controlled trials have compared these two options, but oral contraceptives are **less expensive** and have **fewer side effects**.
- The effect of oral estrogen therapy on the growth of microadenomas: patients treated with oral contraceptives and estrogen/progesterone replacement for 2 years do not show increase in tumor size.

25. c. Severe side effects of the agonists precluding their use

Ref: Diagnosis and Treatment of Hyperprolactinemia: An Endocrine Society Clinical Practice Guideline 2011

Dopamine Agonist Resistance

- Failure to achieve a normal prolactin level on maximally tolerated doses of dopamine agonist and a failure to achieve a 50% reduction in tumor size.
- Failure to restore fertility in patients receiving standard doses of dopamine agonist may also be reflective of treatment resistance.
- Some patients may have **discordant responses**, i.e. reduction in tumor size without normalization of prolactin levels and vice versa, and others may be partially resistant and require higher than typical doses of dopamine agonists to achieve a response.
- Dopamine agonist resistance differs from **intolerance**, where side effects of the agonists preclude their use.

26. c. Women are more likely than men to be dopamine agonist resistant

Ref: Diagnosis and Treatment of Hyperprolactinemia: An Endocrine Society Clinical Practice Guideline 2011

- The mechanism of dopamine agonist resistance is not completely understood. There is **decreased number of D2 receptors** expressed on resistant prolactinomas, but this finding is not invariable. Dopamine receptor binding is normal, and no dopamine receptor mutation has been identified in prolactinomas.
- Microadenomas are less resistant to dopamine agonists than are macroadenomas.
- 10% of patients with microadenomas and 18% of patients with macroadenomas do not achieve normal prolactin levels on cabergoline.
- **Men are more likely than women to be dopamine agonist resistant**.
- Increasing the cabergoline dose to as much as 11 mg/week has been necessary in a few patients to overcome resistance.
- Patients with Parkinson's disease receiving at least 3 mg of cabergoline daily are at risk for moderate to severe cardiac valve regurgitation.

27. a. Continuation of dopamine agonist therapy in microadenomas

Ref: Diagnosis and Treatment of Hyperprolactinemia: An Endocrine Society Clinical Practice Guideline 2011

- Guidelines recommend that women with prolactinomas be instructed to discontinue dopamine agonist therapy as soon as they discover that they are pregnant.
- In selected patients with macroadenomas who become pregnant on dopaminergic therapy and who have not had prior surgical or radiation therapy, it may be prudent to continue dopaminergic therapy throughout the pregnancy, especially if the tumor is invasive or is abutting the optic chiasm.

28. b. Quinagolide

Ref: Diagnosis and Treatment of Hyperprolactinemia: An Endocrine Society Clinical Practice Guideline 2011

Drugs and Pregnancy

- Bromocriptine
  - It crosses the placenta, fetal drug exposure is likely for up to the first 4 weeks after conception, a critical period for early organogenesis.
  - The incidence of congenital malformations or abortions is not increased.
  - Long-term follow-up of up to 9 year in a limited number of children who were exposed to the drug in utero also showed no harmful effects.
- Cabergoline
  - It appears to be safe when used to treat infertility in women with hyperprolactinemia, but there is far less published experience with this drug.
  - In a prospective study of 85 women, of whom 80 achieved pregnancy while receiving cabergoline, the drug was withdrawn at 5 weeks gestation, all babies were born healthy, and no mothers experienced tumor expansion.
- Quinagolide
  - It has a poor safety profile in the relatively small number of pregnancies that have been reported, and it should not be prescribed to women desirous of becoming pregnant.

29. c. Serum prolactin measurements during pregnancy are recommended to monitor microadenomas

Ref: Diagnosis and Treatment of Hyperprolactinemia: An Endocrine Society Clinical Practice Guideline 2011

- During pregnancy, serum prolactin levels increase **10-fold**, reaching levels of 150 to 300 ng/mL by term.
- Pituitary gland increases in volume more than 2-fold, primarily due to estrogen-stimulated increase in the number of lactotrophs.
- When dopamine agonists are discontinued at the start of pregnancy, serum prolactin levels increase, and subsequent increases in prolactin levels do not accurately reflect changes in tumor growth or activity.
- Moreover, serum prolactin levels may not increase during pregnancy in all patients with prolactinomas.

- So, guideline recommendation is to **refrain from measuring serum prolactin during pregnancy** in patients with prolactinomas.

30. a. 30%

    Ref: Gillam MP et al, Advances in the Treatment of Prolactinomas. Endocr Rev 27:485-534

- Patients with macroadenoma who did not undergo surgery or irradiation before pregnancy, the risk of symptomatic pituitary tumor enlargement was 31%.
- In those patients who had undergone debulking pituitary surgery or pituitary irradiation before pregnancy, the risk of symptomatic growth was only 2.8%.

31. b. Bromocriptine

    Ref: Diagnosis and Treatment of Hyperprolactinemia: An Endocrine Society Clinical Practice Guideline 2011

Dopamine Agonist Therapy in Pregnancy

- Bromocriptine in divided doses is the **recommended dopamine agonist** of choice because of the larger published experience.
- In patients who cannot tolerate bromocriptine, cabergoline may be administered.
- If reinitiation of dopamine agonist therapy does not decrease tumor size and lead to improved symptoms, surgical resection may be indicated.
- There are no published data to assess a comparative risk of dopaminergic therapy and surgical resection during pregnancy; however, some endocrinologists prefer dopaminergic therapy in this circumstance.
- If the fetus is near term, it may be reasonable to induce delivery before neurosurgical intervention is undertaken.

CHAPTER 11

Endocrinology of Hirsutism

Multiple Choice Questions

1. Hirsutism, defined as excessive male-pattern facial and body hair, affects between 5 and 10% of reproductive age women. Which of the following is incorrect regarding hirsutism?
   a. Hirsutism can be the initial or only sign of androgen excess and usually is a consequence of chronic anovulation
   b. The length of hair is determined primarily by the duration of the telogen phase
   c. Activins and bone morphogenetic proteins are involved in hair follicle development
   d. One's total endowment of hair follicles is determined by 22 weeks of gestation

2. Which of the following does not hold true for hirsutism?
   a. Hypertrichosis can be associated with certain drugs, systemic illness or malignancy
   b. Hirsutism implies a transformation from vellus to terminal hair
   c. Hypertrichosis is characterized by a generalized increase in terminal body hair
   d. Scalp hair growth is asynchronous

3. Sexual hair is that which responds to sex steroids. What does not hold true for effects of steroid hormones on hair growth?
   a. Androgens stimulate hair growth all over body
   b. Estrogens leads to growth of finer and lighter hair
   c. Progestins have little or no direct effect on hair growth
   d. Pregnancy can induce greater synchrony among hair follicles

4. Which of the following is not a pre-hormone?
   a. DHEA-S   b. DHEA
   c. DHT   d. Androstenedione

5. Androgen produced exclusively by adrenal gland:
   a. DHEA   b. DHEA-S
   c. Androstenedione   d. Testosterone

6. Free testosterone in women:
   a. 1%   b. 2%
   c. 3%   d. 4%

7. Circulating protein to which testosterone maximally binds?
   a. Albumin   b. Prealbumin
   c. Transthyretin   d. SHBG

8. Which of the following conditions increase SHBG production?
   a. Estrogen
   b. Testosterone
   c. Glucocorticoids
   d. Insulin

9. Which of the following is correct?
   1. Testosterone—measure of ovarian and adrenal activity
   2. DHEAS—measure of adrenal activity
   3. 3a—androstanediol glucuronide—measure of peripheral target tissue activity

   a. 1, 2 & 3   b. 1 and 2 only
   c. 2 and 3 only   d. 1 only

10. Hyperinsulinemia leads to hyperandrogenism by?
    a. Inhibiting hepatic SHBG synthesis
    b. Inhibiting IGFBP-1 synthesis
    c. Increasing thecal cell androgen production
    d. All

11. Ovarian stromal hyperthecosis is a hyperandrogenic state characterized by:
    1. Distinct clusters of luteinized thecal cells scattered throughout the ovarian stroma
    2. Serum testosterone concentrations often less than 150 ng/dL
    3. Severe insulin resistance
    4. Can be seen in postmenopausal women

    a. 1, 3 and 4   b. 1, 2, 3 and 4
    c. 2 and 4   d. 1, 2 and 3

12. Idiopathic hirsutism is one of the most common causes of hirsutism after anovulation. What holds true regarding it?
    a. Regular menstrual cycles
    b. Normal serum androgen levels
    c. Increased sensitivity to androgens
    d. All

13. Which of the following is not true about hirsutism?
    a. Significant reduction in hair growth occur within 6 months of start of treatment
    b. Methods and frequency of hair removal provide the most practical and clinically relevant measure to assess severity of hirsutism
    c. Serial measurements of serum androgen levels during treatment are not necessary
    d. Repeated evaluation of serum androgen is indicated when hirsutism progresses despite treatment

14. How oral contraceptive pills are effective in treating hirsutism?
    1. Suppress ovarian androgen production
    2. Stimulates hepatic SHBG production
    3. Decrease adrenal DHEA-S secretion
    4. Inhibit 5a-reductase activity in skin
    a. All
    b. 1, 2 and 3
    c. 2 and 4
    d. 2, 3 and 4

15. Which androgen concentration provides the best overall measure of androgen production?
    a. Serum free testosterone concentration
    b. Serum total testosterone concentration
    c. Serum DHEAS
    d. Serum androstenedione

16. False about plasma testosterone levels:
    a. Testosterone levels are elevated significantly during normal pregnancy
    b. Laboratory testing for elevated androgen levels should begin with a serum total testosterone concentration
    c. Serum total testosterone > 150 ng/dL have high positive predictive value for detecting androgen producing tumors
    d. Normal serum testosterone levels for females ranges from 20–80 ng/dL

17. Upper limit of testosterone beyond which evaluation for tumor should start in postmenopausal women:
    a. 100 ng/dL
    b. 150 ng/dL
    c. 200 ng/dL
    d. 250 ng/dL

18. What is false about pregnancy luteoma as a cause of hirsutism?
    a. Hyperplastic mass of luteinized ovarian cells
    b. Only one-third of pregnancy luteomas have been associated with maternal hirsutism
    c. Solid masses ranging between 6 and 10 cm in size
    d. Develop in women with gestational trophoblastic disease

19. False about clitoromegaly:
    a. Clitoral length > 5 mm
    b. Clitoral index > 35 mm^2
    c. Clitoral length > 10 mm
    d. Clitoral index is length times width

20. Which of the following is not true for DHEAS?
    a. Derives exclusively from the adrenal gland
    b. Direct measure of adrenal androgen activity
    c. Biologically potent androgen
    d. The upper limit of normal is 350 mg/dL

21. Mechanism of action of spironolactone:
    a. Androgen receptor antagonist
    b. Inhibition of ovarian and adrenal androgen synthesis
    c. 5a-reductase inhibitor
    d. All

22. Following manifestations reflect progressively higher serum androgen levels:
    a. Acne > hirsutism > increased libido > clitoromegaly > virilization
    b. Increased libido > hirsutism > clitoromegaly > virilization
    c. Increased libido > acne > clitoromegaly > virilization
    d. Hirsutism > increased muscle mass > clitoromegaly > virilization

23. Percentage of testosterone derived from ovary, adrenal and peripheral conversion from androstenedione, respectively:
    a. 25, 25, 50
    b. 25, 50, 25
    c. 50, 25, 25
    d. 0, 25, 75

24. How many percent anovulatory women with hirsutism have elevated serum testosterone levels?
    a. 50%
    b. 25%
    c. 70%
    d. 90%

25. Autosomal recessive disorder?
    a. Congenital adrenal hyperplasia
    b. Androgen insensitivity syndrome
    c. Marfan syndrome
    d. Myotonic dystrophy

26. **Not true about 17-hydroxyprogesterone:**
    a. Offers a cost effective means to detect late onset CAH
    b. Values >200 ng/dL warrants ACTH stimulation test
    c. Values >800 ng/dL are diagnostic of late onset CAH
    d. Late afternoon measurements are taken

27. **What is not true about ACTH stimulation test?**
    a. Synthetic ACTH is administered intravenously in a dose of 250 mcg
    b. Test yields one hour value that is plotted on nomogram and predicts the genotype of forms of 21-hydroxylase deficiency
    c. An abnormal 17-hydroxypregnenolone/17-OHP ratio is suggestive of 3b-hydroxysteroid dehydrogenase deficiency
    d. Can be done anytime during the day or during the menstrual cycle

28. **Ovarian endocrine tumors causing virilization, all *except*:**
    a. Luteomas
    b. Granulosa cell tumors
    c. Hyper-reaction luteinalis
    d. Sertoli-Leydig cell tumors

Questions Based on Recent Guidelines

29. **Long-term treatment options for hirsutism all *except*:**
    a. GnRH agonist therapy alone
    b. Cyproterone
    c. Oral contraceptives
    d. Progestational agents

30. **First line drug therapy for hirsutism:**
    a. OCPs
    b. Antiandrogens
    c. OCPs in combination with antiandrogens
    d. Metformin

31. **Which antiandrogen is not recommended by Endocrine society for management of hirsutism?**
    a. Finasteride
    b. Flutamide
    c. Spironolactone
    d. Cyproterone acetate

Answer with Explanations

1. **b. The length of hair is determined primarily by the duration of the telogen phase**
   Ref: Speroff 8th/ed p 534

Hirsutism
- Defined as excessive male-pattern facial and body hair, affects between **5 and 10%** of reproductive age women.
- Hirsutism can be the initial or only sign of androgen excess and usually is a consequence of chronic anovulation.

Virilization
- Describes the signs and symptoms of **more severe androgen excess**, which include deepening of the voice, temporal balding (androgenic alopecia), breast atrophy, changes in body habitus, and clitoromegaly.
- Virilization is rare and most commonly results from congenital adrenal hyperplasia or androgen-producing tumors of the ovary or adrenal.

Embryology of Hair Follicle
- Hair follicles develop at approximately **8–10 weeks** of gestation from a small group of epidermal cells overlying undifferentiated mesenchyme.
- Members of the transforming growth factor beta superfamily, activins and bone morphogenetic proteins in particular, play an important role in the communication between the epithelial and mesenchymal compartments during normal hair follicle development.
- One's total endowment of hair follicles is determined by **22 weeks** of gestation and no new hair follicles develop de novo thereafter.
- Differences in hair growth among races and ethnic groups probably also reflect **differences in the local levels of 5a-reductase** activity.
- Hair growth is cyclic, rather than continuous, and exhibits three distinct phases, known as **telogen** (quiescent phase), **anagen** (growth phase), and **catagen** (involution phase).
- The length of hair is determined primarily by the duration of the growth phase.
- Scalp hair remains in anagen for **2–5 years** and spend only a relatively short time in telogen. Elsewhere, such as on the forearm, the hair cycle has a short anagen and a long telogen, yielding a short hair of relatively stable length.

2. **c. Hypertrichosis is characterized by a generalized increase in terminal body hair**
   Ref: Endocrine society clinical practice guidelines 2018, p 1237

Hair is categorized as:
- **Vellus**—fine, soft, short, and unpigmented
- **Terminal**—long, coarse, and pigmented
- **Lanugo**—vellus hair that covers the body of infants

Hypertrichosis
- Uncommon condition characterized by a generalized increase in **vellus** body hair.
- It may be associated with certain drugs (e.g., phenytoin, penicillamine, diazoxide, minoxidil, cyclosporin), systemic illness (e.g., hypothyroidism, anorexia nervosa, malnutrition, porphyria, dermatomyositis) or malignancy (as a paraneoplastic syndrome).
- Hirsutism implies a transformation from vellus to terminal hair.

3. **a. Androgens stimulate hair growth all over body**
   Ref: Kamini A Rao 2nd/ed p 159
- Sexual hair is that which responds to sex steroids and grows primarily on the face, chest, lower abdomen, the pubis, and in the axillae.
- In androgen-sensitive areas, androgen stimulates hair follicles, inducing the growth of thicker, longer, and darker hairs.
- Because androgen stimulation of hair follicles requires the conversion of testosterone to DHT, the sensitivity of hair follicles to androgens is determined by the local level of 5α-reductase activity, helping to explain the varying extent of hirsutism observed in women with similar levels of androgen excess.
- Effects of steroid hormones on hair growth:
    - Androgens, particularly testosterone, stimulate growth and increase the diameter and pigmentation of hair. Androgens also increase the proportion of time terminal hairs spend in anagen, **except on the scalp**, where androgen decreases the duration of anagen. (So, not whole body!)
    - Estrogens have actions opposite those of androgens, generally resulting in slower growth of finer and lighter hair.

- Progestins have little or no direct effect on hair growth.
- Pregnancy, characterized by high levels of both estrogen and progesterone, can induce greater synchrony among hair follicles, leading to periods of growth or shedding.

4. **c. DHT**

Ref: Kamini A Rao 2nd/ed p 159

- Hirsutism reflects the interaction between circulating androgen levels and the sensitivity of hair follicles to androgen stimulation.
- In women, the major circulating androgens (in descending order of serum concentration) are: DHEA-S > DHEA > Androstenedione > Testosterone > DHT
- DHEA-S, DHEA, and androstenedione can be considered **pre-hormones** because they have little or no intrinsic androgenic activity and require conversion to testosterone to exert androgenic effects.

5. **b. DHEA-S**

Ref: Speroff 8th/ed p 536

Hormone	Ovary %	Adrenal %	Peripheral %
DHEA-S	-	100	-
DHEA	20	50	30
Androstenedione	50	50	-
Testosterone	25	25	50

- **DHEA-S**
  - Produced almost exclusively by the adrenal glands, at a rate ranging between 3.5 and 20 mg/day.
  - The normal serum concentration is 100–350 mg/dL in most laboratories.
- **DHEA** production:
  - Adrenals—50%
  - Ovaries—20%
  - Peripheral conversion of DHEA-S—30%
- **Androstenedione** production:
  - Ovaries—50%
  - Adrenals—50%
- **Testosterone** production:
  - Adrenals—25%
  - Ovaries—25%
  - Peripheral conversion of androstenedione—50%

The production rate ranges between 0.1 and 0.4 mg/day and the normal serum concentration is 20–80 ng/dL.

6. **a. 1%**

Ref: Yen & Jaffe's 8th ed/p 550

Testosterone

- The production rate ranges between 0.1 and 0.4 mg/day and the normal serum concentration is **20–80 ng/dL**.
- Levels do not fluctuate widely, but are **lowest during the early follicular phase**, and approximately 20% higher at midcycle.
- In normal women, about 80% of circulating testosterone is bound to SHBG, another 19% is loosely bound to albumin, leaving only about 1% unbound or free.
- Routine serum immunoassays for testosterone measure the total testosterone concentration, including both bound and unbound hormone. However, the androgenic actions of testosterone relate primarily to the amount of free hormone and, to a limited extent, to the fraction associated with albumin.
- Anything that affects the SHBG concentration also affects the concentration of free/active testosterone.

7. **d. SHBG**

Ref: Yen & Jaffe's 8th ed/p 897

- Calculated free testosterone levels in women have been found to be nearly identical with corresponding values determined by equilibrium dialysis.
- The calculation is made using the ratio between testosterone and SHBG (in units of nmol/L): **T (ng/mL) × 3.467/SHBG × 100**

In normal women, about 80% of circulating testosterone is bound to SHBG, another 19% is loosely bound to albumin, leaving only about 1% unbound or free.

8. **a. Estrogen**

Ref: Yen & Jaffe's 8th ed/p 98

- **Factors decreasing SHBG production:**
  - Androgens
  - Insulin
  - Glucocorticoids
  - Liver diseases
  - Testosterone binding capacity in men is lower than in normal women due to high androgen levels in men; approximately 3% of total testosterone circulates in the free, active form in men.
- **Factors increasing SHBG production:**
  - Estrogens
  - Thyroid hormone
  - Binding capacity is increased in women with hyperthyroidism, in pregnancy, and during treatment with estrogens.

9. a. 1, 2 & 3

Ref: Speroff 8th/ed p 538

The three principal laboratory measurements of potential clinical use for evaluation of androgen excess:
1. Testosterone—measure of ovarian and adrenal activity
2. DHEAS—measure of adrenal activity
3. 3a-androstanediol glucoronide- measure of peripheral target tissue activity

3a-androstanediol is the peripheral tissue metabolite of DHT, and its glucuronide conjugate, 3a-androstanediol glucuronide (3a-AG), can be used as a **marker of peripheral androgen metabolism**.

Serum 3a-AG levels correlate highly with levels of 5a-reductase activity in genital skin and are elevated almost uniformly in hirsute women, including those with normal serum androgen levels, indicating that **"idiopathic" hirsutism** likely results from increased peripheral 5a-reductase activity.

10. d. All

Ref: Kamini A Rao. 2nd/ed p 485

Hyperinsulinemia leads to hyperandrogenism by:
- Increasing thecal cell androgen production—because of similarity between the receptors for insulin and IGF-1.
- Inhibiting hepatic SHBG synthesis—increased free testosterone.
- Inhibiting IGFBP-1 synthesis—increased IGF-1, thus stimulating thecal androgen synthesis.

11. a. 1, 3 & 4

Ref: Yen & Jaffe's 8th/ed p 549; Braithwaite SS et al. Postmenopausal virilization due to ovarian stromal hyperthecosis. J Clin Endocrinol Metab 46:295–300, 1978

Ovarian Stromal Hyperthecosis

- It is a **histologic diagnosis**, based on the observation of distinct clusters of luteinized thecal cells scattered throughout the ovarian stroma.
- Patients with hyperthecosis typically are obese, severely hirsute, and often virilized.
- Most have serum testosterone concentrations greater than 150 ng/dL.
- Exhibit severe insulin resistance and hyperinsulinemia.
- It is likely that most, if not all, patients with the HAIR-AN syndrome have ovarian hyperthecosis.
- The extent of theca cell involvement may vary from minimal to extensive.
- Severe hyperthecosis may be accompanied by extensive and dense fibroblast growth resulting in an enlarged ovary of extremely firm texture, findings that are clearly distinct from those found in PCOS.
- The degree of hyperthecotic transformation in the ovary is not correlated to the severity of disease.
- Hyperthecosis also can arise in postmenopausal women.
- GnRH agonist treatment can avoid surgery because insulin-induced steroidogenic activity in ovary is still LH dependent.

12. d. All

Ref: Yen & Jaffe's 8th/ed p 898; Kamini A Rao 2nd/ed p 159

Idiopathic Hirsutism

- In about 10% to 15% of hirsute women, serum androgen levels are in the normal range and with the occurrence of normal menstrual cycles, the diagnosis of "idiopathic hirsutism" is made.
- **Increased sensitivity** to androgens is seen, mediated by:
  - Increased peripheral 5a-reductase activity
  - Alteration in the androgen receptor function.

13. a. Significant reduction in hair growth occur within 6 months of start of treatment

Ref: Kamini A Rao 2nd/ed p 164; Endocrine society clinical practice Guidelines. J Clin Endocrinol Metab, April 2018, 103(4):1233-57

- No significant reduction in hair growth may occur for up to 6 months, which approximates the half-life of a hair follicle growth cycle.
- Change in dose, drug, or the addition of a second drug should be considered **only after 6 months** if the patient judges her response inadequate.
- The severity of hirsutism should be defined before treatment begins to provide the means for monitoring response; the methods and frequency of hair removal provide the most practical and clinically relevant measure.
- Serial measurements of serum androgen levels during treatment are neither necessary nor helpful, but repeated evaluation is indicated when hirsutism progresses despite treatment.

14. a. All

Ref: Speroff 8th/ed p 545

Estrogen-progestin contraceptives have number of complementary non-contraceptive actions that make them a logical and effective treatment for hirsutism:
- Androgen production in hirsute women usually is an LH-dependent process. Estrogen-progestin contraceptives suppress pituitary LH secretion and thus also suppress ovarian androgen production.
- The high level of estrogen in combination contraceptives stimulates hepatic SHBG production, thereby increasing binding capacity for circulating androgens and decreasing the amount of free/active androgen.

- Directly or indirectly, estrogen-progestin contraceptives can decrease adrenal DHEA-S secretion.
- Contraceptive progestins inhibit 5a-reductase activity in skin, which decreases the production of dihydrotestosterone (DHT), the major nuclear androgen in hair follicles and sebaceous glands.

Although the progestin suppresses gonadotropins secretion to a lesser extent than estrogen-progestin regimens, LH still is suppressed sufficiently to cause a significant decrease in ovarian androgen production. In addition, testosterone clearance increases during treatment with medroxyprogesterone acetate, due to induction of hepatic enzyme activity.

15. b. Serum total testosterone concentration

Ref: Speroff 8th/ed p 513

Following points to be kept in mind regarding laboratory evaluation of androgens in patients with hirsutism:
- Laboratory evaluation is indicated for many but not all women with hirsutism.
- The **primary aim** is to identify those having potentially serious endocrine disorders requiring specific treatment (nonclassical CAH, androgen-secreting tumors, Cushing syndrome).
- Thyroid disorders and hyperprolactinemia should be excluded in women with menstrual dysfunction.
- Laboratory evaluation is recommended for women with:
  - Moderate or severe hirsutism
  - Hirsutism that is sudden in onset, rapidly progressive
  - Associated with symptoms or signs of virilization
- The **serum total testosterone concentration** provides the best overall measure of androgen production and is the only hormone that need be measured in most women with hirsutism who merit evaluation.
- Testing for nonclassical CAH can be safely reserved for
  - Patients with an early onset of hirsutism (pre- or peri-menarcheal onset, including those with premature adrenarche)
  - Women with a family history of the disorder
  - Those in high-risk ethnic groups (Hispanic, Mediterranean, Slavic, or Ashkenazi Jewish heritage)
- Additional evaluation also is indicated for
  - Those with hirsutism having onset before puberty or after age 25
  - Rapidly progressive hirsutism
- Hirsutism that is accompanied by signs of virilization or hypercortisolism (Cushing syndrome).

16. c. Serum total testosterone > 150 ng/dL have high positive predictive value for detecting androgen producing tumors

Ref: Speroff 8th/ed p 545; Yen & Jaffe's 8th/ed p 550

Serum Testosterone

- A serum total testosterone concentration greater than 150 ng/dL identifies almost all women with a potential androgen-producing tumor.
- The suggested threshold value has very **high sensitivity and negative predictive value**, indicating that it captures virtually all women with tumors and can effectively exclude the diagnosis.
- The positive predictive value of a serum total testosterone greater than 150 ng/dL is quite low, indicating that few women who meet the criterion will, in fact, have a tumor, primarily because such tumors are very rare; the large majority will have PCOS or hyperthecosis.
- Except for high serum T values in the adult-male range, a moderate increase of this androgen is a poor predictor of androgenic tumors. Instead, the clinical finding of virilization (i.e., voice change, male pattern androgenic alopecia, clitoromegaly, or rapid onset of symptoms) is the best predictor of these neoplasms.
- It also is important to remember that testosterone levels are elevated significantly during normal pregnancy. Concentrations are greater than 100 ng/dL during the first trimester and can reach 500–800 ng/dL by term, primarily due to the estrogen-induced increase in SHBG.
- Mother and fetus normally are protected from virilization because free testosterone levels rise only modestly and are rapidly converted to estrogen via placental aromatization.

17. a. 100 ng/dL

Ref: Kamini A Rao 2nd/ed p 162

- Free androgen index: testosterone/SHBG × 100

Normal serum testosterone levels ranges from 20–80 ng/dL.

Because testosterone levels normally are lower in postmenopausal women, concentrations greater than **100 ng/dL** should raise suspicion for a tumor.

Hormonal evaluation of hirsutism	
Parameter	Normal value in females (ng/dL)
Total testosterone	20–80
Free testosterone	0.3–1.9
Bioavailable testosterone	0.8–10
Free androgen index	0.7–1
Androgen producing tumors premenopausal	>150
Androgen producing tumors postmenopause	>100

18. **d. Develop in women with gestational trophoblastic disease**

Ref: Speroff 8th/ed p 363

Pregnancy Luteoma

- Hyperplastic mass of luteinized ovarian cells.
- Not a true tumor.
- Most luteomas produce little androgen or have little or no androgenic effect, serum concentrations of androstenedione, testosterone, and dihydrotestosterone can be increased, sometimes dramatically.
- Only approximately one-third of reported pregnancy luteomas have been associated with maternal hirsutism or virilization, probably because any increase in serum free testosterone is limited by the large increase in SHBG levels that occurs during pregnancy.
- Luteomas are solid masses ranging between 6 and 10 cm in size
- Half of cases are bilateral.
- Pregnancy luteomas typically regress promptly after delivery.
- In contrast, functional androgen-producing **theca-lutein cysts (hyperreactio luteinalis)** can develop in women with multiple pregnancies, isoimmunized or diabetic mothers, and those with molar pregnancies or gestational trophoblastic disease, all of which are associated with increased maternal serum hCG concentrations.

19. **a. Clitoral length > 5 mm**

Ref: Speroff 8th/ed p 542

Clitoromegaly generally is defined by:
- Clitoral length > 10 mm
- Clitoral index (length times width) > 35 mm^2.

20. **c. Biologically potent androgen**

Ref: Speroff 8th/ed p 545; Yen & Jaffe's 8th/ed p 603

Salients points regarding DHEA-S:
- DHEA-S circulates in higher concentration than any other steroid.
- Derives exclusively from the adrenal gland.
- Direct measure of adrenal androgen activity.
- The upper limit of normal in most laboratories is approximately **350 mg/dL**.
- DHEA-S is primarily as a pre-hormone, providing substrate for conversion to testosterone and dihydrotestosterone in the periphery.

21. **d. All**

Ref: Basic & clinical pharmacology. Katzung 14th/ed p 265-66

Spironolactone is an **aldosterone antagonist** having structural similarity to progestins.

Mechanism of action:
- Androgen receptor antagonist, competing with dihydrotestosterone (DHT) for binding to the androgen receptor
- Inhibition of ovarian and adrenal androgen synthesis
- 5-a reductase inhibitor

Receptor blocking action is most important mechanism.

22. **a. Acne > hirsutism > increased libido > clitoromegaly > virilization**

Ref: Speroff 8th/ed p 542

- Virilization or masculinization are terms reserved for extreme androgen effects characterized by development of:
  - Male hair pattern
  - Deepening of voice
  - Increased muscle mass
  - General male body habitus

Following manifestations reflect progressively higher serum androgen levels:

Acne > hirsutism > increased libido > clitoromegaly > virilization

23. **a. 25, 25, 50**

Ref: Speroff 8th/ed p 537

About 50% testosterone is derived from peripheral conversion of androstenedione, while adrenal gland and ovary contribute equal amounts, 25% each.

In midcycle, ovarian contribution increases by 10-15%.

24. **c. 70%**

Ref: Speroff 8th/ed p 544; Kamini A Rao 2nd/ed p 160

Serum testosterone levels (normal 20-80 ng/dL) are elevated in most (70%), but not all, women with chronic anovulation and hirsutism.

25. **a. Congenital adrenal hyperplasia**

Ref: Endocrinology: adult & pediatric. Larry Jameson, Leslie J De Groot 7th/ ed p 57.

Nonclassical 21-hydroxylase deficiency is one of the most common autosomal recessive diseases and, as in the classical form of the disorder, prevalence varies with ethnicity.

Non-classical 21-hydroxylase deficiency affects between 1 in 100 and 1 in 1,000 Caucasians.

Most common cause is 21-hydroxylase deficiency.

26. **d. Late afternoon measurements are taken**

Ref: Endocrinology: adult & pediatric. Larry Jameson, Leslie J De Groot 7th/ ed p 1818

17-hydroxyprogesterone

- Must be measured in **morning** to avoid later elevations due to diurnal pattern of ACTH secretion.
- In nonclassically affected individuals, because of pulsatile and diurnal variations in 17-OHP secretion, midmorning and afternoon concentrations may be normal. Of all single measurements, early morning measurement of serum 17-OHP concentration is the most likely to show an elevation.
- Its measurement offers a cost effective means to detect late onset CAH, avoiding ACTH stimulation test.
- The baseline values are <200 ng/dL
- Levels >200 ng/dL, but less than 800 ng/dL warrants ACTH stimulation test
- Values >800 ng/dL are diagnostic of late onset CAH
- In hirsute patients with a high risk of congenital adrenal hyperplasia (positive family history, member of a high-risk ethnic group), endocrine society suggest this screening even if serum total and free testosterone are normal.

27. d. Can be done anytime during the day or during the menstrual cycle

Ref: Yen & Jaffe's 8th/ed p 420

ACTH Stimulation Test

- Testing must be performed in the **morning**, but it can be scheduled any time during the menstrual cycle.
- A pharmacological dose of synthetic ACTH (0.25 mg cosyntropin) is administered after a basal blood sample has been obtained.
- A second sample is collected 30 to 60 minutes later.
- Stimulated 17-OHP responses of < 500 ng/dL at 30 minutes are within normal limits.
- Responses > 1500 ng/dL are consistent with 21-hydroxylase deficiency.
- Intermediate responses, 500 to 1500 ng/dL, are consistent with heterozygosity for 21 hydroxylase deficiency.
- Test yields one hour value that is plotted on nomogram and predicts the genotype of homozygote and heterozygote forms of 21-hydroxylase deficiency.
- Dexamethasone pretreatment is not necessary.
- Heterozygote carriers for 21-hydroxylase deficiency have ACTH-stimulated levels of 17-OHP up to 1000 ng/dL: patients with late onset deficiency have stimulated levels above 1200 ng/dL.
- An abnormal 17-hydroxypregnenolone/17-OHP ratio is suggestive of 3b-hydroxysteroid dehydrogenase deficiency.

28. b. Granulosa cell tumors

Ref: Yen & Jaffe's 8th/ed p 697

Ovarian endocrine tumors causing virilization:
- Luteomas
- Gestational theca-lutein cysts (hyperreaction luteinalis)
- Sertoli-Leydig cell tumors (arrhenoblastomas)

All are associated with markedly elevated levels of testosterone, dihydrotestosterone, and androstenedione.

Luteomas

- Derived from luteinization and hyperplasia of theca interna cells.
- Bilateral in approximately 45% of cases.
- Maternal virilization or hirsutism occurs in approximately 35% of such women, and the risk of virilization of a female fetus is high.

Theca-Lutein Cysts

- These are associated with a lower risk of virilization of a female fetus.
- This disorder occurs typically in conditions with elevated circulating levels of hCG (such as gestational trophoblastic tumors, diabetes, and Rh isoimmunization), which directly stimulates ovarian steroid production.
- In majority of cases, the cysts are bilateral.

Sertoli-Leydig Cell Tumors

- The risk of both maternal and fetal virilization is highest with Sertoli-Leydig cell tumors.
- These tumors are usually unilateral. Fortunately, such tumors are usually associated with chronic anovulation and infertility and are therefore rarely seen in pregnancy.

29. a. GnRH agonist therapy alone

Ref: Yen & Jaffe's 8th/ed p 637; Endocrine Society Clinical Practice Guidelines. J Clin Endocrinol Metab, April 2018, 103(4):1233-57

Long-term agonist therapy cannot be used alone without add back therapy due to risk associated.

GnRH agonist therapy should be an effective treatment for women with ovarian hyperthecosis who typically have severe hyperandrogenism. However, the impact of treatment on their hirsutism can be less than expected, even when gonadotropin secretion is suppressed profoundly, because most also have severe insulin resistance, with hyperinsulinemia driving their androgen production.

30. a. OCPs

Ref: Endocrine Society Clinical Practice Guidelines. J Clin Endocrinol Metab, April 2018, 103(4):1233-57

- For majority of women with hirsutism who are not seeking fertility, guidelines suggest OCPs as initial therapy for treating patient-important hirsutism.
- For most women with hirsutism, they suggest against antiandrogen monotherapy as initial therapy (because of the teratogenic potential of these medications) unless these women use adequate contraception.
- However, for women who are not sexually active, have undergone permanent sterilization, or who are using long-acting reversible contraception, they suggest using either OCPs or antiandrogens as initial therapy.
- No specific OCP is suggested over another as initial therapy, as all OCPs appear to be equally effective for hirsutism, and the risk of side effects is low.
- If hirsutism remains despite 6 months of monotherapy with an OCP, addition of antiandrogens is suggested.
- Guidelines do not suggest one antiandrogen over another. However, they recommend against the use of flutamide because of its potential hepatotoxicity.
- For all pharmacologic therapies for hirsutism, guidelines suggest a trial of at least 6 months before making changes in dose, switching to a new medication, or adding medication.

Metformin for Hirsutism

Updated systematic review of nine trials have shown metformin was no more effective than placebo for lowering hirsutism scores.

Other insulin sensitizers, troglitazone and rosiglitazone, had no significant effect on hirsutism.

So, guidelines are against using insulin-lowering drugs for the sole indication of treating hirsutism.

31. b. Flutamide

Ref: Endocrine Society Clinical Practice Guidelines. J Clin Endocrinol Metab, April 2018, 103(4):1233-57

Antiandrogens used for the treatment of hirsutism	
Cyproterone acetate	50–100 mg/d on menstrual cycle days 5–15, with EE 20–35 mg on days 5–25
Spironolactone	100–200 mg/d [given in divided doses (twice daily)]
Finasteride	2.5–5 mg/d
Flutamide	250–500 mg/d (high dose) 62.5 to #250 mg/d (low dose)

Flutamide

- Pure antiandrogen with a dose response inhibition of the androgen receptor.
- The major concern with flutamide is its propensity for **hepatic toxicity**.

CHAPTER 12

Endocrinology of Obesity

Multiple Choice Questions

1. **Obesity is an excess of body fat. Overweight is a body weight that includes:**
   a. Muscle
   b. Water
   c. Fat
   d. All

2. **Most accurate method of determining body fat:**
   a. Skinfold measurement
   b. Hydrodensitometry
   c. Body mass index nomogram
   d. Quetelet index

3. **Obesity is associated with which of the following?**
   a. Hypertension
   b. Diabetes
   c. Hypertriglyceridemia
   d. All

4. **BMI of 32 will be labelled as:**
   a. Overweight
   b. Class I obesity
   c. Class II obesity
   d. Class III obesity

5. **What is optimal BMI?**
   a. 19-24.9
   b. 18-25
   c. 19-25
   d. 18.5-24.5

6. **Which of the following is not correct for obesity?**
   a. Women have lower metabolic rate
   b. Obesity is excess storage of triglycerides in adipose cells
   c. Men have greater prevalence
   d. Basal metabolic rate decreases with age

7. **Which of the following is incorrect regarding fat metabolism?**
   a. Body weight is directly correlated with level of alcohol consumption
   b. Production and availability of glycerophosphate is rate limiting in lipogenesis
   c. Chief metabolic products produced from fat are free fatty acids
   d. 4 calories are there in one gram of triglyceride

8. **What is not true about free fatty acids released from adipose tissue?**
   a. Retrobulbar and perirenal fat is first to mobilize
   b. Omental, mesenteric and subcutaneous fat is more easily mobilized
   c. Free fatty acid release is stimulated by physical exercise
   d. Circulating free fatty acids are derived from endogenous triglycerides

9. **Major physiologic antagonist of lipase enzyme activity:**
   a. ACTH
   b. TSH
   c. Insulin
   d. Growth hormone

10. **The hypothalamic location of the appetite center:**
    a. Ventromedial nucleus
    b. Ventral noradrenergic bundle
    c. Arcuate nucleus
    d. Preoptic area

11. **Neuropeptides that inhibit appetite include all except:**
    a. Corticotropin-releasing hormone (CRH)
    b. Neurotensin
    c. Ghrelin
    d. Oxytocin

12. **Leptin leads to:**
    a. Decreased appetite
    b. Increase in heat production and activity
    c. Decrease in the hypothalamic peptide neuropeptide Y (NPY)
    d. All

13. **NPY causes:**
    a. Stimulates food intake
    b. Decreases heat production
    c. Increases insulin
    d. Increases cortisol

14. What of the following is not correct?
    a. Fasting and exercise decrease leptin secretion
    b. The neurons that respond to NPY originate in the arcuate nucleus
    c. Caloric restriction decreases the expression of NPY
    d. The NPY neurons stimulate feeding and inhibit heat production

15. All of the following inhibit food intake, *except:*
    a. NPY
    b. CRH
    c. Urocortin
    d. Leptin

16. Ghrelin is a complex hormone. What is not correct regarding ghrelin?
    a. It stimulate the release of growth hormone
    b. Promotes gonadotropin secretion
    c. Regulation of food intake and energy metabolism
    d. Expressed in the ovaries and placenta

17. Ghrelin circulating in the blood predominantly comes from:
    a. Gastrointestinal tract
    b. Hypothalamus
    c. Pituitary
    d. Ovaries

18. In all of the following, ghrelin levels will be higher, *except:*
    a. Anorexia
    b. Bulimia
    c. Cachexia
    d. Obesity

19. Weight loss in obese and lean people produces the following response:
    a. Decreased leptin
    b. Decreased insulin
    c. Increased ghrelin
    d. All

20. All of the following are correct for congenital leptin deficiency, *except:*
    a. Macrosomic at birth
    b. Autosomal recessive disorder
    c. Hyperphagia
    d. Early onset obesity

21. Which of the following is not component of metabolic syndrome?
    a. High HDL-cholesterol
    b. Hypertension
    c. Diabetes mellitus
    d. Hypertriglyceridemia

22. Which statement is not correct regarding obesity?
    a. Hypothyroidism does not cause obesity
    b. Waist circumference >88 cm is predictor of metabolic dysfunction
    c. Gynoid obesity is associated with more cardiovascular risk factors than android obesity
    d. Circulating insulin level is proportional to volume of body fat

Newer Questions from Recent Guidelines

23. Which of the following is a lipase inhibitor used in management of obesity?
    a. Rimonabant
    b. Orlistat
    c. Amphetamines
    d. Sibutramine

24. BMI after which pharmacotherapy for weight reduction is indicated along with lifestyle modifications in a person without any comorbidities:
    a. 30 kg/m^2
    b. 27 kg/m^2
    c. 25 kg/m^2
    d. 40 kg/m^2

25. BMI after which bariatric surgery for weight reduction is indicated along with lifestyle modifications in a person without any comorbidities:
    a. 30 kg/m^2
    b. 25 kg/m^2
    c. 35 kg/m^2
    d. 40 kg/m^2

26. Which of the following medications given to reduce weight do not target appetite mechanisms?
    a. Locaserin
    b. Liraglutide
    c. Orlistat
    d. Phentermine

27. Injectable GLP-1 agonist, FDA approved for weight reduction:
    a. Liraglutide
    b. Topiramate
    c. Locaserin
    d. Bupropion

28. The modifications of gastrointestinal function after bariatric surgeries in increasing order:
    a. RYGB > BPD > AGB
    b. AGB > RYGB > BPD
    c. BPD > RYGB > AGB
    d. AGB > BPD > RYGB

29. Hormone seen to decrease post-bariatric surgery:
    a. Ghrelin and GLP-1
    b. Ghrelin and peptide YY
    c. Ghrelin and Leptin
    d. GLP-1 and peptide YY

Answer with Explanations

1. **d. All**

   Ref: Speroff 8th/ed p 860
   - Obesity is an excess storage of **triglycerides** in adipose cells. There is a difference between obesity and overweight.
   - Obesity is an excess of body fat.
   - Overweight is a body weight, including muscle, bone, fat, and body water, in excess of some standard or ideal weight.

2. **b. Hydrodensitometry**

   Ref: Speroff 8th/ed p 860
   - The most accurate method of determining body fat is to determine the density of the body by underwater measurement known as **hydrodensitometry**.
   - It certainly is not practical to measure density by submerging individuals in water; therefore, skinfold measurements with calipers have become popular as an index of body fat, or expensive imaging techniques can be utilized.
   - It is far simpler to utilize the body mass index nomogram, a method that corresponds closely to densitometry measurements.

3. **d. All**

   Ref: Yen & Jaffe's 8th/p 548
   - Overweight individuals have a higher prevalence of hypertension at every age, and the risk of developing hypertension is related to the amount of weight gain after age 25.
   - The two in combination (hypertension and obesity) increase the risk of heart disease, cerebrovascular disease, and death.

   Obesity is associated with four major risk factors for atherosclerosis:
   - Hypertension
   - Diabetes
   - Hypercholesterolemia
   - Hypertriglyceridemia

4. **b. Class I obesity**

   Ref: BMI Classification. World Health Organization, 2014

   The body mass index (**Quetelet index**) is the ratio of weight divided by the height squared (in metric units).
   - BMI = kilograms/meters^2
   - <18.9—underweight
   - 19.0–24.9—normal
   - 25.0–29.9—overweight
   - 30.0–34.9—class I obesity
   - 35.0–39.9—class II obesity
   - >40.0—class III obesity

5. **a. 19–24.9**

   Ref: BMI Classification. World Health Organization, 2014

   Optimal BMI is 19.0 to 24.9 kg/m^2

6. **c. Men have greater prevalence**

   Ref: Speroff 8th/ed p 862

   Salient points regarding obesity:
   - Women have a greater prevalence of obesity compared with men because women have a **lower metabolic rate** than men.
   - Postmenopausal loss of the increase in metabolic rate that is associated with the luteal phase of the menstrual cycle.
   - The difference between men and women is even greater in older age.
   - Basal metabolic rate decreases with age.

7. **d. 4 calories are there in 1 gram of triglyceride**

   Ref: Speroff 8th/ed p 862
   - Each cell of adipose tissue can be regarded as a package of triglyceride, the most concentrated form of stored energy. There are **8 calories/g of triglyceride** compared to 1 calorie/g of glycogen.
   - Because alcohol diverts fat from oxidation to storage, body weight is directly correlated with the level of alcohol consumption.
   - The production and availability of glycerophosphate (required for reesterification of fatty acids and their storage as triglycerides) are considered rate limiting in lipogenesis, and this process depends on the presence of glucose.
   - The chief metabolic products produced from fat are the circulating **free fatty acids**. Their availability is controlled by adipose tissue cells.
   - When carbohydrate is in short supply, a flood of free fatty acids can be released. The free fatty acids in the peripheral circulation are almost wholly derived from endogenous triglycerides that undergo rapid hydrolysis to yield free fatty acid and glycerol.
   - The glycerol is returned to the liver for resynthesis of glycogen.

8. **a. Retrobulbar and perirenal fat is first to mobilize**
   Ref: Speroff 8th/ed p 863

- Areas from which energy is not easily mobilized are retrobulbar and perirenal fat where the tissue serves a structural function.

Free fatty acid release from adipose tissue is stimulated by physical exercise, fasting, exposure to cold, nervous tension, and anxiety.

The release of fatty acids by lipolysis varies from one anatomic site to another. Omental, mesenteric, and subcutaneous fat is more labile and easily mobilized than fat from other sources.

9. **c. Insulin**
   Ref: Speroff 8th/ed p 864

Adipose tissue lipase is sensitive to stimulation by both epinephrine and norepinephrine. Other hormones that activate lipase are adrenocorticotropic hormone (ACTH), thyroid-stimulating hormone (TSH), growth hormone, thyroxine (T4), 3,5,3'-triiodothyronine (T3), cortisol, glucagon, as well as vasopressin and human placental lactogen (hPL).

Lipase enzyme activity is inhibited by insulin, which appears to be alone as the **major physiologic antagonist** to the array of stimulating agents.

When both glucose and insulin are abundant, transport of glucose into fat cells is high, and glycerophosphate production increases to esterify fatty acids.

10. **b. Ventral noradrenergic bundle**
    Ref: Yen & Jaffe's 8th/p 4; Speroff 8th/ed p 865

Lesions of the ventromedial nucleus produced by radiofrequency current fail to cause obesity. These lesions lead to overeating and obesity only when they extend beyond the ventromedial nucleus. Selective destruction of the **ventral noradrenergic bundle** results in hyperphagia.

A sudden onset of hyperphagia can be due to a hypothalamic lesion. Possible causes include tumors, trauma, inflammatory processes, and aneurysms.

11. **c. Ghrelin**
    Ref: Yen & Jaffe's 8th/p 408

Neuropeptides that inhibit appetite include
- Corticotropin-releasing hormone (CRH)
- Neurotensin
- Oxytocin
- Cyclo (HisPro), a peptide derived by proteolysis of thyrotropin-releasing hormone.

Ghrelin

- It is a small peptide, secreted predominantly by the stomach, which circulates in two forms.
- The active form is acetylated and promotes GH secretion.
- Ghrelin influences food intake, sleep, body weight, gastrointestinal mobility, and reproduction.
- Ghrelin suppresses LH pulsatility in the pituitary.
- Circulating ghrelin concentrations are higher during fasting, and decrease after food intake, indicating that ghrelin signals energy deficient states and modulates appetite and carbohydrate metabolism.

12. **d. All**
    Ref: Yen & Jaffe's 8th/ed p 905

Leptin

- It is a 146-amino acid protein produced primarily by adipocytes.
- It is a key regulator of satiety and body mass index.
- Its levels reflect the amount of energy stores and nutritional state.
- It decreases food intake and body weight via its hypothalamic receptors.
- It coordinates body mass status with reproductive function. Leptin acts as a permissive factor in reproductive-pulsatile hypothalamic GnRH secretion does not occur unless leptin levels reach a threshold value. Such a mechanism ensures that energy stores are sufficient to support a pregnancy.
- It may be measured by RIA or ELISA and in adult women with normal body weight, leptin values are between 10 and 30 pg/mL. Serum levels of leptin increase in obese subjects, probably because in obesity there is a condition of leptin resistance.

13. **a. Stimulates food intake**
    Ref: Speroff 8th/ed p 867; Yen & Jaffe's 8th/p 472

- NPY stimulates food intake, decreases heat production, and increases insulin and cortisol secretion.

NPY is a 36-amino acid polypeptide that is a potent stimulator of eating when injected directly into the rodent brain.

14. **c. Calorie restriction decreases the expression of NPY**
    Ref: Speroff 8th/ed p 868; Yen & Jaffe's 8th/p 472

- Just remember one simple rule: when food supply or storage is excess, leptin level will increase, when food supply or storage is less, NPY level will increase.
- Circulating levels of leptin are correlated with the percent body fat. In other words increased body fat increases the expression of the LEP gene in fat cells.

(more fat, more leptin, just remember like that). The amount of leptin in the circulation, therefore, is a measure of the amount of adipose tissue in the body.
- Fasting and exercise decrease leptin secretion and increase NPY gene expression in the arcuate nucleus.
- The NPY neurons stimulate feeding and inhibit heat production.
- Caloric restriction increases the expression of NPY in the arcuate nucleus and the release of NPY in the paraventricular nucleus.

15. a. NPY

Ref: Speroff 8th/ed p 869; Yen & Jaffe's 8th/p 472

CRH inhibits food intake and increases energy expenditure. The specific food and energy response associated with CRH may also be mediated by urocortin, a CRH-related peptide.

Urocortin is very potent in reducing food intake.

16. b. Promotes gonadotropin secretion

Ref: Speroff 8th/ed p 870; Yen & Jaffe's 8th/p 408

Ghrelin is a complex hormone, named for its ability to stimulate the release of growth hormone. Ghrelin participates in the following functions:
- Regulation of food intake and energy metabolism
- Affects sleep and behavior
- **Inhibits gonadotropin secretion**
- Expressed in the ovaries and the placenta
- Involved in gastric motility and acid secretion
- Involved in activity of the pancreas
- Secretion of growth hormone, prolactin, and ACTH

17. a. Gastrointestinal tract

Ref: Speroff 8th/ed p 870; Yen & Jaffe's 8th/p 408

Ghrelin

- 28-amino acid peptide
- Secreted mainly in the **upper portion of the stomach**, but in other tissues as well, including the intestine, pituitary, hypothalamus, kidney, ovary, testis, and placenta.
- The ghrelin circulating in the blood is predominantly from the stomach and intestine, and its target is the energy-regulating centers in the hypothalamus.
- Given to rodents, ghrelin acutely increases food intake and causes obesity.

18. d. Obesity

Ref: Speroff 8th/ed p 870; Yen & Jaffe's 8th/p 408

The circulating level of ghrelin is lower in obese individuals, reduced with food intake and increased with fasting. Thus, ghrelin levels are higher in individuals with anorexia, bulimia, or cachexia.

19. d. All

Ref: Speroff 8th/ed p 870

Weight loss in obese and lean people produces the same response, decreased leptin and insulin, and an increase in ghrelin.

20. a. Macrosomic at birth

Ref: Speroff 8th/ed p 872; Paz-Filho G, et al: Congenital leptin deficiency: diagnosis and effects of leptin replacement therapy. Arq Bras Endocrinol Metabol 54(8):690-97, 2010.

Congenital Leptin Deficiency

- Children have **normal birth weights**, but immediately began gaining excessive weight with marked increases in appetites.
- Display suppression of gonadal function.
- Congenital leptin deficiency is now recognized as a rare **recessive inherited disorder**, the result of mutations at various sites on the *LEP* gene and associated with **hyperphagia** and the onset of obesity at an early age.

21. a. High HDL- cholesterol

Ref: Speroff 8th/ed p 707; Kamini A Rao 2nd/ed p 491

Diagnostic criteria for metabolic syndrome according to National Cholesterol Education Program (NCEP III) expert panel on detection, evaluation and treatment of high blood cholesterol in adults. 3 of the following 5 suggests metabolic syndrome.

1.	Central obesity (waist circumference in cm)	
	Male	>102
	Female	>88
2.	Elevated triglycerides (mg/dL)	>150
3.	Decreased HDL cholesterol (mg/dL)	
	Male	<40
	Female	<50
4.	Elevated arterial BP (mm Hg)	>130/85
5.	Elevated fasting blood glucose (mg/dL)	>110

22. c. Gynoid obesity is associated with more cardiovascular risk factor than android obesity

Ref: Speroff 8th/ed p 878; Yen & Jaffe's 8th/p 548

- Contrary to popular misconception, hypothyroidism does not cause obesity. Weight gain due to hypothyroidism is confined to the fluid accumulation of myxedema.

Endocrine Effects of Insulin on Obesity

- The most important endocrine change in obesity is elevation of the basal blood insulin level.

- The circulating insulin level is proportional to the volume of body fat.
- Overweight individuals are characterized by insulin resistance.
- At least one mechanism for the increased resistance to insulin observed with increasing weight is down-regulation of insulin receptors brought about by the increase in insulin secretion.
- The increase in insulin resistance affects the metabolism of carbohydrate, fat, and protein.
- Circulating levels of free fatty acids increase as a result of inadequate insulin suppression of the fat cell.
- Insulin resistance results in decreased catabolism of triglycerides, yielding a decrease in HDL-cholesterol and an increase in LDL-cholesterol.
- Hyperinsulinemia is also directly associated with hypertension.

Gynoid obesity (the pear shape) refers to fat distribution in the **lower body** (femoral and gluteal regions), whereas **android obesity** (the apple shape) refers to **central body** distribution.

Gynoid fat is more resistant to catecholamines and **more sensitive to insulin** than abdominal fat; thus, extraction and storage of fatty acids easily occur, and fat is accumulated more readily in the thighs and buttocks. This fat is associated with minimal fatty acid flux, and, therefore, the negative consequences of fatty acid metabolism are less.

Gynoid fat is principally stored fat.

The clinical meaning of all this is that women with gynoid obesity are less likely than women with android obesity to develop diabetes mellitus and coronary heart disease.

23. b. Orlistat

Ref: Kamini A Rao 2nd/ed p 497; Pharmacological Management of Obesity: An Endocrine Society Clinical Practice Guideline 2015

Orlistat

- It is a **lipase inhibitor**, acts by reducing intestinal absorption of fats.
- Dose of 120 mg three times a day with meals is given.
- It decreases absorption of fat soluble vitamins, especially vitamin D.
- Major side effects are related to gastrointestinal tract.

24. a. 30 kg/m²

Ref: Pharmacological Management of Obesity: An Endocrine Society Clinical Practice Guideline 2015

Endocrine society guidelines recommend:
- Diet, exercise, and behavioural modification be included in all obesity management approaches or body mass index (BMI) >25 kg/m²
- Pharmacotherapy is indicated along with lifestyle modifications when BMI > 27 kg/m² with comorbidity or BMI over 30 kg/m² without comorbidities
- Bariatric surgery is indicated in patients with BMI > 35 kg/m² in presence of comorbidities or BMI over 40 kg/m² without comorbidities

BMI for intervention	Without comorbidities	With comorbidities
Pharmacotherapy	30	27
Bariatric surgery	40	35

25. d. 40 kg/m²

Ref: Pharmacological Management of Obesity: An Endocrine Society Clinical Practice Guideline 2015

26. c. Orlistat

Ref: Pharmacological Management of Obesity: An Endocrine Society Clinical Practice Guideline 2015

- Orlistat is a pancreatic and gastric lipase inhibitor
- FDA approved in 1999 for chronic weight management
- Adverse effects:
  - Decreased absorption of fat-soluble vitamins, steatorrhrea, oily spotting, flatulence with discharge, fecal urgency, oily evacuation, increased defecation, fecal incontinence.

27. a. Liraglutide

Ref: Pharmacological Management of Obesity: An Endocrine Society Clinical Practice Guideline 2015

Liraglutide

- GLP-1 agonists
- Other from same family is exenatide
- Helps weight reduction
- Dose recommended is, 3.0 mg SC QD
- FDA approved in 2014 for chronic weight management
- Nausea, vomiting, pancreatitis Medullary thyroid cancer history, multiple endocrine neoplasia type 2 history.

28. b. AGB > RYGB > BPD

Ref: Endocrine and Nutritional Management of the Post-Bariatric Surgery Patient: An Endocrine Society Clinical Practice Guideline 2010

Bariatric Surgery

- Common operations include various banding procedures, which restrict the amount of food entering the stomach, the Roux-en-Y Gastric bypass (RYGB), the duodenal switch/ Gastric sleeve (DS/GS), or the biliopancreatic diversion (BPD).

- The modifications of gastrointestinal function after these surgeries are **least with banding**, greater with RYGB, and greatest with BPD or DS/GS.

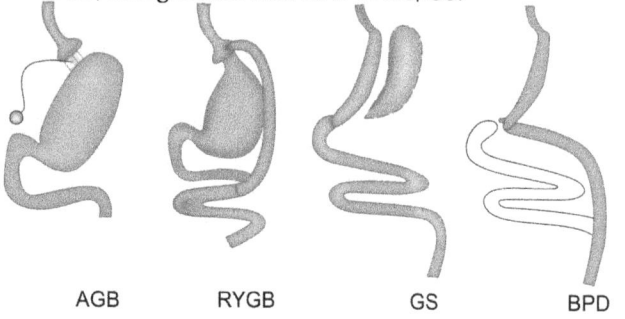

AGB　　RYGB　　GS　　BPD

29. c. Ghrelin and leptin

Ref: Endocrine and Nutritional Management of the Post-Bariatric Surgery Patient: An Endocrine Society Clinical Practice Guideline 2010

Various hormones may be involved in postoperative weight homeostasis in case of bariatric surgeries.

Hormones involved in homeostasis post-bariatric surgery	
Decreased	Increased
Ghrelin	Glucagon-like peptide-1
Leptin	Peptide YY
Insulin	

CHAPTER 13

Endocrinology of Reproduction and Thyroid

Multiple Choice Questions

1. Most common cause of hypothyroidism in areas with normal iodine intake:
   a. Autoimmune
   b. Pituitary failure
   c. Hypothalamic failure
   d. Post radiation

2. The full response of TSH to changes in T4 is slow. How much minimum time is needed to show changes in order to adjust the dose?
   a. 2–4 weeks
   b. 4–6 weeks
   c. 8–10 weeks
   d. 10–12 weeks

3. Risk factors associated with TSH suppressive doses of thyroxine:
   a. Iron deficiency anemia
   b. Cardiac arrest
   c. Sedation
   d. Osteoporosis

4. Which of the following is not true for aging patient and thyroid?
   a. Decreased response of TSH to TRH
   b. Increased TSH levels
   c. Decreased conversion of T4 to T3
   d. Slightly decreased TBG concentrations

5. What is not true regarding synthetic thyroxine T4?
   a. Requires minimum of 8 weeks before dose change
   b. Mixtures of T4 and T3 is as useful as synthetic thyroxine T4
   c. Standard replacement therapy irrespective of age
   d. Natural thyroid preparations are inferior

6. Which is not true regarding T3?
   a. Removal of one iodine from the phenolic ring of T4 yields T3
   b. Removal of one iodine from nonphenolic ring yields reverse T3
   c. One third of T4 is converted to T3
   d. Reverse T3 is more potent than T3

7. Most common cause of thyrotoxicosis in pregnancy:
   a. Graves' disease
   b. Trophoblastic disease
   c. Multinodular goitre
   d. TSH hypersecretion

8. Arrange according to potency with highest potent first:
   a. T3 > RT3 > T4
   b. T4 > T3 > RT3
   c. T3 > T4 > RT3
   d. RT3 > T3 > T4

9. Most commonly used assay to assess thyroid function:
   a. Free thyroxine assay (FT4)
   b. Total thyroxine assay (TT4)
   c. Free thyroxine index (FTI)
   d. Total T3 and Reverse T3

10. Which of the following statement is incorrect?
    a. Thyroid hormone treatment does not help infertility in euthyroid women
    b. Maternal TSH levels reach nadir at 10 weeks
    c. For patients with elevated TSH but normal free T4, no need to undergo any further testing
    d. Primary cause of hyperthyroidism is Graves' disease

11. Carbohydrate calories appear to be the primary determinant of T3 levels in adults. Which of the following condition is not associated with low T3 and elevated RT3?
    a. Recovery from illness
    b. Febrile diseases
    c. Burn injuries
    d. Anorexia nervosa

12. Circulating thyroid hormones are present in the circulation mainly bound to proteins. Which of the following statement is incorrect regarding binding proteins?
    a. 70% of thyroid hormones are bound to thyroxine-binding globulin (TBG)
    b. Binding proteins have a greater affinity for T3

c. 30% is bound to thyroxine-binding prealbumin and albumin
d. TBG is synthesized in the liver

13. **The measurement of which hormones provide the most accurate assessment of thyroid function?**
    a. T4 and TSH
    b. T3 and TSH
    c. TSH only is enough
    d. T3 and T4

14. **Which of the following is true for TRH?**
    a. TRH stimulates prolactin secretion by the pituitary
    b. Estrogen increases the TRH receptor content of the pituitary
    c. TSH response to TRH is inhibited by dopamine agonists and glucocorticoids
    d. All

15. **Which statement regarding TSH is not correct?**
    a. Levels of TSH falls with age
    b. Measured by highly sensitive assays using monoclonal antibodies
    c. Ultrasensitive TSH assay can detect concentrations as low as 0.01 mIU/mL
    d. Nearly all women with elevated TSH have hypothyroidism

16. **A 24-year-old patient comes with low TSH and normal T4. T3 is ordered which comes out to be normal. What holds true for above condition?**
    a. She is in compensated state called subclinical hyperthyroidism
    b. High risk of true hyperthyroidism
    c. TSH suppression by general illness and drugs often extend below 0.1 mIU/mL
    d. She is suffering from overt hyperthyroidism

17. **Not true for subclinical hyperthyroidism:**
    a. Runs risk of osteoporosis
    b. Atrial fibrillation is common cardiovascular problem
    c. Normal T4, elevated T3
    d. Most common cause is overtreatment with thyroxine

18. **In most cases of hypothyroidism, a specific cause is not apparent. Which of the following statement is incorrect regarding hypothyroidism?**
    a. When goiter formation is present along with autoimmune reaction, it is called Hashimoto's thyroiditis
    b. More common in men
    c. Can be a cause of recurrent miscarriages
    d. Increases with aging

19. **Subclinical hypothyroidism is a risk factor for:**
    a. Coronary heart disease
    b. Iron deficiency anemia
    c. Recurrent pregnancy loss
    d. All

20. **Not part of Graves's disease triad:**
    a. Anasarca
    b. Hyperthyroidism
    c. Ophthalmopathy
    d. Pretibial myxedema

21. **Which of the following is not correct regarding changed thyroid gland physiology in pregnancy?**
    a. Increase in TBG
    b. TSH levels nadir at 10 weeks
    c. Increase in free T3 and free T4
    d. Increased renal iodine clearance

22. **Which of the following statements is true?**
    1. A sensitive TSH assay is the initial screening assay
    2. If TSH is low or high, a free T4 should be obtained
    3. If TSH is low and free T4 is normal, a free T3 level is measured
    4. If the T3 is also normal, this compensated state is called subclinical hyperthyroidism
    5. If TSH is low and free T4 is normal, a high free T3 would confirm hyperthyroidism
    a. 1, 2 and 5
    b. 1, 3 and 4
    c. 2, 3, 4
    d. All

Questions Based on Newer Guidelines

23. **As per American Thyroid Association guidelines, how should levothyroxine administration be timed with respect to meals and beverages in order to maintain maximum, consistent absorption:**
    a. 1 hour prior breakfast or 3 hour post dinner
    b. 2 hour prior breakfast or 3 hour post dinner
    c. 1 hour prior breakfast or 1 hour post dinner
    d. 2 hour prior breakfast or 2 hour post dinner

24. **Which of the following statements is correct as per recent guidelines for LT4 replacement?**
    I. Evaluation for gastrointestinal disorders is indicated in patients with higher than expected LT4 requirements.
    II. LT4 should be separated from other potentially interfering medications.
    III. A change in an identifiable formulation of levothyroxine (brand name or generic) should be followed by re-evaluation of serum TSH at steady state.
    a. I only
    b. I, II and III
    c. II and III
    d. None

25. Which of the following factors is not associated with decreased LT4 absorption?
    a. Helicobacter pylori gastritis
    b. Autoimmune atrophic gastritis
    c. Lactose intolerance
    d. Gastric bypass surgeries

26. Which of the following is false about the factors which determine the levothyroxine dose required by a hypothyroid patient for reaching the appropriate serum TSH goal?
    a. There is consistent evidence that lean body weight can influence dose requirement
    b. The etiology of a patient's hypothyroidism affects their LT4 dose
    c. Older patients require higher doses of LT4
    d. Pregnancy typically require an increase in their LT4 dose early in the first trimester

27. What are the potential deleterious effects of inadequate levothyroxine?
    a. Dyslipidemia
    b. Atherosclerotic cardiovascular disease
    c. Congestive heart failure
    d. All of the above

28. What is the appropriate management of perceived allergy to the constituents of levothyroxine or intolerance to levothyroxine?
    a. Reduce the LT4 dose and advance it slowly
    b. Changing the product
    c. Treating concomitant iron-deficiency anemia
    d. All of the above

29. The TSH range for each trimester as outlined in ATA guidelines for the management of thyroid disease during pregnancy:
    I. 0.1–2.5 mIU/L for the first trimester
    II. 0.2–3.0 mIU/L for the second trimester
    III. 0.3–3.0 mIU/L for the third trimester
    a. I, II and III
    b. I and II
    c. II and III
    d. None

30. What is the recommended daily iodine intake in women planning pregnancy, women who are pregnant, and women who are breastfeeding?
    a. 150, 250, 250 mcg
    b. 250, 250, 250 mcg
    c. 150, 200, 250 mcg
    d. 200, 250, 200 mcg

31. What is the safe upper limit for iodine consumption in pregnant and breastfeeding women?
    a. 100 mcg
    b. 300 mcg
    c. 500 mcg
    d. 1000 mcg

32. Which of the following is not recommended by American Thyroid Association?
    a. Evaluation of serum TSH concentration is recommended for all women seeking care for infertility
    b. LT4 treatment is recommended for infertile women with overt hypothyroidism who desire pregnancy
    c. Good evidence exist to treat subclinical hypothyroidism in women with thyroid autoantibody-negative attempting natural conception
    d. Insufficient evidence exists to treat thyroid autoantibody-positive euthyroid women who are attempting natural conception

Answer with Explanations

1. **a. Autoimmune**

   Ref: Yen & Jaffe's 8th/ed p 688

   - Hypothyroidism can occur due to pituitary failure in which case the TSH will be inappropriately low for the T4.
   - The most common cause is **autoimmune thyroid disease**—Hashimoto disease (elevated titers of antithyroid antibodies) in areas with normal iodine intake.
   - However, making an etiologic diagnosis in women adds little to the clinical management.

2. **b. 4–6 weeks**

   Ref: American thyroid association guidelines 2014; p 1688

   ## Levothyroxine Replacement

   - The treatment of hypothyroidism involves replacement of thyroid hormone with synthetic T4 (levothyroxine).
   - A general guide for replacement is a weight-based dose of **1.6 μg/kg** once daily, but actual requirements may vary.
   - To minimize problems with absorption, levothyroxine should be taken without other drugs, especially calcium or iron-containing tablets.
   - Recovery of hypothalamic-pituitary axis usually requires **4–6 weeks** at which time TSH and free T4 levels can be measured.

3. **d. Osteoporosis**

   Ref: American thyroid association guidelines 2014; p 1688

   ## Levothyroxine and Bone Loss

   - Excess levels of thyroid hormones, especially levels that lead to serum **TSH < 0.1 mIU/L**, have been shown in many studies to be associated with adverse outcomes, especially related to the cardiovascular system and the skeleton in older persons or postmenopausal women.
   - The use of hormone therapy, exercise programs and possibly bisphosphonate treatment must be considered.

4. **a. Decreased response of TSH to TRH**

   Ref: Speroff 8th/ed p 887; Guidelines for the Treatment of Hypothyroidism. American Thyroid Association Task Force on Thyroid Hormone Replacement 2014; p 1690

   ## Thyroid and Aging

   - Thyroxine metabolism and clearance decrease in older people, and thyroxine secretion decreases in compensation to maintain normal serum thyroxine concentrations.
   - Conversion of T4 to T3 decreases, and TSH levels increase.
   - TSH response to TRH is normal in older women.
   - TBG concentration decreases slightly.
   - Because of risk of coronary heart disease, initial dose should be 25–50 mg/day for about 5 weeks, followed by dose adjustment as per clinical and biochemical assessment
   - Average final dose is 70% of that of younger patients.

5. **c. Standard replacement therapy irresepective of age**

   Ref: Speroff 8th/ed p 892; Guidelines for the Treatment of Hypothyroidism. American Thyroid Association Task Force on Thyroid Hormone Replacement 2014; p 1707

   ## Synthetic Thyroxine

   - Initial therapy is started with synthetic thyroxine, T4, given daily.
   - Mixtures of T4 and T3, such as dessicated thyroid, provides T3 in excess of normal thyroid secretion. So, its better to provide T4 and allow peripheral conversion process to provide T3.
   - **Natural thyroid preparations are not better**, rather potentially detrimental. So patients taking biologic preparations are switched to synthetic thyroxine.

6. **d. Reverse T3 is more potent than T3**

   Ref: Speroff 8th/ed p 886

   You must remember following salient points regarding T3:
   - Removal of one iodine from phenolic ring of T4 yields T3
   - Removal of one iodine from nonphenolic ring yields reverse T3
   - RT3 is **biologically inactive**
   - One third of T4 is converted to T3, in peripheral tissues, largely liver and kidney. About 40% is converted to inactive, RT3.
   - T4 serves as prohormone of T3 with little intrinsic activity of its own.

7. **a. Grave's disease**

   Ref: Yen & Jaffe's 8th/ed p 605

   The most common cause of thyrotoxicosis in pregnancy is **Graves' disease**.
   - Most patients with Graves' disease will have detectable levels of TSH-receptor antibodies, TRAb.

- The clinician should always keep in mind that trophoblastic disease can cause hyperthyroidism due to the TSH property inherent in human chorionic gonadotropin.
- The maternal changes with pregnancy can make diagnosis difficult.
- Tachycardia on awakening from sleep and a failure to gain weight should make a clinician suspicious.

8. **c. T3 > T4 > RT3**

Ref: Speroff 8th/ed p 886; Guidelines for the Treatment of Hypothyroidism. American Thyroid Association Task Force on Thyroid Hormone Replacement 2014; p 1678

T3 > T4 > RT3

- T3 is **3-5 times more potent** than T4 because the nuclear thyroid receptor has a ten-fold greater affinity for T3 compared to T4.
- T4 is secreted at 20 times the rate of T3, but it is T3 which is responsible for most actions in the body.

9. **a. Free thyroid assay (FT4)**

Ref: Speroff 8th/ed p 888

Free thyroxine assay: Assays that measure free T4 are usually **displacement assays** using an antibody to T4. The result is not affected by changes in TBG and binding.

10. **c. For patients with elevated TSH but normal free T4, no need to undergo any further testing**

Ref: Guidelines for the Treatment of Hypothyroidism. American Thyroid Association Task Force on Thyroid Hormone Replacement 2014; p 1693

- For patients with elevated TSH but normal free T4, it is worth measuring **antithyroid antibodies**. A positive test identifies those who are likely to become clinically hypothyroid.
- Presence of thyroid peroxidase antibodies (TPOAb) increases the risk of developing overt hypothyroidism by 3.4-fold.
- Reasons to treat subclinical hypothyroidism:
  - To avoid appearance of goiter
  - Some patients feel improved physical and mental well-being

Two primary causes of hyperthyroidism are Graves' disease (toxic diffuse goiter) and Plummer's disease (toxic nodular goiter).

Plummer's disease is usually encountered in postmenopausal women who have had a long history of goiter.

11. **a. Recovery from illness**

Ref: Speroff 8th/ed p 886

- Carbohydrate calories appear to be the primary determinant of T3 levels in adults.
- A **reciprocal relationship** exists between T3 and RT3.
- During periods of stress, when a decrease in metabolic rate would conserve energy, the body produces more RT3 and less T3.

Following conditions are associated with low T3 but high RT3:
- Febrile diseases
- Burn injuries
- Malnutrition
- Anorexia nervosa

On recovery, this process reverses, and metabolic rate increases.

12. **b. Binding protein have a greater affinity for T3**

Ref: Yen & Jaffe's 8th/ed p 604

Salient features regarding binding proteins:
- Approximately 70% of thyroid hormones are bound to thyroxine-binding globulin (TBG)
- TBG is major determining factor in the total thyroid hormone concentration in the circulation.
- 30% is bound to thyroxine-binding prealbumin and albumin.
- The binding proteins have a **greater affinity for T4** and, thus, allow T3 to have greater entry into cells.
- TBG is synthesized in the **liver**, and this synthesis is increased by estrogens.

Protein	Percentage bound %
TBG	70
Prealbumin (Transthyretin)	20
Albumin	10

13. **a. T4 and TSH**

Ref: Speroff 8th/ed p 887

- The measurement of T4 and TSH, provides the most accurate assessment of thyroid function.

Pituitary secretion of TSH is very sensitive to changes in the circulating levels of thyroid hormone; a slight change in the circulating level of T4 will produce a many-fold greater response in TSH.

14. **d. All**

Ref: Yen & Jaffe's 8th/ed p 605

Thyrotropin-releasing Hormone (TRH)

- The thyroid axis is stimulated by the hypothalamic factor, thyrotropin-releasing hormone (TRH) and inhibited by somatostatin and dopamine.

- Estrogen increases the TRH receptor content of the pituitary; hence, the TSH response to TRH is greater in women than in men, and greater in women taking estrogen-progestin contraceptives.
- The TSH response to TRH is influenced mainly by the thyroid hormone concentration in the circulation; however, lesser effects are associated with dopamine agonists and glucocorticoids.

15. a. Levels of TSH fall with age

Ref: Speroff 8th/ed p 887

Elderly people normally have slightly higher TSH levels with normal upper limit going as high as 7.5 uIU/mL.

16. a. She is in compensated state called subclinical hyperthyroidism

Ref: Speroff 8th/ed p 892; American Thyroid Association guidelines 2017

Subclinical Hyperthyroidism

- Compensated state with low TSH, normal T4 and T3.
- TSH suppression by general illness and drugs **does not extend below 0.1 uU/mL.**
- Most common cause is **overtreatment** with thyroxine.
- All patients treated with thyroid hormone should have their TSH levels assessed every year.
- Atrial fibrillation is common cardiovascular problem associated with subclinical hyperthyroidism, especially in older women when TSH is less than 0.1 mIU/mL
- Progression to overt hyperthyroidism is uncommon.
- Patients with hyperthyroidism are at risk of osteoporosis.
- The biochemical diagnosis of overt hyperthyroidism is confirmed in the presence of a suppressed or undetectable serum TSH and inappropriately elevated serum TT4/FT4, or T3.

17. c. Normal T4, elevated T3

Ref: Speroff 8th/ed p 892

Compensated state is associated with low TSH, normal T4 and T3.

18. b. More common in men

Ref: Yen & Jaffe's 8th/ed p 604

Salient points for hypothyroidism:
- In most cases of hypothyroidism, a specific cause is not apparent.
- It is believed that hypothyroidism is usually secondary to an autoimmune reaction, and, when goiter formation is present, it is called Hashimoto's thyroiditis.
- Thyroid hormone treatment does not help infertility in euthyroid women.
- Hypothyroidism can be a cause of **recurrent miscarriages**, and an assessment of thyroid function is worthwhile in these patients.
- Hypothyroidism increases with aging and is more common in **women**.
- Up to 45% of thyroid glands from women older than age 60 show evidence of thyroiditis. In women admitted to geriatric wards, 2-4% have clinically apparent hypothyroidism.

19. d. All

Ref: Speroff 8th/ed p 891

Subclinical hypothyroidism is a strong risk factor for coronary heart disease. In addition, **iron deficiency anemia** is common in patients with subclinical hypothyroidism and responds better when levothyroxine is added to iron treatment.

20. a. Anasarca

Ref: Yen & Jaffe's 8th/ed p 607

Graves' Disease

- 5 to 10 times more common in **women** than men.
- Characterized by the triad of hyperthyroidism, ophthalmopathy, and pretibial myxedema.
- Caused by autoantibodies that have TSH properties and, therefore, bind to and activate the TSH receptor.
- TSH-receptor antibodies can distinguish Graves' disease from toxic goitre.
- Menstrual changes associated with hyperthyroidism are unpredictable, ranging from amenorrhea to oligomenorrhea to normal cycles.

21. c. Increase in free T3 and free T4

Ref: Speroff 8th/ed p 898

Thyroid Gland Physiology in Pregnancy

- Increased renal iodine clearance leading to increased risk of iodine deficiency in pregnancy in iodine deficient areas.
- Increase in TBG leads to **decrease in free T3 and free T4.**
- Increase in TBG is due to increased hepatic TBG synthesis and increased TBG glycosylation.
- TSH reaches nadir at the same time that hCG reaches a peak at **10 weeks** of pregnancy.

22. d. All

Ref: Speroff 8th/ed p 889

- If the initial TSH is low, especially less than 0.08 mIU/mL, then measurement of a high T4 will confirm the diagnosis of hyperthyroidism.

- If the T4 is normal, the T3 level is measured, because some patients with hyperthyroidism will have predominantly T3 toxicosis.
- If the T3 is normal, this compensated state is called subclinical hyperthyroidism.

23. **a. 1 hour prior breakfast or 3 hours post dinner**
Ref: Guidelines for the Treatment of Hypothyroidism. American Thyroid Association Task Force on Thyroid Hormone Replacement 2014

Levothyroxine: ATA Guidelines for Drug Intake

- Because co-administration of food and levothyroxine is likely to impair levothyroxine absorption, ATA recommends that, if possible, levothyroxine be consistently taken either **60 minutes before breakfast or at bedtime (3 or more hours after the evening meal)** for optimal, consistent absorption.
- Absorption of LT4 occurs in the **jejunum and ileum**.
- An acidic pH in the stomach, as occurs during fasting conditions, appears to be important for subsequent intestinal absorption.
- The absorption of an orally administered dose of LT4 is about 70–80% under optimum fasting conditions.
- Therefore, if a patient is unable to take oral medications, the appropriate intravenous dose is approximately 75% of the oral dose.

24. **b. I, II and III**
Ref: Guidelines for the Treatment of Hypothyroidism. American Thyroid Association Task Force on Thyroid Hormone Replacement 2014

- In patients in whom levothyroxine dose requirements are much higher than expected, evaluation for gastrointestinal disorders such as **Helicobacter pylori–related gastritis**, atrophic gastritis, or celiac disease should be considered. Several gastrointestinal disorders appear to affect either LT4 absorption or serum TSH levels, possibly mediated through an impact on gastric acidity.
- Levothyroxine should be separated from other potentially interfering medications and supplements (e.g., calcium carbonate and ferrous sulfate). A **4-hour** separation is traditional.
- Because use of different levothyroxine products may sometimes be associated with altered serum TSH values, a change in an identifiable formulation of levothyroxine (brand name or generic) should be followed by re-evaluation of serum TSH at steady state.

25. **d. Gastric bypass surgeries**
Ref: Guidelines for the Treatment of Hypothyroidism. American Thyroid Association Task Force on Thyroid Hormone Replacement 2014

Factors associated with decreased LT4 absorption:

- Full stomach
- Gastrointestinal diseases
- Helicobacter pylori gastritis
- Autoimmune atrophic gastritis
- Celiac disease
- Lactose intolerance
- Intestinal giardiasis
- Obesity
- Advancing age

Although there are case reports of increased LT4 requirements after intestinal bypass surgery, when studied directly LT4 absorption appears to be preserved after Roux-en-Y surgery and in patients undergoing various other gastric bypass procedures. Such reports are consistent with **the ileum being the main site** of LT4 absorption.

26. **c. Older patients require higher doses of LT4**
Ref: Guidelines for the Treatment of Hypothyroidism. American Thyroid Association Task Force on Thyroid Hormone Replacement 2014

- Declining lean body mass or alterations in body composition and/or changes associated with menopause accounted for the reduced LT4 requirement with age.
- Sick patients older than 65 years, who are taking other medications in addition to LT4 for a variety of comorbidities, require lower weight-based doses of LT4 to normalize their serum TSH than do healthy controls of a similar age who are taking only LT4.
- The daily LT4 dose is more dependent on **lean body mass** than total body weight, which explains why the elderly often require lower doses of LT4.

27. **d. All of the above**
Ref: Guidelines for the Treatment of Hypothyroidism. American Thyroid Association Task Force on Thyroid Hormone Replacement 2014

The guidelines say that the adverse effects of thyroid hormone deficiency include:

- Detrimental effects on the serum lipid profile
- Progression of cardiovascular disease

Guidelines recommend that patients with overt hypothyroidism be treated with doses of levothyroxine that are adequate to normalize serum thyrotropin levels, in order to reduce or eliminate these undesirable effects.

28. d. All of the above

Ref: Guidelines for the Treatment of Hypothyroidism. American Thyroid Association Task Force on Thyroid Hormone Replacement 2014

Perceived allergy or intolerance to levothyroxine can be managed by:
- Changing the dose, starting with slow dose and increasing slowly
- Changing the product
- Consideration of gel capsules
- Treating concomitant iron-deficiency anemia
- Consultation with an allergist.

29. a. I, II and III

Ref: Stagnaro-Green A et al; 2011 Guidelines of the American Thyroid Association for the diagnosis and management of thyroid disease during pregnancy and postpartum. Thyroid 21:1081-1125.

The TSH range for each trimester as outlined in the ATA guidelines for the management of thyroid disease during pregnancy:

Trimester	TSH value (mIU/L)
I	0.1–2.5
II	0.2–3.0
III	0.3–3.0

Reference ranges should be defined in healthy TPOAb-negative pregnant women with optimal iodine intake and without thyroid illness.

30. a. 150, 250, 250 mcg

Ref: American Thyroid Association guidelines 2017

- The US Institute of Medicine recommends dietary allowances to be used as goals for individual total daily iodine intake (dietary and supplement) are:
    - 150 mcg/d for women planning a pregnancy
    - 220 mcg/d for pregnant women
    - 290 mcg/d for women who are breastfeeding

The WHO recommends 250 mcg/d for pregnant and lactating women

- This is optimally started 3 months in advance of planned pregnancy.
- In low-resource countries and regions where neither salt iodization nor daily iodine supplements are feasible, a single annual dose of 400 mg of iodized oil for pregnant women and women of childbearing age can be used as a temporary measure to protect vulnerable populations.
- This should not be employed as a long-term strategy or in regions where other options are available.

31. c. 500 mcg

Ref: American Thyroid Association guidelines 2017

Sustained iodine intake from diet and dietary supplements exceeding **500 mcg** daily should be avoided during pregnancy due to concerns about the potential for fetal thyroid dysfunction.

32. c. Good evidence exist to treat subclinical hypothyroidism in women with thyroid autoantibody-negative attempting natural conception

Ref: American Thyroid Association Guidelines 2017

- Evaluation of serum TSH concentration is recommended for all women seeking care for infertility.
- LT4 treatment is recommended for infertile women with overt hypothyroidism who desire pregnancy.
- **Insufficient evidence** exist to determine if LT4 therapy improves fertility in subclinically hypothyroid, thyroid autoantibody-negative women who are attempting natural conception (not undergoing ART). However, administration of LT4 may be considered in this setting given its ability to prevent progression to more significant hypothyroidism once pregnancy is achieved.
- Insufficient evidence exists to determine whether LT4 therapy improves the success of pregnancy following ART in TPOAb-positive euthyroid women. However, administration of LT4 to TPOAb-positive euthyroid women undergoing ART may be considered given its potential benefits in comparison to its minimal risk. In such cases, 25–50 mcg of LT4 is a typical starting dose.
- Insufficient evidence exists to determine if LT4 therapy improves fertility in nonpregnant, thyroid autoantibody-positive euthyroid women who are attempting natural conception.
- Subclinically hypothyroid women undergoing IVF or intracytoplasmic sperm injection (ICSI) should be treated with LT4. The goal of treatment is to achieve a TSH concentration <2.5 mU/L.
- Glucocorticoid therapy is not recommended for thyroid autoantibody-positive euthyroid women undergoing ART.

CHAPTER 14

Endocrinology of Endometriosis

Multiple Choice Questions

1. Which of the following statements is incorrect regarding endometriosis?
   a. Overall prevalence is 3–10%
   b. Mean age at diagnosis 25-35 years
   c. Smoking decreases risk
   d. There is direct relationship between endometriosis and BMI

2. All of the following can lead to endometriosis in a teenager, an age when endometriosis is rare, *except:*
   a. Turner syndrome
   b. Mullerian anomalies
   c. Transverse vaginal septum
   d. Imperforate hymen

3. Risk factors for endometriosis, all *except:*
   a. Early menarche   b. Menorrhagia
   c. Polymenorrhea   d. Nulliparity

4. Which theory holds that endometrial tissue shed during menstruation is transported via fallopian tubes into peritoneal cavity where it is implanted on the surface of pelvic organs?
   a. Sampson's theory
   b. Halban theory
   c. Induction theory
   d. Direct implantation theory

5. Which of the following can not be explained by Sampson's theory?
   a. Endometriosis in Mullerian anomalies
   b. Endometriomas
   c. Endometriosis in premenarcheal girls
   d. Rectovaginal endometriosis

6. Prevalence of endometriosis in 1st degree relative of affected women over general population is increased by how many folds?
   a. 7 times   b. 5 times
   c. Doubles   d. No genetic relation

7. Which of the following statements is incorrect?
   a. Endometriosis is associated with changes in both cell mediated and humoral immunity
   b. Ectopic endometrium is resistant to apoptosis
   c. Impaired scavenger function is seen in endometriosis
   d. There is no difference in ectopic and eutopic endometrium

8. Ectopic endometriotic tissue shows progesterone resistance and is characterized by:
   a. High local aromatase activity, low 17β HSD activity
   b. High local aromatase activity, high 17β HSD activity
   c. Low local aromatase activity, low 17β HSD activity
   d. Low local aromatase activity, high 17β HSD activity

9. Most common symptom associated with endometriosis:
   a. Menorrhagia   b. Dysmenorrhea
   c. Dyspareunia   d. Dyschezia

10. The pain associated with endometriosis has been attributed to:
    a. Focal bleeding from endometriotic implants
    b. Action of inflammatory cytokines in peritoneal cavity
    c. Infiltration of nerves in pelvic floor
    d. All

11. Which of the following is incorrect regarding dysmenorrhea observed in endometriosis?
    a. Dysmenorrhea begins before onset of menstrual flow and persists throughout menses
    b. Deeply infiltrating disease may be associated with dyschezia
    c. The severity of symptoms correlate with severity of endometriosis
    d. It is the most common complaint

12. Which of the following is least likely the characteristic of ovarian endometrioma?
    a. Cystic structure with internal septations
    b. Low level internal echoes
    c. Crisp echogenic capsule
    d. Solid areas

13. Gold standard for diagnosis of endometriosis:
    a. Laparoscopy with histologic examination
    b. Laparoscopy
    c. MRI
    d. Transrectal sonography

14. Progestins act as powerful antiestrogen by one of the following mechanisms *except*:
    a. Inhibition of 17β-hydroxysteroid dehydrogenase
    b. Stimulation of sulfotransferase
    c. Inhibiting estrogen's induction of its own receptors
    d. Suppression of estrogen mediated transcription of oncogenes

15. OCPs prevent relapse in case of endometriosis when given postoperatively by one of the following mechanisms:
    I. Ovulation inhibition
    II. Reduction in amount of menstrual flow
    III. Inhibition of uterine contractility
    IV. Modifications in tubal function, thickening of endosalpingeal mucous
    a. I, II & III
    b. I, II, III & IV
    c. I & II
    d. I only

16. Which of the following support coelomic metaplasia theory?
    1. Endometriosis in men
    2. Endometriosis in adolescent girl in absence of Mullerian anomalies
    3. Endometriosis in prepubertal girl
    4. Endometriosis in women who never menstruated
    a. 1, 2, 3
    b. 1, 2, 3, 4
    c. 2 and 4
    d. 1 only

17. Which of the following statements not true regarding endometriosis?
    a. Medical therapies are effective against endometriosis in patients with infertility
    b. Continuous OCP treatment has been dubbed "pseudopregnancy"
    c. GnRH treatment has been dubbed "pseudomenopause" or "medical oophorectomy"
    d. Luteinized unruptured follicle syndrome can be seen in endometriosis

18. Which of the following theory does not explain etiology of endometriosis?
    a. Coelomic metaplasia
    b. Retrograde menstruation
    c. Mendelian theory
    d. Vascular or lymphatic transport

19. Which of the following statements is incorrect regarding CA-125 measurements in endometriosis?
    a. CA-125 has sensitivity of 80% in detecting endometriosis
    b. Cell surface antigen expressed by derivatives of the coelomic epithelium
    c. Levels over 65 IU/mL are more likely to be associated with dense omental adhesions, ruptured endometriomas, or cul-de-sac obliteration.
    d. A sustained elevation of serum CA-125 after surgical treatment predicts a relatively poor prognosis

20. Occult vaginal bleeding is thought to be the antecedent event for pelvic endometriosis which occurs in majority of neonates but in how many neonates overt bleeding is observed?
    a. 15%
    b. 10%
    c. 5%
    d. 1%

21. Which of the following is not source of estradiol for endometriotic tissue?
    a. Ovary
    b. Adrenal gland
    c. Fat and skin
    d. Local production in endometriotic tissue

22. Which of the following is most common complaint in adolescent endometriosis?
    a. Acyclic pain only
    b. Cyclic pain only
    c. Both acyclic and cyclic pain
    d. Gastrointestinal pain

23. Which of the following is correct about deep endometriosis?
    a. Rapidly progressive disease
    b. Recurrent disease
    c. Mostly present as single nodule
    d. Also known as adenomyosis interna

24. First line drug therapy for pain management in endometriosis:
    a. NSAIDs
    b. OCPs
    c. Progestins
    d. GnRH analogues

Questions Based on Recent Guidelines

25. Which of the following is correct regarding endometriosis as per ESHRE?
    a. Usefulness of 3D sonography to diagnose rectovaginal endometriosis is not well established
    b. Usefulness of MRI to diagnose peritoneal endometriosis is not well established
    c. Use of immunological biomarkers, including CA-125, in plasma, urine or serum to diagnose endometriosis is not recommended
    d. All are true

26. Which of the following is incorrect regarding GnRH analogue usage in endometriosis?
    a. GnRH agonists can be used as one of the options for reducing endometriosis-associated pain
    b. Hormonal add-back therapy should be added to GnRH agonist therapy, to prevent bone loss and hypoestrogenic symptoms
    c. Hormone add-back therapy is known to reduce the effect of GnRH agonist therapy
    d. No specific GnRHa can be recommended over another in relieving endometriosis-associated pain

27. Orally active, non-peptide GnRH antagonist used for endometriosis associated pain:
    a. Elagolix   b. Cetrorelix
    c. Ganirelix   d. Rimonabant

28. Which does not hold true regarding surgery in endometriosis?
    a. Ablation and excision of peritoneal disease are thought to be equally effective for treatment of endometriosis-associated pain
    b. LUNA is recommended as an additional procedure to conservative surgery to decrease pain
    c. Presacral neurectomy (PSN) is effective additional procedure to conservative surgery to reduce endometriosis-associated midline pain
    d. When endometriosis is identified at laparoscopy, surgical treatment is recommended

29. Which of the following are true for endometriotic cystectomy?
    a. Cystectomy is recommended instead of drainage and coagulation
    b. Cystectomy is preferred over CO_2 laser vaporization
    c. Bilateral cystectomy runs risk of premature ovarian insufficiency
    d. All

30. False statement related to endometriosis surgery:
    a. Use of oxidised regenerated cellulose prevents adhesion formation
    b. Icodextrin after operative laparoscopy for endometriosis to prevent adhesion formation is not recommended
    c. Preoperative hormonal treatment improves outcome of surgery for pain in women with endometriosis
    d. Postoperative hormonal therapy prolong symptom-free interval and prevent recurrence of symptoms

31. Which of the following is not an indication for cystectomy prior to ART?
    a. Inaccessible ovary
    b. To improve fertility
    c. Pain
    d. Suspected rupture or torsion of cyst

32. Which of the following is incorrect regarding dienogest in endometriosis?
    a. Steroidal fourth-generation selective progestin
    b. Anti-proliferative and anti-inflammatory effects on endometriotic lesions
    c. More adverse effect on metabolic profile
    d. At a dose of 2 mg per day, ovulation is inhibited but ovarian hormone production is not completely suppressed

33. Which of the following is incorrect regarding medical management of endometriosis?
    a. DMPA-SC 104 is effective in reducing endometriosis-associated pain
    b. DMPA-SC 104 is associated with greater decline in BMD as compared to DMPA-IM 150
    c. Ovulation may be inhibited for up to 12 months with DMPA-IM 150
    d. LNG-IUS may be specially useful for deep infiltrating rectovaginal endometriosis

34. SERMs have tissue-selective effects, acting as ER agonists in bone, but as ER antagonists in breast and uterus. Which of the following is selective estrogen receptor modulator?
    a. Bazedoxifene   b. Asoprisnil
    c. Fulvestrant   d. Resveratrol

35. Endometriosis is a multifactorial disease in which angiogenesis seems to be involved. Which of the following are antiangiogenic agents that can be of help in medical management of endometriosis?
    a. Parecoxib   b. Rapamycin
    c. Cabergoline   d. All

Answer with Explanations

1. **d. There is direct relationship between endometriosis and BMI**

    Ref: Speroff 8th/ed p 1221; Yen & Jaffe's 8th/ed p 610
    - The true overall prevalence of endometriosis is unknown, primarily because surgery is the only reliable method for diagnosis.
    - The prevalence of asymptomatic endometriosis is:
        - Women seeking elective sterilization: 1-7%
        - Women of reproductive age with pelvic pain: 12-32%
        - Infertile women: 9-50%
        - Teens with chronic pelvic pain or dysmenorrhea: 50%
        - The overall prevalence of endometriosis in reproductive aged women probably is between 3% and 10%.
    - The mean age at time of diagnosis of endometriosis ranges between 25 and 35 years.
    - The prevalence of endometriosis is **inversely** related to body mass index.

2. **a. Turner syndrome**

    Ref: Speroff 8th/ed p 1221

    Endometriosis is rare in premenarcheal girls but may be identified in half or more of the adolescents and young women under 20 with complaints of chronic pelvic pain or dyspareunia. Most cases in young women are associated with
    - Mullerian anomalies
    - Cervical agenesis
    - Vaginal obstruction

    Fewer than 5% of women who require surgery for endometriosis are postmenopausal. Most have history of receiving estrogen therapy.

3. **b. Menorrhagia**

    Ref: Speroff 8th/ed p 1222

    ## Risk Factors for Endometriosis
    - Early menarche
    - Polymenorrhea
    - Black race
    - Low BMI
    - Low parity
    - Number of years since last childbirth
    - Alcohol
    - Caffeine
    - Exposure to polychlorinated biphenyl or dioxin
    - Prenatal exposure to DES

    ## Protective Factors
    - High parity
    - Prolonged periods of lactation
    - Regular exercise
    - Smoking

    The correlation between the risk of disease and volume or duration of menses is less consistent.

4. **a. Sampson's theory**

    Ref: Speroff 8th/ed p 1222

    Sampson's theory also known as retrograde menstruation and implantation theory holds that endometrial tissue shed during menstruation is transported via fallopian tubes into peritoneal cavity where it implants on the surface of pelvic organs.

5. **c. Endometriosis in premenarcheal girls**

    Ref: Yen & Jaffe's 8th/ed p 615
    - The coelomic metaplasia theory holds that endometriosis results from spontaneous metaplastic change in mesothelial cells derived from coelomic epithelium (located in peritoneum and pleura).
    - The induction theory is a variation on the same theme and envisions that coelomic metaplasia is induced by exposure to menstrual effluent or other stimuli.
    - Endometriosis in premenarcheal girls can be explained by spontaneous or induced coelomic metaplasia.

6. **a. 7 times**

    Ref: Malinak LR et al. Am J Obstet Gynecol 1980
    - Endometriosis is **six to seven times** more prevalent among the first degree relatives of affected women than in general population.
    - Predisposition to the disease is inherited as a **complex genetic trait** for which the phenotype reflects interactions between allelic variants of susceptibility genes and environmental factors.

7. **d. There is no difference in ectopic and eutopic endometrium**

    Ref: Yen & Jaffe's 8th/ed p 615
    - Endometriosis is associated with changes in both cellular and humoral immunity, suggesting that

impaired immune function may contribute to development of the disease.
- Macrophages are a normal inhabitant of peritoneal fluid and their numbers and activity is much increased in endometriosis.
- Instead of acting as scavengers to eliminate ectopic endometrial cells, activated peritoneal macrophages and circulating monocytes appear to promote disease by secreting growth factors and cytokines that stimulate proliferation of ectopic endometrium and inhibit their scavenger functions.
- Compared to normal endometrium (eutopic), ectopic endometrium differs in 3 distinct ways.
- It produces:
  - High local estrogen (due to presence of aromatase enzyme)
  - High local prostaglandin (due to presence of COX-2 enzyme)
  - Resistant to actions of progesterone.

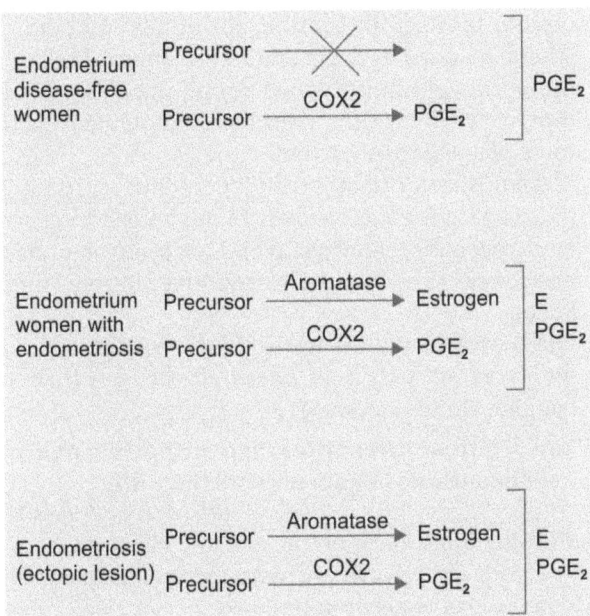

8. a. High local aromatase activity, low 17β HSD activity

Ref: Yen & Jaffe's 8th/ed p 625

In the normal endometrium, progesterone acts as an anti-estrogen in a paracrine fashion, by stimulating retinoic acid production in the stroma, which then induces 17β HSD activity in the epithelium, resulting in the conversion of estradiol to the less potent estrogen, estrone.

However, in endometriotic stromal cells, progesterone does not induce retinoic acid production, and epithelial **17β HSD activity remains low**; tissue estradiol levels are elevated, because **high local aromatase** activity drives production and low 17β HSD activity impairs its metabolism.

9. b. Dysmenorrhea

Ref: Dysmenorrhea and endometriosis. ACOG Committee opinion 2018

Pain is the most common symptom associated with endometriosis.

10. d. All

Ref: Dysmenorrhea and endometriosis. ACOG Committee opinion 2018

Tender nodularity in the cul-de-sac and along the uterosacral ligaments has approximately 85% sensitivity and 50% specificity as a clinical criterion for the diagnosis of deeply infiltrating endometriosis.

The pain associated with endometriosis has been attributed to three primary mechanisms.
1. The direct and indirect effects of focal bleeding from endometriotic implants.
2. The actions of inflammatory cytokines in the peritoneal cavity.
3. Irritation or direct infiltration of nerves in the pelvic floor.

Severe dysmenorrhea and deep dyspareunia are commonly associated symptoms; those having disease adjacent to or within the rectal wall also may have dyschezia.

11. c. The severity of symptoms correlate with severity of endometriosis

Ref: Speroff 8th/ed p 1230

The intensity of pain associated with deeply infiltrating endometriosis relates to the depth of penetration and to the proximity or direct invasion of nerves.

The severity of endometriosis **does not correlate** with the number and severity of symptoms; women with advanced disease may have few or no symptoms and those with minimal or mild disease may have incapacitating pain.

12. d. Solid areas

Ref: NICE guidelines 2017

- Transvaginal ultrasonography can detect ovarian endometriomas, but can not image pelvic adhesions or superficial peritoneal foci of disease.
- Endometriomas can have varying ultrasonographic features but appear typically as cystic structures with diffuse low-level internal echoes surrounded by a **crisp echogenic capsule**. Some have internal septations or thickened nodular walls.

- Solid areas are not seen.
- The GDG recommends that clinicians base the diagnosis of ovarian endometrioma in premenopausal women on the following ultrasound characteristics:
- Ground glass echogenicity.
- One to four compartments.
- No papillary structures with detectable blood flow.

13. a. Laparoscopy with histologic examination

Ref: NICE guidelines 2017

Laparoscopy with histologic examination of excised lesions is the **gold standard** for the diagnosis of endometriosis.

Biopsy is helpful for:
- To confirm the diagnosis of endometriosis
- To exclude malignancy

The optimal time during the menstrual cycle to perform laparoscopy is not clear, but to avoid under-diagnosis, surgery generally should not be performed during or within 3 months after hormonal medical treatment.

The GDG recommends that clinicians perform a laparoscopy to diagnose endometriosis, although evidence is lacking that a positive laparoscopy without histology proves the presence of disease.

The GDG recommends that clinicians confirm a positive laparoscopy by histology, since positive histology confirms the diagnosis of endometriosis, even though negative histology does not exclude it.

The GDG recommends that clinicians obtain tissue for histology in women undergoing surgery for ovarian endometrioma and/or deep infiltrating disease, to exclude rare instances of malignancy.

14. a. Inhibition of 17β hydroxysteroid dehydrogenase

Ref: Speroff 8th/ed p 1229

Progestins act as powerful antiestrogen by the following mechanisms:
- **Stimulate 17β-hydroxysteroid dehydrogenase** and **sulfotransferase** activity, the enzymes that work in concert to convert estradiol to estrone sulfate which is rapidly cleared from the body.
- It antagonize estrogen action by inhibiting estrogen's induction of its own receptors.
- Suppression of estrogen mediated transcription of oncogenes

Together, these actions explain anti-mitotic, growth limiting effects of progesterone and progestins on endometrium.

15. b. I, II, III & IV

Ref: Yen & Jaffe's 8th/ed p 635

OCPs work by:
- Ovulation inhibition
- Reduction in amount of menstrual flow
- Inhibition of uterine contractility
- Modifications in tubal function, thickening of endosalpingeal mucous

Ovulation should be inhibited until conception is desired.

16. b. 1, 2, 3, 4

Ref: Speroff 8th/ed p 1223

Endometriosis in following conditions can be explained by coelomic metaplasia theory:
- Endometriosis in a premenarcheal girl
- In women who never have menstruated
- In adolescent girls having had relatively few menstrual cycles
- Because intact endometrial cells have no access to the thorax in the absence of an anatomical defect, the implantation theory cannot explain cases of pleural and pulmonary endometriosis (almost all of which occur on the right side)
- Metaplasia in the pleura (derived from the coelomic epithelium, like the peritoneum and the Müllerian ducts), induced by steroid hormones or chemical stimuli released by degenerating endometrial cells into the peritoneal fluid (which communicates with the thoracic cavity via the right hemi-diaphragm), is the more plausible explanation.
- Metaplasia in misintegrated coelomic epithelium (adjacent to the mesenchymal limb buds during early embryogenesis) can explain endometriosis in unusual peripheral sites like the extremities (thumb, thigh, knee).
- Rare cases of endometriosis have been observed in men treated with high doses of estrogen (urinary bladder, abdominal wall)

17. a. Medical therapies are effective against endometriosis in patients with infertility

Ref: NICE guidelines 2017

Medical therapies have no measurable effect on fertility and are not an effective treatment for patients with endometriomas or pelvic adhesions.

18. c. Mendelian theory

Ref: Yen & Jaffe's 8th/ed p 615

Endometriosis does not show Mendelian inheritance.

19. a. CA-125 has sensitivity of 80% in detecting endometriosis

Ref: Yen & Jaffe's 8th/ed p 615

- CA-125 is **transmembrane glycoprotein**, initially identified in serous ovarian carcinomas, circulates at elevated concentrations in women with endometriosis.
- Cutoff values that provide 90% overall specificity have less than 30% sensitivity, and if adjusted to achieve even 50% sensitivity, specificity falls to 70%.

- As a screening test for advanced stages of endometriosis, values associated with 90% specificity have less than 50% sensitivity.
- Overall, the serum CA-125 concentration does not have the necessary sensitivity to be an effective screening test for the diagnosis of endometriosis.
- CA-125 may have utility in monitoring the progression of disease or recurrence during therapy.
- Other biomarkers:
  - IL-6
  - Monocyte chemoattractant protein (MCP-1)
  - Interferon-γ (IFN-γ)
  - ICAM-1

NICE 2017 do not recommend CA125 to diagnose endometriosis.

20. c. 5%.

Ref: Human Reproduction Vol 28; 2013, p 2893-97

Occult vaginal bleeding occurs in majority of neonates, although overt bleeding is estimated to occur in only **5%** of neonates.

- The pathogenetic mechanisms may be different in adolescents and premenarchal girls than in adult.
- Neonates have relatively long cervix in comparison to uterine body.
- Cervix is plugged with mucus.
- The hypothesis: Retrograde neonatal bleeding (due to cervical obstruction by thick mucus in the long neonatal cervix) > The fragments of shed endometrial tissue contain an endometrial epithelial progenitor cell, perivascular mesenchymal stem/stromal cell and niche cells > Rapid adherence to neonatal mesothelium > Invade > Become contiguous with the mesothelial lining > Remain in a quiescent state for ~10 years > Rising estrogen levels during puberty > Reactivation of stem/progenitor cells to initiate growth of endometriosis lesions.

21. b. Adrenal gland

Ref: Yen & Jaffe's 8th/ed p 623

The three sources of estradiol in endometriotic tissue.
1. Ovary,
2. Fat and skin which has aromatase activity,
3. Local production in endometriotic tissue.

22. c. Both acyclic and cyclic pain.

Ref: Laufer et al, J Pediatr Adolesc Gynecol 1997; 10:199

Clinical manifestations in adolescent endometriosis:
- Both **acyclic and cyclic pain**—most common, seen in 63% of the patients
- Acyclic pain only
- Cyclic pain only
- Gastrointestinal pain
- Urinary symptoms
- Irregular menses
- Vaginal discharge

23. c. Mostly presents as single nodule

Ref: Deep endometriosis. Fertil Steril 2012; 98:564-71

Deep Endometriosis

- Defined as **adenomyosis externa**, mostly presents as a **single nodule**, larger than 1 cm in diameter, in the vesicouterine fold or close to the lower 20 cm of the bowel.
- When diagnosed, most nodules are **no longer progressive**.
- In >95% of cases, it is associated with very severe pain and is probably a cofactor in infertility.
- Its prevalence is estimated to be **1-2%**.
- Deep endometriosis is suspected clinically and can be confirmed by ultrasonography or magnetic resonance imaging.
- Contrast enema is useful to evaluate the degree of sigmoid occlusion.
- Excision is feasible in over 90% of cases often requiring suture of the bowel muscularis or full-thickness defects.
- Segmental bowel resections are rarely needed except for sigmoid nodules.
- Deep endometriosis often involves the ureter causing hydronephrosis in some 5% of cases. The latter is associated with 18% ureteral lesions.
- Deep endometriosis surgery is associated with late complications such as late bowel and ureteral perforations, and recto-vaginal and uretero-vaginal fistulas.
- Recurrence of deep endometriosis is rare.

24. a. NSAIDs

Ref: NICE Guidelines 2017

Consider a short trial (3 months) of paracetamol or a NSAID alone or in combination for first line management of endometriosis related pain.

25. d. All are true

Ref: ESHRE Endometriosis Guideline Development Group 2013

26. c. Hormone add-back therapy is known to reduce the effect of GnRH agonist therapy

Ref: ESHRE Endometriosis Guideline Development Group 2013

- Clinicians are recommended to use GnRH agonists (nafarelin, leuprolide, buserelin, goserelin or triptorelin), as one of the options for reducing

endometriosis-associated pain, although evidence is limited regarding dosage or duration of treatment.
- Clinicians are recommended to prescribe hormonal add-back therapy to coincide with the start of GnRH agonist therapy, to prevent bone loss and hypoestrogenic symptoms during treatment.
- This is **not known to reduce the effect** of treatment on pain relief.
- The GDG recommends clinicians to give careful consideration to the use of GnRH agonists in young women and adolescents, since these women may not have reached maximum bone density.

27. **a. Elagolix**
    Ref: *Reproductive Sciences 2014, Vol. 21(11) 1341-51*

Elagolix

- Short-acting, **nonpeptide**, GnRH antagonist, administered **orally**, that unlike injectable depot GnRH agonists and antagonists, produces a **dose-dependent suppression** of ovarian estrogen production, that is, from partial suppression at lower doses to full suppression at higher doses.
- This attribute may provide reduction in endometriosis-associated pain, while minimizing the hypoestrogenic side effects that limit long-term treatment with GnRH agonists.
- Oral administration and a **short half-life** (~6 hours) allows for rapid elimination of elagolix from the body, if treatment needs to be discontinued for any reason.
- ELAGOLIX was approved by FDA for management of moderate-to-severe pain associated with endometriosis on July 23, 2018

Advantages of elagolix over GnRHa
- No flare effect
- Orally active
- Rapid onset (within 24 hours)
- Availability of two doses for individual tailoring of therapy.

28. **b. LUNA is recommended as an additional procedure to conservative surgery to decrease pain**
    Ref: *ESHRE Endometriosis Guideline Development Group 2013*

- When endometriosis is identified at laparoscopy, it is recommended to surgically treat endometriosis, as this is effective for reducing endometriosis-associated pain i.e. **'see and treat'**.
- Ablation or Excision?
    - Ablation and excision of peritoneal disease are thought to be **equally effective** for treatment of endometriosis-associated pain.
    - Excision of lesions could be preferred with regard to the possibility of retrieving samples for **histology**.
    - Ablative techniques are unlikely to be suitable for advanced forms of endometriosis with deep endometriosis component.
- Laparoscopic uterosacral nerve ablation (LUNA) is **not recommended** as an additional procedure to conservative surgery to reduce endometriosis-associated pain
- Presacral neurectomy (PSN) is effective as an additional procedure to conservative surgery to reduce endometriosis-associated midline pain, but it requires a high degree of skill and is a potentially hazardous procedure.

29. **d. All**
    Ref: *ESHRE Endometriosis Guideline Development Group 2013*
- Cystectomy is superior to drainage and coagulation in women with ovarian endometrioma (≥3 cm) with regard to the recurrence of endometriosis-associated pain and the recurrence of endometrioma.
- Cystectomy is probably more effective than CO_2 laser vaporization in women with ovarian endometrioma (≥3 cm) with regard to recurrence of endometrioma.

30. **c. Preoperative hormonal treatment improves outcome of surgery for pain in women with endometriosis**
    Ref: *ESHRE Endometriosis Guideline Development Group 2013*

Preoperative Hormonal Therapy

- The role of preoperative hormonal treatment has been assessed in a Cochrane review that concluded that there was **no evidence of a benefit of preoperative medical therapy** on the outcome of surgery.
- This conclusion is shared by the GDG, but it also acknowledges that in clinical practice, surgeons prescribe preoperative medical treatment with GnRH analogues as this **can facilitate surgery** due to reduced inflammation, vascularization of endometriosis lesions and adhesions.
- From a patient perspective, medical treatment should be offered before surgery to women with painful symptoms **in the waiting period** before the surgery can be performed, with the purpose of reducing pain before, not after, surgery.

Postoperative Hormonal Therapy
- Postoperative hormonal therapy may not improve the outcome of surgery but is an important adjunct to surgery to prolong the symptom-free interval and prevent recurrence of symptoms.

31. **b. To improve fertility**

    ESHRE Endometriosis Guideline Development Group 2013

- Laparoscopic ovarian cystectomy in women with unilateral endometriomas before ART may not be useful in improving cycle outcome.
- In women with endometrioma larger than 3 cm, the GDG recommends clinicians only to consider cystectomy prior to assisted reproductive technologies to improve endometriosis-associated **pain** or the **accessibility** of follicles.
- The GDG recommends that clinicians counsel women with endometrioma regarding the risks of **reduced ovarian function** after surgery and the possible loss of the ovary.
- The decision to proceed with surgery should be considered carefully if the woman has had previous ovarian surgery.

32. **c. More adverse effect on metabolic profile**

    Ref: Fertility and sterility Vol 107, March 2017

Dienogest

- Steroidal **fourth-generation** selective progestin
- Anti-proliferative and anti-inflammatory effects on endometriotic lesions
- **Less** adverse effect on metabolic profile due to **lack of androgenic side effects**
- At a dose of **2 mg per day**, ovulation is inhibited but ovarian hormone production is not completely suppressed.

33. **b. DMPA-SC 104 is associated with greater decline in BMD as compared to DMPA-IM 150**

    Ref: Fertil Steril 2006;85:314 –25

DMPA-SC 104

- Reduces endometriosis-associated pain as effectively as leuprolide with less decline in BMD.
- Compared with DMPA-IM 150, DMPA-SC 104 users experience **smaller** median percentage declines in BMD.
- Ovulation may be inhibited for up to 12 months with DMPA-IM 150 usage.

LNG-IUS

- LNG-IUS reduces endometrial proliferation and stimulates apoptosis in endometriotic tissue.
- LNG-IUS offers advantages that it does not provoke hypoestrogenism and requires only a single medical intervention every 5 years.
- It may be specially useful in cases of deep infiltrating rectovaginal endometriosis.
- LNG-IUS reduced cell proliferation, PRA and ER-a expression and increased Fas expression in eutopic and ectopic endometrium of patients with endometriosis.

34. **a. Bazedoxifene**

    Ref: Flores VA et al. Obstet Gynecol. 2018.

- SERMs have **tissue-selective effects**, acting as ER agonists in bone, but as ER antagonists in breast and uterus.

SERM bazedoxifene antagonizes estrogen-induced uterine endometrial tissue.

These drugs can also be associated with an increased incidence of venous thromboembolic events, vasomotor symptoms and sometimes stroke, reinforcing need of safety studies before their introduction to endometriosis therapeutic arsenal.

35. **d. All**

    Ref: Human Reproduction Update. Vol 18, 2012, p 682-702

Endometriosis is a multifactorial disease in which angiogenesis seems to be involved.

VEGF may be involved in progress of ectopic lesions in endometriosis.

- Romidepsin—inhibitor of VEGF gene transcription
- Parecoxib—a selective COX-2 inhibitor
- Rapamycin—antiangiogenic agent
- Epigallocatechin Gallate (EGCG)—major component of green tea, antiangiogenic agent
- Bevacizumab
- Lodamin—oral potent angiogenesis inhibitor
- Cabergoline—VEGFR-2 endocytosis

CHAPTER 15

Fibroids and Reproduction

Multiple Choice Questions

1. **Most common tumor of the reproductive tract:**
   a. Fibromyomas
   b. Adenomyomas
   c. Endometriomas
   d. Tuberculomas

2. **Which of the following statements false about fibroids?**
   a. Mostly benign tumors
   b. Polyclonal origin
   c. More common in African decent people
   d. Incidence of 70% in women of reproductive age

3. **Fibroid associated with maximum adverse effects on IVF outcomes:**
   a. FIGO 3
   b. FIGO 6
   c. FIGO 2
   d. FIGO 0

4. **FIGO Type 3 fibroid corresponds to:**
   a. Extracavitary but abutting the endometrium
   b. Extracavitary but not reaching the endometrium
   c. Intramural with submucosal component
   d. Intramural with subserosal component

5. **Fibroids are estimated to be the sole factor for infertility in how many percent cases?**
   a. 1%   b. 5%
   c. 10%   d. 15%

6. **Infertility is associated with myomas in how many percent cases?**
   a. 1-5%   b. 5-10%
   c. 10-15%   d. 15-20%

7. **Mechanisms by which myomas may affect reproductive outcomes, all *except*:**
   a. Interference with sperm transport
   b. Altering endometrial receptivity
   c. Increasing expression of HOXA 10
   d. Altering uterine contractility

8. **Mechanism by which submucosal myomas affect reproductive outcomes?**
   a. Local inflammation caused by mucus ulceration would alter the biochemical characteristics of intrauterine fluids
   b. Submucosal fibroids create a hostile environment for the spermatozoa
   c. Disrupt the endometrial blood supply affecting embryo nidation
   d. All

9. **Which of the following is not true with respect to fibroids?**
   a. Women interested in pregnancy should not be offered uterine artery embolization as a treatment option for uterine fibroids
   b. Posterior uterine incision is preferred to remove fibroids during myomectomy to minimize formation of postoperative adhesions
   c. In unexplained infertility, submucosal fibroids should be removed in order to improve conception and pregnancy rates
   d. A hysterosalpingogram is not an appropriate test to evaluate and classify fibroids

10. **Expression of which of the following genes is altered in endometrial tissue in patients with fibroids?**
    1. HOXA 10
    2. HOXA 11
    3. LIF
    4. Integrin b3
    a. 1, 2 and 4 only   b. 1 only
    c. 1 and 2 only   d. 1, and 3 only

11. **Hereditary leiomyomatosis are most commonly associated with which cancer?**
    a. Breast cancer
    b. Renal cell carcinoma
    c. Endometrial carcinoma
    d. No association with any cancer

12. Incidence of leiomyosarcomas in patients with leiomyomas:
    a. 1%
    b. 5%
    c. 10%
    d. <1%

13. All of the following are associated with less risk of myomas, *except*:
    a. Obesity
    b. Exercise
    c. Smoking
    d. Multiparity

14. Which is the least sensitive method to detect submucosal myomas?
    a. Hysterosalpingo-contrast sonography
    b. Saline infusion sonography
    c. Transvaginal sonography
    d. Hysteroscopy

15. Which of the following is false about red degeneration of fibroids?
    a. Central hemorrhagic infarction of the myoma
    b. Pain is the hallmark of this condition
    c. Associated with leucocytosis
    d. Infectious pathology

16. A 35-year-old multiparous woman presents with complaints of menorrhagia and dysmenorrhea since two years. On per vaginum examination her uterus is uniformly enlarged, 10 weeks size of gravid uterus, tender, firm in consistency. You make diagnosis of fibromyoma uterus. Which of the following go against your diagnosis?
    a. Tender uterus
    b. Uniformly enlarged uterus
    c. Size 10 weeks
    d. Multiparity

17. Which of the following is incorrect for uterine artery embolization as treatment for fibroid uterus?
    a. Ischemic necrosis of myomas
    b. Choice treatment for nulligravida with fibroids
    c. Post-embolization syndrome may present as fever, nausea and vomiting
    d. Day care procedure

18. Hamartomatous polyposis syndrome characterized by leiomyomas as well as other benign tumors like lipomas and hamartomas:
    a. Cowden disease
    b. Bowen disease
    c. Reed disease
    d. Dubowitz disease

19. Cytogenetic rearrangements seen in leiomyomas:
    a. t (12;14)
    b. Trisomy 12
    c. Deletion of 3q
    d. All

20. Which is the best possible way to treat 3 cm FIGO 1 fibroid diagnosed on saline infusion sonography placed in lower one third of uterine cavity with base extending to less than one third of cavity?
    a. Low complexity hysteroscopic myomectomy
    b. High complexity hysteroscopic myomectomy
    c. Open myomectomy
    c. GnRH analogues

21. Which of the following is not true about junctional zone?
    a. Composed of longitudinal and circular smooth-muscle fibers
    b. Hormone dependent zone
    c. Ontogenetically similar to outer myometrium
    d. Thickened in adenomyosis

22. Which of the following hormones play role in growth of fibroids?
    a. Estrogen
    b. Progesterone
    c. Prolactin
    d. All

Answer with Explanations

1. a. Fibromyomas

Ref: Fertil Steril_2017; 108:416-25

Uterine myomas (leiomyomata, fibroids) are the most common tumor of the reproductive tract, with a cumulative incidence of 70% in women of reproductive age.

2. b. Polyclonal origin

Ref: Fertil Steril_2017; 108:416-25

- Fibroids are benign **monoclonal tumors**.
- They are associated with the most severe symptoms in women of **African descent**.
- Compared with Caucasian women with symptomatic myomas, women of African descent typically present at a **younger age** and with a significantly worse myoma burden (larger size and number).

3. d. FIGO 0

Ref: Fertil Steril_ 2018; 109:817-22.

- FIGO 0 is pedunculated submucosal fibroid.
- It is widely recognized that submucosal fibroids are associated with decreased pregnancy rates and implantation rates after IVF treatment.
- Conversely, subserosal fibroids do not appear to affect IVF outcomes.
- The impact of intramural fibroids on the outcome of IVF-ICSI treatment remains incompletely understood, with studies yielding conflicting results.

4. a. Extracavitary but abutting the endometrium

Ref: FIGO Classification system for fibroids 2011

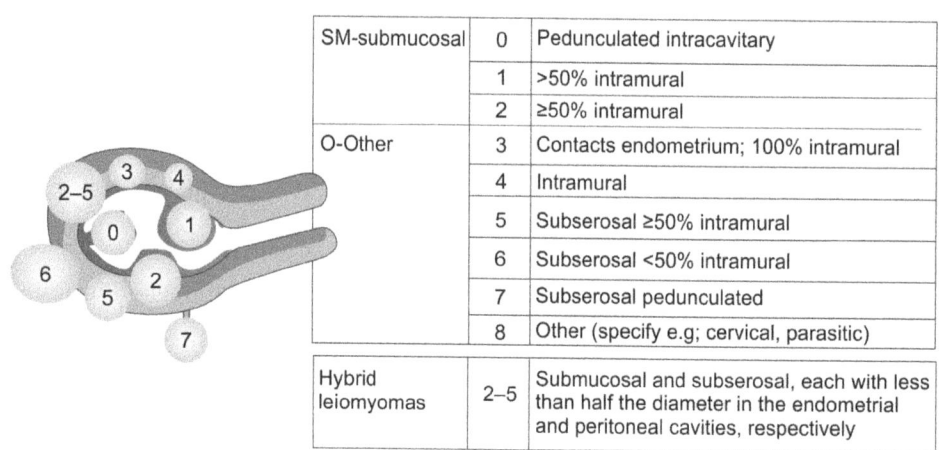

SM-submucosal	0	Pedunculated intracavitary
	1	>50% intramural
	2	≥50% intramural
O-Other	3	Contacts endometrium; 100% intramural
	4	Intramural
	5	Subserosal ≥50% intramural
	6	Subserosal <50% intramural
	7	Subserosal pedunculated
	8	Other (specify e.g; cervical, parasitic)
Hybrid leiomyomas	2-5	Submucosal and subserosal, each with less than half the diameter in the endometrial and peritoneal cavities, respectively

5. a. 1%

Ref: Obstet Gynecol Clin N Am 33 (2006) 145-52

5% to 10% of cases of infertility are associated with myomas. Myomas are estimated to be the **sole factor** for infertility in only **1% to 3%** of cases.

6. b. 5-10%

Ref: Obstet Gynecol Clin N Am 33 (2006) 145-52

5% to 10% of cases of infertility are associated with myomas.

7. c. Increasing expression of HOXA 10

Ref: Obstet Gynecol Clin N Am 33 (2006) 145-52

The mechanisms by which myomas may affect reproductive outcome are as follows:
- Interference with sperm transport or access by:
  - Anatomic distortion of the cervix;
  - Enlarging or deforming the endometrial cavity;
  - Altering the uterine contractility; and
  - Obstructing tubal ostia.
- Implantation failure by:
  - Physically changing the shape of the endometrium;
  - Preventing discharge of intrauterine blood or clots; and
  - Altering the normal endometrial development.

HOXA Genes

- HOXA-10 is a member of the abdominal B subclass of homeobox genes.
- HOXA-10 mRNA expression is necessary for successful endometrial receptivity.

In the secretory phase at the time of implantation, endometrial HOXA-10 mRNA expression is upregulated and improves the endometrial receptivity.

HOXA-10 mRNA expression regulates downstream target genes, which are involved in implantation including integrin b3.

Similar to HOXA-10 mRNA, endometrial HOXA-11 mRNA expression has an important role in endometrial development and implantation.

Concept of Increased Peristalsis

Yoshino et al. using Cine mode, MRI demonstrated **accelerated mid-luteal uterine peristalsis** (defined as ≥2 peristaltic movements in 3 min) in the presence of intramural fibroids and achieved 40% pregnancy rate in this population over 1 year following restoration of normal peristalsis by myomectomy.

8. d. All

Ref: Gynecological Endocrinology, February 2006; 22(2): 106–109

Submucosal fibroids may cause infertility for another series of reasons apart from the one mentioned above.
1. Local inflammation caused by mucus ulceration would alter the biochemical characteristics of intrauterine fluids, creating a hostile environment for the spermatozoa.
2. Submucosal fibroids may disrupt the endometrial blood supply, thus affecting nidation of the embryo.
3. Reduction in levels of certain cytokines mainly IL10 and glycodelin in the midluteal uterine washings of women with submucosal fibroids.

Glycodelin is a progesterone-regulated glycoprotein secreted into uterine luminal cavity by secretory/decidualized endometrial glands and has properties like promoting angiogenesis and suppressing natural killer (NK) cells.

9. b. Posterior uterine incision is preferred to remove fibroids during myomectomy to minimize formation of postoperative adhesions

Ref: SOGC clinical practice guidelines. J Obstet Gynaecol Can 2015;37(3):277–85

SOGC clinical practice guidelines 2015
1. In women with infertility, an effort should be made to adequately evaluate and classify fibroids, particularly those impinging on the endometrial cavity, using transvaginal ultrasound, hysteroscopy, hysterosonography, or magnetic resonance imaging (III-A)
2. Preoperative assessment of submucosal fibroids should include, in addition to an assessment of fibroid size and location within the uterine cavity, evaluation of the degree of invasion of the cavity and thickness of residual myometrium to the serosa. A combination of hysteroscopy and transvaginal ultrasound or hysterosonography are the modalities of choice. (III-B)
3. Submucosal fibroids are managed hysteroscopically. The fibroid size should be <5 cm, although larger fibroids have been managed hysteroscopically, but repeat procedures are often necessary. (III-B)
4. A hysterosalpingogram is not an appropriate exam to evaluate and classify fibroids. (III-D)
5. In women with otherwise unexplained infertility, submucosal fibroids should be removed in order to improve conception and pregnancy rates. (II-2A)
6. Removal of subserosal fibroids is not recommended. (III-D)
7. There is fair evidence to recommend against myomectomy in women with intramural fibroids (hysteroscopically confirmed intact endometrium) and otherwise unexplained infertility, regardless of their size. (II-2D) If the patient has no other options, the benefits of myomectomy should be weighed against the risks, and management of intramural fibroids should be individualized.
8. If fibroids are removed abdominally, efforts should be made to use an **anterior uterine incision** to minimize the formation of postoperative adhesions. (II-2A)
9. Widespread use of the laparoscopic approach to myomectomy may be limited by the technical difficulty of this procedure. Patient selection should be individualized based on the number, size, and location of uterine fibroids and the skill of the surgeon. (III-A)
10. Women, fertile or infertile, seeking future pregnancy should not generally be offered uterine artery embolization as a treatment option for uterine fibroids. (II-3E)

10. a. 1, 2 and 4 only

Ref: Unlu et al. Reproductive Sciences 2015:1-11

- Integrins are heterodimeric integral membrane proteins composed of an α and β chains.
- ITGAV gene encodes the aV protein that is a member of the integrin family.
- Integrin aV has heterodimerized with β3 chain (ITGB3) that is expressed on the luminal and glandular epithelium of the endometrium where facilitates angiogenesis and embryo attachment.
- Its aberrant expression in a variety of reproductive disorders including luteal phase defect, endometriosis, polycystic ovarian syndrome, and tubal disease suggests a critical role for this protein.
- In humans, endometrial leukemia inhibitory factor (LIF) mRNA expression is essential for blastocyst

implantation, and its expression increases in the secretory phase.

Expression of HOXA-10, HOXA-11, ITGB3, ITGAV, and LIF mRNA expression are altered in infertile women with fibromyomas.

11. b. Renal cell carcinoma

Ref: Yen & Jaffe's 8th/ed p 646

Hereditary Leiomyomatosis and Renal Cell Cancer

- This syndrome is **autosomal dominant**.
- Affected families manifest cutaneous leiomyomas and **papillary renal cell carcinoma** (RCC).
- Affected women can have uterine leiomyomas as well as uterine leiomyosarcomas.
- Both malignancies (sarcomas and RCCs) are atypical in their presentation compared with their sporadic counterparts; uterine sarcomas can appear in young premenopausal women, and the papillary RCC is often metastatic at presentation and more likely to be seen in women.
- Two other syndromes with cutaneous and uterine leiomyomas have been described, but lessons from molecular genetics suggest that these are incomplete forms of the hereditary leiomyomatosis and renal cell cancer (HLRCC) syndrome and should be of historical interest only (Reed syndrome or multiple cutaneous and uterine leiomyomas [MCUL]).
- **Fumarate hydratase** (FH), an enzyme that is part of the Krebs tricarboxylic acid cycle, is the gene mutation at 1q 42-43 responsible for HLRCC syndrome.
- Germline mutations appear to result in absent or nonfunctional proteins; thus FH appears to act as a tumor suppressor.
- FH appears to play a role in a small percentage of nonsyndromic leiomyomas seen in white women.

12. d. <1%

Ref: Speroff 8th/ed p 148

- Least common degeneration in leiomyomas: leiomyoma changing to leiomyosarcoma

It is not certain whether leiomyosarcomas arise independently or from leiomyomas. However, the incidence of leiomyosarcomas in patients with leiomyomas is very low (less than 1%).

Gene profiling has not discovered shared abnormalities or a common molecular pathway comparing myomas with leiomyosarcomas.

13. a. Obesity

Ref: Yen & Jaffe's 8th/ed p 643

- Any condition which increases estrogen is associated with increased risk for fibroids.
- Caffeine consumption is **not** noted to be a risk factor for fibroids.

Factors associated with decreased risk	Factors associated with increased risk
Increased parity	Obesity
Increased age at last term birth	Nulligravida
Women with at least two full-term pregnancies	Late childbirth
Smoking	Black race
Leanness	Early menarche
Exercise	Postmenopausal HRT
OCPs	Alcohol, especially beer
Vegetable and fruit intake	Increased red meat or ham consumption
Dietary vitamin A	• In utero DES exposure • Consumption of soy formula in infancy • Low childhood socioeconomic status • Premature birth • Maternal prepregnancy or gestational diabetes

OCPs and Risk of Myomas

The use of oral contraceptives is not associated with an increased risk of uterine myomas, although the Nurses' Health Study reported a slightly increased risk when oral contraceptives were first used in early teenage years.

14. c. Transvaginal sonography

Ref: Vohra R et al. Int J Reprod Contracept Obstet Gynecol. 2017 Oct;6(10):4437-40

Saline infusion sonography is especially helpful for intracavitary abnormalities. So TVS could be supplemented with SCSH for better diagnosis.

Preoperative visualization is important, and mapping of myomas by sonohysterography or magnetic resonance imaging (MRI) is superior to TVS. It is difficult to distinguish between submucosal myomas and endometrial polyps with ultrasonography.

15. d. Infectious pathology

Ref: Speroff 8th/ed p 151

- Red degeneration is due to central infarction of fibroid, so infection is not the etiology, hence antibiotics are not required.
- Main mode of management is fluids and analgesics

Red Degeneration of Fibroid

- Observed during late pregnancy.
- Associated with central hemorrhagic infarction of the myoma.
- Pain is the hallmark of this condition, occasionally associated with rebound tenderness, mild fever, leukocytosis, nausea, and vomiting.
- Usually pain is the only symptom and resolution follows rest and analgesic treatment.

16. a. Tender uterus.

- Uniformly enlarged **tender** uterus goes more in favour of adenomyosis

Adenomyosis

- Ectopic presence of endometrial glands within the myometrium.
- Usually seen in multiparous women.
- Chief presenting complaints are menorrhagia and congestive dysmenorrhea.
- On examination, uterus is mostly less than 12 weeks size, although it can be larger too.
- Uterus is tender in adenomyosis while mostly fibromyomas are nontender, which makes this a differential point.
- Uterus can be uniformly enlarged in both conditions, although most fibromyomas present with irregularly enlarged uterus.

17. b. Choice treatment for nulligravida with fibroids

Ref: Speroff 8th/ed p 154

- UAE should not be offered to women interested in retaining fertility as it decreases chances of conception and increases pregnancy complications in case woman conceives.

Uterine Artery Embolization

- It effectively reduces bleeding, pain, and fibroid size.
- UAE is done under local anesthesia that takes about one hour.
- A catheter is advanced from the femoral artery to the uterine arteries to allow direct injection of polyvinyl particles or gelatin microspheres that occlude the blood flow.
- Myomas undergo necrosis in response to the **transient ischemia**, but normal tissue generates fibrinolysis and survives.
- The procedure is not recommended for large fibroids.
- After 5 years, recurrence of symptoms is about 10% to 25%.
- Post-embolization syndrome—Most patients experience pain, nausea, and low-grade fever with a very high white blood count for 1 to 2 days following the procedure.
- Serious complications include complication-related hysterectomy, amenorrhea, premature menopause, septicemia from uterine infection, bowel obstruction, and pulmonary embolus.
- A significant number of patients with larger myomas acquire intra-abdominal adhesions after the procedure.
- The general recommendation is that embolization should not be performed in women who desire to retain their fertility.

18. a. Cowden disease

Ref: Yen & Jaffe's 8th/ed p 647

Cowden Disease

- This disease is a type of hamartomatous polyposis syndrome characterized by leiomyomas as well as other benign tumors, including lipomas and hamartomas.
- It is **autosomal dominant** in inheritance and involves the candidate gene phosphatase and tensin homologue (PTEN).
- Patients with Cowden disease are at increased risk for endometrial, thyroid, kidney, and colorectal cancers.
- Around 40% of women with Cowden disease are reported to have fibroids.
- Finally, deletions of collagen genes COL4A5 and COL4A6 have also been shown to be associated with a familial syndrome known as diffuse leiomyomatosis with Alport syndrome and rarely with nonsyndromic fibroids.

19. d. All

Ref: Yen & Jaffe's 8th/ed p 646

- Leiomyomas are monoclonal, and each tumor is an independent clonal event.

Cytogenetic Rearrangements and Leiomyomas

Although 40% of fibroids have 46,XX karyotypically normal cells, there are specific karyotypic abnormalities that have been consistent in a number of studies:

Translocations	t(12;14);
Trisomy	12
Rearrangements	6p, 10q, and 13q
Deletion	3q, 7q, and 1p

High-mobility-group protein A2 (HMGA2, formerly called HMGI-C) is an architectural transcription factor located on chromosome 12 that is involved in the pathogenesis of fibroids with t(12;14).

20. a. Low complexity hysteroscopic myomectomy

Ref: Kamini Rao. 2nd/ed p 384

Lasmar Presurgical Classification or STEP-W Classification

	Size (cm)	Topography	Extension of the base	Penetration	Lateral wall	Total
0	>2 to 5	Low	≤1/3	0		
1	>2 to 5	Middle	>1/3 to 2/3	≤50%	+1	
2	>5	Upper	>2/3	>50%		
Score	+	+	+	+	+	

Score	Group	Complexity and therapeutic options
0 to 4	I	Low complexity hysteroscopic myomectomy
5 to 6	II	High complexity hysteroscopic myomectomy. Consider GnRH use? Consider Two-step hysteroscopic myomectomy.
7 to 9	III	Consider alternatives to the hysteroscopic technique

(STEP-W: Size, Topography, Extension, Penetration, Wall)

Information given in question:
- 3 cm-score 1
- FIGO 1 fibroid- score 1
- Placed in lower one third of uterine cavity—score 0
- Base extending to less than one third of cavity—score 0
- No comment on wall in the question.
- Total score: 2

So, this comes under group I; means treatment of choice is low complexity hysteroscopic myomectomy.

21. c. Ontogenetically similar to outer myometrium

Ref: Chassang et al. American Journal of Roentgenology · May 2011

- Ontogenetically, JZ has similar origin as endometrium.

Junctional Zone (JZ)

- Also referred to as inner myometrium, archimyometrium or stratum subvasculare is visible as a hypoechogenic subendometrial halo.
- This layer is composed of longitudinal and circular closely packed smooth-muscle fibers.
- It is a hormone dependent zone located between the endometrium and myometrium passing through cyclical changes in its thickness.
- The effect of the hormonal cycle on this zone of muscular tissue is explained in part by the uterine ontogeny; that is, it appears that cells of the endometrium and cells of the junctional zone have a common Müllerian origin, whereas the outer myometrium is of a non-Müllerian, mesenchymal origin. As a result, the outer myometrium presents little or no dependence on hormonal stimulation and there is no significant variation in its thickness during the reproductive cycle.
- In adenomyosis, the junctional zone is significantly thicker, passing over its hallmark—12 mm.
- In the non-pregnant uterus, contractions commence exclusively from the junctional zone and participate in the regulation of various reproductive events, such as menstrual shedding, transport of the sperm and embryos.

22. d. All

Ref: Yen & Jaffe's 8th/ed p 647

- **Prolactin** appears to play an important role in myoma pathogenesis.
- In vitro studies suggest that it is mitogenic for leiomyoma and myometrial smooth muscle cells and that the prolactin receptor is present in these tissues, setting up an autocrine or local endocrine system.
- Additionally, agents that appear to cause clinical regression of uterine leiomyomas also appear to decrease prolactin production in vitro.

CHAPTER 16

Infertility

Multiple Choice Questions

1. Evaluation for infertility must be started after how many months of unprotected intercourse for women age <35, 35–40 and > 40, respectively?
   a. 12, 6, 3
   b. 24, 6, 6
   c. 12, 12, 6
   d. 24, 3, 3

2. Which of the following statement is correct about infertility?
   a. Fecundity is the probability of achieving a pregnancy in one menstrual cycle
   b. Fecundability is approximately 0.25 in healthy young couples
   c. Fecundability is the ability to achieve a pregnancy that results in a live birth
   d. Occult pregnancy is defined when there is only biochemical evidence of pregnancy without clinical evidence

3. Which of the following is incorrect regarding reproductive aging?
   a. Follicular phase inhibin B levels increase with reproductive aging
   b. Follicular phase becomes shorter with reproductive aging
   c. Rise in FSH levels precedes any apparent rise in LH
   d. Rise in FSH levels precedes any measurable decrease in estradiol levels

4. Which of the following do not have clear cause effect relationship with infertility?
   a. Azoospermia
   b. Bilateral tubal block
   c. Endometriosis
   d. Anovulation

5. Initial infertility evaluation of an infertile couple involves all *except*:
   a. Documentation of competent ovulation
   b. Semen analysis
   c. Documentation of tubal patency
   d. Laparoscopy

6. Recent definition of unexplained infertility includes all *except*:
   a. Normal ovulatory function
   b. Normal semen analysis
   c. At least one patent Fallopian tube
   d. Normal uterine cavity

7. Tests to assess the ovarian follicle pool include:
   1. Anti-Müllerian hormone (AMH)
   2. Follicle-stimulating hormone (FSH) and estradiol on menstrual cycle day 3
   3. Ovarian antral follicle count (AFC) by ultrasound
   4. FSH and estradiol on cycle days 3 and 10 of a clomiphene citrate challenge test (CCCT)
   a. 1 & 2
   b. 1, 2, 3 & 4
   c. 2 & 3
   d. 1 & 3

8. Which of the following is most important determinant of reproductive outcome?
   a. Age
   b. AMH
   c. AFC
   d. Basal FSH

9. Which of the following does not come under term Assisted reproductive technology?
   a. Intracytoplasmic sperm injection (ICSI)
   b. Assisted hatching (AH)
   c. Preimplantation genetic testing (PGT)
   d. Intrauterine insemination (IUI)

10. Which of the following is poorest prognosis for tubal factor infertility?
    a. Sonologically visible hydrosalpinges
    b. Unilateral hydrosalpinges
    c. Fluid in endometrial cavity
    d. Fluid in POD

11. Which of the following is incorrect regarding endometriosis and infertility?
    a. Aspiration of endometriomas with oocyte retrieval runs increased risk for ovarian abscess
    b. Mild endometriosis can present as unexplained infertility

c. GnRH agonist for 3–6 months before IVF can increase the odds of clinical pregnancy
d. Cumulative pregnancy rates after surgery are more for women with complete cul-de-sac obliteration than in those with endometriomas

12. **Mechanisms by which hydrosalpinx impair implantation, all *except*:**
    a. Embryotoxic properties of hydrosalpinx fluid
    b. Decreased expression of integrin αvβ3
    c. Leakage of hydrosalpinx fluid leading to embryo disposal
    d. Reflux phenomenon leading to increased cervix to fundus peristalsis

13. **Advantages of natural cycle IVF include all *except*:**
    a. Requires little medications
    b. Less risks for multiple pregnancy
    c. Less risk for ovarian hyperstimulation syndrome
    d. Less cancellation rates

14. **Which is incorrect about Bologna criteria?**
    a. Age > 35 years
    b. History of prior poor response to gonadotropins using a conventional stimulation protocol (≤3 oocytes)
    c. AMH below 0.5 to 1.1 ng/mL
    d. AFC less than 5 to 7 follicles

15. **Which of the following are adjunctive medications for poor responders?**
    a. DHEA
    b. Coenzyme Q10
    c. Growth hormone
    d. All

16. **In which of the following conditions natural conception can be allowed in HIV serodiscordant couple?**
    a. HIV-positive man on HAART for over six months
    b. Undetectable levels of HIV RNA in the plasma (<50 copies/mL)
    c. Sexual intercourse limited to peak fertility period
    d. All

17. **Which antiretroviral medication has maximal adverse effects on semen parameters?**
    a. Zidovudine
    b. Efavirenz
    c. Abacavir
    d. Emtricitabine

18. **Which of the following is incorrect regarding empty follicle syndrome?**
    a. Rates of EFS after GnRHa are 1.4% to 3.5%
    b. Rates of EFS with hCG trigger is 0.1–2%
    c. Repeat trigger with hCG and oocyte retrieval 35 hours later can be done
    d. EFS is likely when LH <35 IU/L and progesterone ≤3.5 ng/mL measured 8–12 hours after GnRHa trigger

19. **In GnRH-agonist cycles, pituitary downregulation is confirmed with serum estradiol and progesterone levels after menses has begun as following, respectively:**
    a. 50 pg/mL and < 1.0 ng/mL
    b. 100 pg/mL and < 1.0 ng/mL
    c. 50 pg/mL and < 1.5 ng/mL
    d. 30 pg/mL and < 1.5 ng/mL

20. **In which of the following conditions GnRH agonist trigger will be preferred?**
    a. Endometriosis
    b. PCOS
    c. DOR
    d. Previous poor responder

21. **In which of the following conditions hCG trigger will be preferred?**
    a. Hypothalamic dysfunction
    b. Prolonged OCP usage
    c. Baseline LH <0.1 MIU/mL
    d. All

22. **In which of the following conditions GnRH agonist trigger will not be preferred over hCG trigger?**
    a. PCOS
    b. Ovum donor cycles
    c. Hypogonadotropic hypogonadism
    d. Fertility preservation cycles

23. **Oligospermia below which genetic testing for karyotyping and Y chromosome microdeletions must be done?**
    a. < 15 million/mL
    b. < 10 million/mL
    c. < 5 million/mL
    d. <1 million/mL

24. **Life-threatening complication of neurostimulatory methods used to induce ejaculation in men with neurogenic anejaculation:**
    a. Stroke
    b. Autonomic dysreflexia
    c. Myocardial ischemia
    d. Paralysis

25. **Sweet spot refers to LH:FSH ratio of:**
    a. 0.3 to 0.6
    b. 0.3 to 0.9
    c. 0.6 to 0.9
    d. 0.1 to 0.3

26. **Which of the following is incorrect regarding kisspeptins?**
    a. Used for ovulation induction
    b. Kisspeptin is a peptide hormone
    c. Acts upstream of GnRH
    d. Prevents OHSS

27. Which of the following is not true as per ASCO guidelines regarding male fertility preservation?
    a. Sperm cryopreservation is effective method of fertility preservation
    b. Hormonal gonadoprotection in men is successful in preserving fertility
    c. There is higher risk of genetic damage in sperm collected after initiation of therapy
    d. Onco TESE is sperm retrieval which testicular surgery for testicular tumors

28. Which of the following methods of fertility preservation in females is considered experimental as per recent ASCO guidelines?
    a. Ovarian tissue cryopreservation
    b. Embryo cryopreservation
    c. Oocyte cryopreservation
    d. Conservative gynecologic surgery

29. Ovarian stimulation protocols used for fertility preservation in females:
    a. Follicular start
    b. Luteal halt protocol
    c. Late follicular start
    d. Any of the protocols can be used

30. Which of the following is not true as per ASCO guidelines regarding female fertility preservation?
    a. Ovarian tissue cryopreservation and transplantation is the only method available in children
    b. Oophoropexy can be offered when pelvic irradiation is performed as cancer treatment
    c. Ovarian suppression with GnRHa is well recognized method for fertility preservation
    d. ASRM no longer deems oocyte cryopreservation experimental

31. Which of the following drugs is given along with gonadotropins while stimulating cancer patients?
    a. Letrozole
    b. Clomiphene
    c. Ecosprin
    d. Prednisone

32. Which of the following is not true about ART and risk of ovarian tumors?
    a. The risk of ovarian cancer after ART treatment differs as per cause of infertility
    b. ART done for male factor or UEI are not associated with increased risk of ovarian cancer
    c. Association of ART and ovarian cancer was strongest in first years after ART
    d. Risk is increased to 10-fold in ART-treated women with endometriosis

33. Organ of Rosenmuller represents:
    a. Cranial end of Wolffian body
    b. Caudal end of Wolffian body
    c. Cranial end of Mullerian duct
    d. Caudal end of Mullerian duct

34. Which of the following is not true regarding Organ of Rosenmuller?
    a. Represents cranial end of the Wolffian body
    b. The tubules are lined by cubical cells
    c. Consists of horizontal tubules in the mesovarium and mesosalpinx
    d. Homologous to epididymis in male

35. Global prevalence of PCOS as per AE-PCOS 2006 criteria:
    a. 1% to 5%
    b. 5% to 10%
    c. 10% to 15%
    d. 15% to 25%

36. Baseline LH levels sufficient to provide maximal stimulation to thecal cells beyond which further increase is not associated with better ovarian stimulation results:
    a. 0.5 to 1 IU
    b. 1 to 1.5 IU
    c. 1 to 5 IU
    d. >5 IU

37. Live birth rates correlate with number of oocytes retrieved and are maximal when.... oocytes are obtained in fresh embryo transfer cycles:
    a. 10
    b. 20
    c. 15
    d. 5

38. Which of the following statements is incorrect regarding ovarian stimulation for IVF cycles?
    a. GnRH antagonist versus agonist cotreatment show no difference in live birth rates
    b. Monitoring of ovarian stimulation with ultrasound only or in combination with serum estradiol show no difference regarding clinical pregnancy rates
    c. Addition of DHEA/T during ovarian stimulation show increased live birth/ongoing pregnancy rates
    d. Luteal phase supplementation is not required following the late follicular phase administration of GnRH antagonist

39. Pregnancy rate per initiated cycle in natural cycle IVF are:
    a. 1–2%
    b. 3–4%
    c. 5–10%
    d. 10–12%

40. Clinical ascites with oliguria in presence of hematocrit 48% is suggestive of:
    a. Mild OHSS
    b. Moderate OHSS
    c. Severe OHSS
    d. Critical OHSS

Answer with Explanations

1. a. 12, 6, 3

Ref: Yen & Jaffe's 8th/ed p 556

- As per ASRM infertility is defined as the inability to conceive after 12 months of frequent coitus.
- **Fertility** is defined as the capacity to conceive and produce offspring.
- **Infertility** is the state of a diminished capacity to conceive and bear offspring.
- In contrast to **sterility**, infertility is not an irreversible state.
- The current clinical definition of infertility is the inability to conceive **after 12 months** of frequent coitus. Infertility prevalence is approximately 13% among women and 10% among men.
- Since the fertility potential of the female partner decreases after 35 years of age, most authorities recommend initiating an infertility evaluation after **6 months** of attempting conception in women 35 to 40 years of age and after **3 months** in women over 40 years of age.
- Women with known causes of infertility, such as amenorrhea, should immediately start an evaluation to assess the cause and plan the treatment.

2. b. Fecundability is approximately 0.25 in healthy young couples

Ref: Yen & Jaffe's 8th/ed p 556-57

- Fecundability, a population estimate of the probability of achieving pregnancy in one menstrual cycle, is a valuable clinical and scientific concept because it creates a framework for the **quantitative analysis** of fertility potential.

A few definitions:

Fecundability: Probability of achieving a pregnancy in one menstrual cycle.

Fecundity: Ability to achieve a pregnancy that results in a **live birth** based on attempts at conception in one menstrual cycle.

Fecundability is approximately **0.25** in healthy young couples just beginning attempts at conception.

Occult pregnancy: Pregnancy that terminates so soon after implantation that there was no clinical suspicion of its existence.

Chemical pregnancy: A blood or urine human chorionic gonadotropin (hCG) assay demonstrates the presence of a pregnancy, but no clinical evidence of the pregnancy is detectable by ultrasound.

Of all clinical pregnancies, approximately 20% result in a spontaneous abortion.

Of all pregnancies, approximately 30% are lost—either as occult, chemical, or clinical spontaneous abortions.

- I always had this confusion between fecund*ability* and fecund*ity*, even this came in my NEET-SS too, so how I remembered this as *ity* word in hindi means *the end*, so fecundity is the end because we have achieved live birth, so it is easy to remember this way.

3. a. Follicular phase inhibin B levels increase with reproductive aging

Ref: Speroff 8th/ed p 1143

- Inhibin B is derived primarily from smaller antral follicles, so as follicle number decreases, inhibin also decreases.
- Circulating follicular phase inhibin B levels decrease as or even before FSH concentrations begin to increase.
- Inhibin A levels also decline, but only in the later stages of reproductive aging, after the onset of menstrual irregularity.
- Both inhibins selectively inhibit pituitary FSH secretion.
- Consequently, FSH levels rise progressively as inhibin production from smaller cohorts of aging follicles decreases.

4. c. Endometriosis

Ref: Yen & Jaffe's 8th/ed p 557

There are two concepts which should be clear

Concept of cause-effect relationship	Concept of association
Some diseases clearly have a **cause-effect relationship** with infertility	Disease processes where there is no clear cause-effect relationship between disease and infertile state
Example azoospermia, bilateral tubal block and anovulatory state	In these situations, it is preferable to state that there is an **association** between disease condition and infertile state, **causality has not been definitively established**
	Example stage I endometriosis

5. d. Laparoscopy

Ref: Yen & Jaffe's 8th/ed p 558

Primary tests for infertility	• **Documentation of competent ovulation**
	  ○ Midluteal progesterone >3 ng/mL
	  ○ Day 3 FSH or clomiphene challenge test (if female partner >35 years old)
	• **Semen analysis**
	  ○ Volume ≥1.5 mL
	  ○ Concentration ≥15 million/mL
	  ○ Motility ≥32%
	  ○ Morphology ≥4% (using "strict" criteria)
	• **Documentation of tubal patency**
	  ○ Hysterosalpingogram or hysterosalpingo-contrast sonography
	• **Assessment of the uterine cavity**
	  ○ Hysterosalpingogram, hysterosalpingo-contrast sonography, or hysteroscopy

Secondary tests for infertility	• Laparoscopy • Hysteroscopy

6. d. Normal uterine cavity

Ref: RBMO Volume 39 Issue 4 2019

It is estimated that 30–50% of couples presenting for the evaluation of infertility have unexplained infertility.

Unexplained infertility is defined as the absence of identifiable causes for the infertility.

The diagnostic testing required to meet the definition:
1. Normal ovulatory function,
2. Normal semen analysis and
3. At least one patent Fallopian tube.

7. b. 1, 2, 3 & 4

Ref: Yen & Jaffe's 8th/ed p 559

Tests to assess the ovarian follicle pool include measurement of:
- Anti-Mullerian hormone (AMH),
- Follicle-stimulating hormone (FSH) and estradiol on menstrual cycle day 3,
- Ovarian antral follicle count (AFC) by ultrasound, and
- FSH and estradiol on cycle days 3 and 10 of a clomiphene citrate challenge test (CCCT).

8. a. Age

Ref: Speroff 8th/ed p 1141

Age is the most important determinant of female reproductive potential. Success rates achieved with ART also decline as age increases.

The numbers of oocytes retrieved and embryos available are lower, embryo fragmentation rates are higher, and implantation rates are lower in older than in younger women.

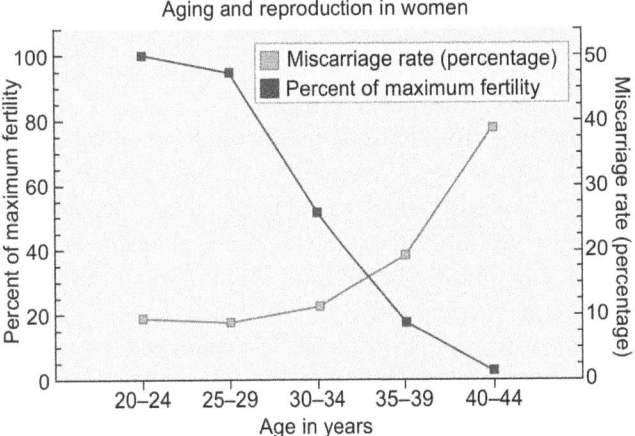

9. d. Intrauterine insemination (IUI)

Ref: Yen & Jaffe's 8th/ed p 779

Assisted reproductive technologies (ART) include
- Intracytoplasmic sperm injection (ICSI)
- In vitro fertilization (IVF)
- Assisted hatching (AH)
- Preimplantation genetic (PGD)
- Gamete or zygote intrafallopian tube transfer (GIFT, ZIFT)
- Tubal embryo transfer (TET)

10. a. Sonologically visible hydrosalpinges

Ref: Textbook of assisted reproductive techniques. D Gardner 5th/ed p 773

- Pregnancy rates are significantly lower (15%) in patients with visible hydrosalpinges compared with patients in whom the hydrosalpinges are not visible (31%).
- Presence of bilateral as opposed to unilateral hydrosalpinx are associated with significantly lower pregnancy (12% vs. 24%) and implantation rates (5% vs. 11%).
- Laparoscopic salpingectomy before IVF is recommended for women with hydrosalpinges.

11. d. Cumulative pregnancy rates after surgery are more for women with complete cul-de-sac obliteration than in those with endometriomas

Ref: Speroff 8th/ed p 1334

Considering all options one by one:
- Aspiration of endometriomas before ovarian stimulation or at time of oocyte retrieval has been associated with an increased risk for developing an ovarian abscess, although the risk appears quite low.

- Treatment options for asymptomatic women with known or suspected minimal or mild endometriosis and no other infertility factors include expectant management, surgical treatment, empiric treatment with clomiphene or exogenous gonadotropins and IUI, and IVF.
- Treatment with a GnRH agonist for 3-6 months before IVF can increase the odds of clinical pregnancy. However, because prolonged treatment with a GnRH agonist also can decrease response to ovarian stimulation, most clinicians do not favor suppressive treatment before IVF.
- Treatment options for infertile women with advanced stages of endometriosis include conservative surgical treatment and IVF.
  - For those with severe symptoms, surgery is the most logical treatment.
  - Data from case series suggest that cumulative pregnancy rates 1-3 years after surgical treatment are approximately 50% for women with endometriomas and about 30% for women with complete cul-de-sac obliteration.
  - Careful surgical technique is important because ovarian function can be compromised by excision of excessive tissue or damage to hilar vessels.
  - The risk of ovarian failure after excision of bilateral ovarian endometriomas is approximately 2.5%.

12. **d. Reflux phenomenon leading to increased cervix to fundus peristalsis**

    Ref: Textbook of assisted reproductive techniques. D Gardner 5th/ed p 776

- Hydrosalpinx fluid may cause an increase in endometrial peristalsis.
- Normal intrauterine peristalsis is from cervix-to-fundus.
- Mathematical simulation model describes a **reflux phenomenon** generated by a pressure gradient from tubal fluid accumulation leading to increased fundus-to-cervix peristalsis.
- It is suggested that this reflux phenomenon could explain the reduced implantation rate associated with hydrosalpinx.

13. **d. Less cancellation rates**

    Ref: Speroff 8th/ed p 1343; Yen & Jaffe's 8th/ed p 795

Natural cycle IVF involves only monitoring the spontaneous cycle and retrieving a single oocyte before the midcycle LH surge occurs.

Advantages	Disadvantages
• It is physically less demanding	• High cancellation rates due to premature LH surges and ovulation
• Requires little or no medication	
• Decreases costs by 75-80%	• Comparatively low success rate
• Eliminates risks for multiple pregnancy	
• Eliminates risks for ovarian hyperstimulation syndrome (OHSS)	• Laboratory to work whole week

Aneuploidy Rates Between Natural and Stimulated Cycles

- One reason offered by advocates of natural cycle IVF is that oocytes derived from stimulated cycles may have an increased rate of aneuploidy; this concern is not supported by evidence, however.
- A recent prospective study demonstrated that there was no difference in the aneuploidy rate of blastocysts derived from natural versus conventional stimulation cycles.
- The delivery rate per euploid transfer was equivalent between natural and stimulated cycles (58.7% vs. 59.0%), but natural cycles were more likely to have no oocytes retrieved, no blastocysts to biopsy or cryopreserve, and no euploid embryos to transfer.

14. **a. Age > 35 years**

    Ref: Younis et al. Journal of Ovarian Research (2015) 8:76

Bologna criteria was proposed to classify patient as expected poor responder.

Two of the following three criteria:
1. Age greater than 40 years;
2. A history of prior poor response to gonadotropins using a conventional stimulation protocol (≤3 oocytes);
3. AMH below 0.5 to 1.1 ng/mL or AFC less than 5 to 7 follicles.

15. **d. All**

    Ref: Yen & Jaffe's 8th/ed p 799

Several supplements, including dehydroepiandrosterone (DHEA), coenzyme Q10 (coQ10), and growth hormone (GH), have been studied as adjunctive medications to help improve follicular development in poor responders.

Dihydroepiandrosterone Supplementation

DHEA, an androgen secreted by both ovaries and the adrenal glands, has been studied as an adjunct to gonadotropins to improve ovarian stimulation in poor responders.

Coenzyme Q10

CoQ10, also known as ubiquinone, is a lipid-soluble antioxidant in the inner mitochondrial membrane that functions as an electron carrier in oxidative phosphorylation.

Growth Hormone Supplementation

GH directly stimulates the development of small antral follicles to gonadotropin dependent stages, as well as promotes maturation of oocytes.

16. d. All

Ref: Recommendations for the use of ART. Aidsinfo.nih. Dec, 2018

Before attempting conception, the partner living with HIV should be on HAART and have achieved sustained suppression of plasma viral load below the limits of detection.

Risk of HIV infection to the partner without HIV is very low when:
- HIV-positive man is on HAART for over six months.
- Undetectable levels of HIV RNA in the plasma (<50 copies/mL).
- Sexual intercourse limited to only 2 to 3 days before ovulation and on the day of ovulation (peak fertility).

17. b. Efavirenz

Ref: Textbook of assisted reproductive techniques. D Gardner 5th/ed p 810

- Studies of HIV-positive men suggest that they have semen parameters below the defined World Health Organization (WHO) normal range.
- There is a significant decrease in volume, count, motility, morphology, and post-wash parameters when CD4 counts drop below median levels (450 cells/mm^3).
- HAART has no significant effect on semen parameters effect other than in those patients on efavirenz, where a reduction in sperm motility was noted.
- The effect of HIV on semen parameters would suggest that HIV-positive men should consider a semen analysis sooner rather than later when attempting to conceive naturally.

18. d. EFS is likely when LH <35 IU/L and progesterone ≤3.5 ng/mL measured 8-12 hours after GnRHa trigger

Ref: Textbook of assisted reproductive techniques. D Gardner 5th/ed p 564

Empty Follicle Syndrome (EFS)

- The "empty follicle syndrome," is characterized by a failure to retrieve oocytes despite apparently normal multifollicular development.
- Rates of EFS after GnRHa trigger: 1.4% and 3.5%
- Rates of EFS with hCG trigger: 0.1-2%
- Patients likely to develop EFS have an LH <15 IU/L and progesterone ≤3.5 ng/mL measured 8-12 hours after trigger.
- The probability of EFS with a post-trigger LH less than 15 IU/L is 18.8%.

How to proceed in case of EFS?
- If there is no LH surge and/or progesterone rise after GnRHa trigger, repeat trigger with hCG and oocyte retrieval 35 hours later have been shown to result in successful retrieval of oocytes.
- If there is a suboptimal LH rise with values less than 15 IU/L, repeat trigger with hCG can be given as soon as possible to proceed with retrieval as planned or the cycle may be cancelled. Alternatively, the patient can proceed with unilateral follicle aspiration and, if there are no oocytes, re-trigger with hCG and repeat oocyte retrieval of the contralateral ovary 34 hours later.
- Addition of a standard or low dose hCG to GnRHa trigger in a "dual trigger" protocol demonstrates an improvement in the number and proportion of mature oocytes. However, adjuvant hCG in addition to GnRHa trigger should be used with caution in patients at high risk of OHSS development.

19. a. 50 pg/mL and < 1.0 ng/mL

Ref: Yen & Jaffe's 8th/ed p 800

In GnRH-agonist cycles, documentation of pituitary downregulation is performed by assessing serum estradiol and progesterone levels after menses has begun; levels should be suppressed with estradiol levels typically less than 50 pg/mL and progesterone less than 1.0 ng/mL.

20. b. PCOS

Ref: Textbook of assisted reproductive techniques. D Gardner 5th/ed p 562

- The use of GnRHa has been advocated as a substitute to hCG for the induction of oocyte maturation and prevention of OHSS during IVF cycles since the late 1980s to early 1990s.
- However, the subsequent widespread use of GnRHa for pituitary downregulation during controlled ovarian stimulation limited its use as an option for triggering oocyte maturation.
- After GnRH antagonists were introduced for prevention of the LH surge during controlled ovarian stimulation in the late 1990s, GnRHa could then be used again for the induction of oocyte maturation.

- GnRH antagonist blocks the GnRH receptors on the pituitary by competitive inhibition.
- Administration of GnRHa will then displace the antagonist on the receptors and activate them to promote a release of gonadotropins stored in the anterior pituitary.
- In patients with increased risk of OHSS, GnRH agonists are preferred for trigger.

21. d. All

Ref: Textbook of assisted reproductive techniques. D Gardner 5th/ed p 562

Some patients are not well suited for use of a GnRHa trigger as it relies on the ability to mount an **endogenous surge** of gonadotropins.

- As a result, patients with hypothalamic dysfunction are not ideal candidates for GnRHa trigger for oocyte maturation.
- Moreover, women who have had long-term suppression of the hypothalamus and pituitary may have a failed or suboptimal response because they may not be able to mount an optimal LH surge after GnRHa trigger.

22. c. Hypogonadotropic hypogonadism

Ref: Textbook of assisted reproductive techniques. D Gardner 5th/ed p 562

Indications for gonadotropin-releasing hormone agonist trigger:
- High risk for ovarian hyperstimulation syndrome development
- Oocyte donors
- Elective cryopreservation of oocytes or embryos
- Fertility preservation for medical reasons (e.g., cancer)
- Fertility preservation for social reasons
- Trophectoderm biopsy for preimplantation genetic testing
- Premature serum progesterone rise prior to induction of oocyte maturation

- Any patient who does not plan to have a fresh embryo transfer may be an ideal candidate for GnRHa trigger.
- A single bolus of GnRHa will interact with the GnRH receptors and cause the endogenous release or "flare" of gonadotropins from the anterior pituitary.
- The resultant surge of LH and FSH resembles the natural mid-cycle surge of gonadotropins seen shortly before ovulation, and thus a bolus of GnRHa can "trigger" ovulation.

- Role of FSH in ovulation:
  - Plays a role in oocyte maturation
  - Resumption of meiosis
  - Plays role in function of the oocyte-cumulus complex
  - Facilitation of its detachment from the follicle wall
  - Generation of LH receptors on granulosa cells
- Thus, there may be advantages to an ovulation trigger that result in a surge of both LH and FSH.
- An important drawback to the GnRH-agonist—only trigger is the resulting luteal phase deficiency, unless rescued by a bolus of hCG or intensive progesterone and estradiol support.

23. c. < 5 million/mL

Ref: Infertility in the male. Cambridge. 4th/ed p 165

In patients with less than 10 million sperm per mL, serum FSH and testosterone should be determined.

Men with non-obstructive azoospermia or severe oligospermia (less than 5 million/mL) should be offered karyotyping and screening for Y chromosome microdeletions.

24. b. Autonomic dysreflexia

Ref: Infertility in the male. Cambridge. 4th/ed p 460

- Autonomic dysreflexia is a risk for any method of sperm retrieval in patients with a level of injury T6 and above.

Autonomic Dysreflexia
- It is a **potentially life-threatening** medical complication
- Result from an **uninhibited sympathetic reflex response** to an irritating stimulus below the level of injury.
- Symptoms: hypertension, bradycardia, sweating, chills, and headache.
- In some cases, autonomic dysreflexia can lead to dangerously high blood pressure levels, and this complication can lead to stroke, seizure, or even death.
- Symptoms can be well managed or prevented by oral administration of **nifedipine**.

25. a. 0.3 to 0.6

Ref: Yen & Jaffe's 8th/ed p 801; Fertility and Sterility Vol. 102, No. 5, November 2014

- Relative proportion of LH and FSH administered have a substantial impact on the outcomes of ovarian stimulation.
- A ratio of LH-to-FSH that falls **between 0.30 and 0.60** during the cycle provides the **lowest risk of a premature increase in P** and represents a target "sweet spot" for clinicians.

- This relationship holds true for low responders, normal responders, and high responders.
- High responders had the greatest risk of a premature increase in P when compared with all other groups.
- Extremes of stimulation that deviated the furthest from the optimal ratio, or sweet spot, of 0.30–0.60, were at the greatest risk of a premature increase in P.
- The relative risk of premature P increase was more pronounced in the lower ranges of the LH-to-FSH ratio spectrum than the >.60 range.

26. **a. Used for ovulation induction**

Ref: Yen & Jaffe's 8th/ed p 802

Kisspeptin

- **Peptide hormone** that acts upstream of GnRH.
- Proteolytic cleavage of kisspeptin gives rise to kisspeptin-54, which binds a G-protein coupled receptor, Kiss1R, in the arcuate nucleus of the hypothalamus and stimulates pulsatile GnRH release.
- A subcutaneous injection of kisspeptin-54 to induce final follicle maturation in a group of high-responders demonstrated proof of concept that this also could be used as a trigger option to reduce the risk of **OHSS**.

27. **b. Hormonal gonadoprotection in men is successful in preserving fertility**

Ref: ASCO Clinical practice guidelines. J Clin Oncol 36. 2018 by American Society of Clinical Oncology

Recommendations for Sperm cryopreservation in adult men:
- Sperm cryopreservation is effective, and health care providers should discuss sperm banking with postpubertal males receiving cancer treatment.
- Hormonal gonadoprotection in men is **not successful** in preserving fertility. It is not recommended.
- Other methods such as testicular tissue cryopreservation and reimplantation or grafting of human testicular tissue, should be performed only as part of clinical trials or approved experimental protocols.
- Post chemotherapy: Men should be advised of a potentially higher risk of genetic damage in sperm collected after initiation of therapy.

It is strongly recommended that sperm be collected **before initiation of treatment** because the quality of the sample and sperm DNA integrity may be compromised after a single treatment.

28. **a. Ovarian tissue cryopreservation**

Ref: ASCO Clinical practice guidelines. J Clin Oncol 36. 2018 by American Society of Clinical Oncology

- Ovarian tissue cryopreservation for the purpose of future transplantation does not require ovarian stimulation and can be performed immediately.
- In addition, it does not require sexual maturity and hence may be the **only method available in children**.
- Finally, this method may also **restore global ovarian function**.
- However, it should be noted further investigation is needed to confirm whether it is safe in patients with leukemias.

29. **d. Any of the protocols can be used**

Ref: ASCO Clinical practice guidelines. J Clin Oncol 36. 2018 by American Society of Clinical Oncology

- More flexible ovarian stimulation protocols for oocyte collection are now available.
- Timing of this procedure no longer depends on the menstrual cycle in most cases, and stimulation can be initiated with less delay compared with old protocols.
- Of special concern in estrogen-sensitive breast and gynecologic malignancies is the possibility that these fertility preservation interventions (e.g. ovarian stimulation regimens that increase estrogen levels) and/or subsequent pregnancy may increase the risk of cancer recurrence.
- Aromatase inhibitor—based stimulation protocols are now well established and may ameliorate this concern.
- Studies do not indicate increased cancer recurrence risk as a result of aromatase inhibitor—supplemented ovarian stimulation and subsequent pregnancy.

30. **c. Ovarian suppression with GnRHa is well recognized method for fertility preservation**

Ref: ASCO Clinical practice guidelines. J Clin Oncol 36. 2018 by American Society of Clinical Oncology

- There is conflicting evidence to recommend GnRHa and other means of ovarian suppression for fertility preservation.
- The Panel recognizes that, when proven fertility preservation methods such as oocyte, embryo, or ovarian tissue cryopreservation are not feasible, and in the setting of young women with breast cancer, GnRHa may be offered to patients in the hope of reducing the likelihood of chemotherapy-induced ovarian insufficiency.
- However, GnRHa should not be used in place of proven fertility preservation methods.

31. **a. Letrozole**

Ref: ASCO Clinical practice guidelines. J Clin Oncol 36. 2018 by American Society of Clinical Oncology

Refer to above explanation.

32. **d. Risk is increased to 10-fold in ART-treated women with endometriosis**

Ref: Human Reproduction pp 1-7, 2019

- Ovarian cancer is a complex, multifactorial disease that is often detected at late stages.
- Use of ovulation-inducing drugs has been hypothesized to increase risk of ovarian cancer.
- There has been concern about long-term effects of fertility drugs.
  Theories related to ovarian cancer
  - Incessant ovulation theory
  - Elevated gonadotropin levels theory
- These two theories suggest that use of fertility drugs
  - Stimulate ovulation and create a condition of high gonadotropin levels, increasing risk of ovarian cancer.
  - Repeated damage and subsequent repair cycles that occur during ovulation on the epithelial surface of the ovary contribute to DNA damage and increases risk of ovarian cancer.
- The risk of ovarian cancer after ART treatment differed substantially according to the **cause** of infertility.
- ART done for male factor or unexplained infertility are not associated with increased risk of ovarian cancer.
- Association of ART and ovarian cancer was strongest in first two years.
- Risk is increased to **4-fold** in ART-treated women with endometriosis.
- Probable explanation for increased risk of ovarian cancer seen in endometriosis
  - Endometriosis is condition of uncontrolled cell proliferation
  - Resistance to apoptosis
  - Higher hormone dosages
  - More treatment attempts to achieve a pregnancy
- It may currently just be too early to determine whether there is an association between fertility drug use and ovarian cancer risk given that many of exposed women are only now beginning to reach ovarian cancer age range.

33. **a. Cranial end of Wolffian body**

Ref: Shaw's Textbook of Gynaecology, 15th/ed p 12

- The epoophoron is a remnant of the mesonephric tubules that can be found next to the ovary and fallopian tube.
- Epoophoron is homologue to epididymis in male.

Organ of Rosenmuller

- Also known as epoophoron represents **cranial end of the Wolffian body**.
- It consists of vertical tubules in the mesovarium and mesosalpinx.
- The tubules are lined by cubical cells.
- Paroophoron sometimes forms paraovarian cyst.

34. **c. Consists of horizontal tubules in the mesovarium and mesosalpinx**

Ref: Shaw's Textbook of Gynaecology, 15th/ed p 12

- Epoophoron consists of **vertical** tubules in the mesovarium and mesosalpinx. (not horizontal)

Paroophoron
- Group of rudimentary tubules in broad ligament the epoophoron and the uterus that constitutes a remnant of lower part of the mesonephros.
- It corresponds to the paradidymis of the male.

Epo = Up = and upright things are vertical too. (So, we can remember that epoophoron represents cranial and not caudal end of wolffian body, and it consists of vertical tubules.)

35. **c. 10% to 15%**

Ref: AE-PCOS 2006

Global prevalence of PCOS varies as per the criteria used.

Criteria	Global prevalence
NIH 1990	5% to 10%
AE-PCOS 2006	10% to 15%
ESHRE/ASRM 2003	6% to 21%

Use of NIH 1990 criteria for PCOS is associated with reduced variability in prevalence across countries

Greater estimates of PCOS prevalence with the Rotterdam 2003 and AE-PCOS 2006 criteria are largely attributed to their more expansive definition and inclusion of additional phenotypes, compared with NIH 1990 diagnostic criteria.

36. **a. 0.5 to 1 IU**

Ref: Yen & Jaffe's 8th/ed p 756

Baseline LH levels of at least **0.5 to 1 IU** are sufficient to provide maximal stimulation to thecal cells beyond which further increase is not associated with better ovarian stimulation results.

37. **c. 15**

Ref: Sunkara et al, Human Reproduction, Volume 26, Issue 7, July 2011, p 1768-1774

Live birth rates correlated with the number of oocytes retrieved across all age groups.
- Maximal when **15 oocytes** were obtained
- Plateaued between **15 and 20 oocytes**
- Lower if more than **40 oocytes** were retrieved.

38. **d. Luteal phase supplementation is not required following the late follicular phase administration of GnRH antagonist**

Ref: Yen & Jaffe's 8th/ed p 771

- Attempts to secure pituitary recovery during the luteal phase by the early follicular phase cessation of GnRH agonist cotreatment all failed because it takes at least 2 to 3 weeks for LH secretion to recover.
- Because of the rapid recovery of pituitary gonadotropin release after discontinuation of GnRH antagonist, it has been speculated that luteal phase supplementation may not be required following the late follicular phase administration of antagonist.
- However, various studies in IVF applying GnRH antagonist cotreatment have now clearly shown that luteolysis is also initiated prematurely resulting in a significant reduction in the length of the luteal phase along with greatly compromised chances for pregnancy.
- High early luteal phase steroid production is primarily responsible for advanced luteolysis due to massive negative feedback resulting in greatly suppressed LH secretion.

39. **b. 3–4%**

Ref: Yen & Jaffe's 8th/ed p 794

Natural Cycle IVF

- Associated with low pregnancy rates: **3–4%**
- IVF is a resource-intensive treatment, and pregnancy rates in the range of 3% to 4% per IVF cycle initiated are not cost-effective.
- There is no difference in the aneuploidy rate of blastocysts derived from natural versus conventional stimulation cycles.
- The delivery rate per euploid transfer was equivalent between natural and stimulated cycles (58.7% vs. 59.0%), but natural cycles were more likely to have no oocytes retrieved, no blastocysts to biopsy or cryopreserve, and no euploid embryos to transfer.

40. **c. Severe OHSS**

Ref: RCOG Green top guideline Number 5, February 2016

Proposed RCOG classification of severity of OHSS

Category	Features
Mild OHSS	• Abdominal bloating • Mild abdominal pain • Ovarian size <8 cm^3
Moderate OHSS	• Moderate abdominal pain • Nausea/Vomiting • Ultrasound evidence of ascites • Ovarian size 8–12 cm^3
Severe OHSS	• Clinical ascites/hydrothorax • Oliguria (<300 mL/day or < 30 mL/hour) • Hematocrit > 45% • Hyponatremia (sodium < 135 nmol/L) • Hypo-osmolality (osmolality < 282 mOsm/kg) • Hyperkalemia (potassium >5 mmol/L) • Hypoproteinemia (serum albumin <35 g/L) • Ovarian size > 12 cm^3
Critical OHSS	• Tense ascites/large hydrothorax • Hematocrit >55% • White cell count > 25,000/mL • Oliguria/anuria • Thromboembolism • Acute respiratory distress syndrome

CHAPTER 17

Embryology

Multiple Choice Questions

1. **A mature human oocyte measure ...... micrometer in diameter:**
   a. 80–100
   b. 100–120
   c. 120–150
   d. 150–180

2. **Which of the following is incorrect regarding physiology of sexual reproduction?**
   a. Binding of sperm to ZP3 initiates the acrosome reaction
   b. Interaction between sperm Izumo1 and its cognate Juno receptor on the oolemma is essential for fertilization
   c. Oocyte derived Phospholipase C (PLC)-zeta mobilizes intracellular Ca^{2+} stores to induce oocyte activation
   d. Cells of the human embryo are likely totipotent through the cleavage stage

3. **Incorrect statement about fertilization:**
   a. A normally fertilized oocyte exhibits two distinct pronuclei and two polar bodies
   b. Polyploidy can be observed in up to 5-10% of embryos
   c. ICSI offers better clinical pregnancy rates than IVF
   d. Conventional IVF achieves fertilization rates between 50% and 70%

4. **Emerging indication for in vitro maturation (IVM) of oocytes:**
   a. OHSS prevention
   b. Fertility preservation
   c. DOR patients
   d. Natural cycle IVF

5. **Which of the following pregnancy complication is seen most frequently in pregnancies achieved by IVM?**
   a. Gestational diabetes
   b. Hypertensive disorders of pregnancy
   c. Preterm birth
   d. Congenital malformations

6. **Ideal pressure which should be kept while retrieving oocytes:**
   a. 200 mm Hg
   b. 150 mm Hg
   c. 120 mm Hg
   d. 250 mm Hg

7. **Which of the following statements incorrect about embryo culture?**
   a. Pre-compaction embryos prefer pyruvate and post-compaction embryos favor glucose as a nutrient
   b. Extended culture is a more reliable test of viability and developmental potential
   c. Implantation rate for blastocysts is significantly higher than for cleavage-stage embryos
   d. Higher risk for cancelled transfer is seen with cleavage-stage embryos

8. **In which of the following conditions assisted hatching procedures are not useful?**
   a. Frozen thawed embryos
   b. Thick zona pellucida
   c. First ART cycles
   d. Age > 38 years

9. **Which of the following holds incorrect for proper technique of embryo transfer?**
   a. Transit time between incubator and uterus < 1 minute
   b. Maintaining steady pressure on plunger to prevent backflow
   c. No blood on the tip of transfer catheter
   d. Ideal volume of media for transfer 100 microlitre

10. **Which of the following is considered as a good quality embryo?**
    1. Number of cells corresponding to the day of its development
    2. Blastomeres of equal size with regular distribution
    3. Less than 10% fragmentation
    4. No evidence of multinucleation
    a. 1, 2 & 3
    b. 1, 2, 3 & 4
    c. 2, 3 & 4
    d. 3 & 4

11. **Which of the following is incorrect regarding human sperm chromatin packaging?**
    a. Highly compact packaging of primary sperm DNA filament is produced by DNA- histone complexes
    b. The fundamental packaging unit of mammalian sperm chromatin is a toroid containing 50-60 kilobases of DNA
    c. Toroids are cross-linked by disulfide bonds
    d. Human sperm contains two types of protamines and type 2 protamine is deficient in cysteine residues

12. **Which of the following methods can be used to assess the oocyte quality?**
    1. Polar body biopsy
    2. Morphologic assessment
    3. Polarized microscope to visualize meiotic spindle
    4. Zona pellucida thickness
    5. Blastomere biopsy
    a. All
    b. 1, 2, 3 & 4
    c. 1, 2 & 3
    d. 2, 3 & 4

13. **Which is incorrect regarding in vitro maturation?**
    a. GV-stage oocytes are retrieved when the follicles reach a diameter of 6 to 12 mm
    b. hCG priming may improve maturation rates following culture
    c. Retrieved oocytes are cultured for 28 to 36 hours to allow time for progression to metaphase II
    d. Smaller needle (19 or 20G) and a higher pressure on the aspiration pump may improve oocyte yield

14. **Morphologic evidence of normal fertilization 18 hours post insemination:**
    a. 2 pronuclei and 2 polar bodies
    b. 2 pronuclei and no polar body
    c. 1 pronuclei and no polar body
    d. 1 pronuclei and 1 polar body

15. **Indications for ISCI include:**
    a. Severe male factor infertility
    b. Prior total fertilization failure (TFF) with conventional IVF
    c. Human immunodeficiency virus serodiscordance
    d. All of the above

16. **Sequential embryo culture medium system, a "back to nature" approach includes:**
    a. First medium, high in lactate and pyruvate; second medium, high in glucose
    b. First medium, high in glucose; second medium, high in lactate and pyruvate
    c. First medium, high in glucose; second medium, high in amino acids
    d. First medium, high in lactate and pyruvate; second medium, high in amino acids

17. **Optimal temperature, pH, and Oxygen Tension for in vitro culture of human embryos:**
    a. 37°C, 7.2 to 7.4, 21% b. 36°C, 7.2 to 7.4, 2%
    c. 37°C, 7.2 to 7.4, 5%   d. 36°C, 7.4 to 7.6, 5%

18. **Which of the following constitute noninvasive methods for evaluation of embryo quality?**
    1. PGT-A
    2. Conventional morphology
    3. Time-Lapse imaging
    4. Metabolomics
    5. NICS
    a. All of the above   b. 1, 2, 3 & 4
    c. 2, 3, 4 & 5   d. 2 & 3

19. **Which of the following parameters is least important predictor of development to blastocyst stage?**
    a. Duration of the first cytokinesis
    b. Time interval between the end of the first cleavage and initiation of the second cleavage
    c. Synchronicity of the blastomeres in the second cleavage division
    d. Time to 2-cell, 3-cell, and 5-cell stages

20. **Fill in the blanks:**

Stage	Days post fertilization	Location in reproductive tract
Pre-zygote	0	Fallopian tubes
2-cell embryo	1	Fallopian tubes
4-cell embryo	2	1....................
8 cell embryo	3	2....................
Morula	4	3....................
Blastocyst	5–6	Intrauterine

a. 1. Fallopian tube, 2. Uterotubal junction, 3. Interstitial portion of fallopian tube
b. 1. Fallopian tubes, 2. Fallopian tubes, 3. Uterotubal junction
c. 1. Fallopian tubes, 2. Fallopian tubes, 3. Fallopian tubes
d. 1. Fallopian tubes, 2, Uterotubal junction, 3. Intrauterine

21. **Which of the following statements is incorrect regarding embryo?**
    a. Blastocyst formation rate may be improved when embryos are cultured together in group
    b. Inner cell mass quality may be more predictive of implantation and live birth than trophoectoderm quality
    c. Soluble human leukocyte antigen (sHLA-G) is the candidate marker of viability in the culture medium
    d. NICS is a noninvasive comprehensive chromosome screening platform in which DNA released from the embryo into spent culture media is analyzed by NGS

22. **Which of the following is incorrect statements regarding ICSI?**
    a. Most powerful micromanipulation procedure for treating male factor infertility
    b. Post retrieval, the oocytes are incubated for four hours
    c. Cumulus–corona cells are removed with help of cumulase prior to insemination
    d. ICSI is performed both in MI as well as MII oocytes with almost equal pregnancy rates

23. **Which is incorrect regarding blastocyst embryo transfer when compared to cleavage stage transfer?**
    a. Better temporal synchronization between embryo and uterus
    b. Developmentally more competent embryos
    c. Decreased risk of monozygotic twinning
    d. Less risk of multiple gestations

24. **Optimal depth of embryo transfer from the fundus of the uterus:**
    a. 0.5 cm
    b. 1.0 cm
    c. 1.5 cm
    d. 2.0 cm

25. **As per ASRM 2017, number of euploid cleavage stage embryos that can be transferred in a woman 37 years of age undergoing her first transfer:**
    a. 1
    b. 2
    c. 3
    d. 4

26. **Luteal phase support with exogenous progesterone is critical following IVF. Optimal window for initiating luteal phase support begins .... oocyte retrieval and ends by .... after oocyte retrieval:**
    a. Before, 3 days
    b. Before, 6 days
    c. After, 3 days
    d. After, 6 days

27. **Temperature of liquid nitrogen used for sperm cryopreservation:**
    a. −196°C
    b. −176°C
    c. −156°C
    d. −296°C

28. **Which of the following is incorrect for embryo cryopreservation?**
    a. Slow freezing methods have been successfully used for freezing blastocysts
    b. Vitrification has shown better post-thaw survival as compared to slow freezing
    c. Clinical pregnancy rates are nor related to development stage at cryopreservation
    d. The amount of time elapsed from a freeze-all cycle does not seem to affect pregnancy rates

29. **Which of the following is germline nuclear transfer technology for prevention of mitochondrial diseases?**
    a. Maternal spindle transfer
    b. Polar body transfer
    c. Germinal vesicle transfer
    d. All of the above

30. **Risks involved with germline nuclear transfer technologies include:**
    a. Karyoplast mtDNA carryover
    b. Incompatibility between donor and recipient
    c. Shifts in mutation copy number during development
    d. All of the above

31. **Most common method used for sperm cryopreservation:**
    a. Slow freezing
    b. Rapid cooling
    c. Vitrification
    d. All are equally used

32. **Gold standard for ovarian tissue cryopreservation:**
    a. Slow freezing
    b. Rapid cooling
    c. Vitrification
    d. All are equally used

33. **Method used for oocyte cryopreservation with maximum post thaw survival:**
    a. Slow freezing
    b. Rapid cooling
    c. Vitrification
    d. All are equal

34. **Ideal macroenvironment to control air quality in IVF laboratory include all *except*:**
    a. High efficiency particulate air (HEPA) filters
    b. High tightness factor
    c. Multiple air exchanges per hour
    d. Under negative pressure

35. **During ICSI, following is suggestive of break in the oolemma:**
    a. Sudden quivering of the convexities at the site of invagination of the oolemma
    b. Proximal flow of the cytoplasmic organelles
    c. Spermatozoon moving upward into the pipette
    d. All of the above

36. **Major component of extracellular matrix secreted by cumulus cells:**
    a. Glucoronic acid
    b. Hyaluronic acid
    c. Sulfonic acid
    d. Nitric acid

37. **Which of the following embryos following ICSI can be transferred?**
    1. 0 PN
    2. 1 PN
    3. 2 PN
    4. 3 PN
    a. All can be transferred
    b. 3 Only
    c. 1 & 3
    d. 2 & 3

38. **Time lapse imaging has shown that timing of pronuclear breakdown (PNB) is a key factor in assessment of embryo selection. When does first cleavage happen normally?**
    a. 16-18 hours post-insemination/ICSI
    b. 25-26 hours post-insemination/ISCI
    c. 42-44 hours post-insemination/ICSI
    d. 66-68 hours post-insemination/ICSI

Answer with Explanations

1. **b. 100–120**

   Ref: Inderbir Singh's Human Embryology 11th/ed p 36

   ### Structure of the Ovum at Ovulation

   - The ovum that is shed from the ovary is not fully mature.
   - It is a secondary oocyte that is undergoing division to shed off the second polar body.
   - It is surrounded by the zona pellucida. Some cells of the corona radiata can be seen sticking to the outside of the zona pellucida.
   - No nucleus is seen, as the nuclear membrane has dissolved for the second meiotic division. A spindle is, however, present.
   - Between the cell membrane (or vitelline membrane) and the zona pellucida, a distinct perivitelline space is seen. The first polar body lies in this space.
   - Ovum is a very large cell and measures more than **100–120 µm** in diameter. In contrast, most other cells of the body measure less than 10 µm (1 µm is 1,000th of a millimeter).
   - Oocytes with a diameter of 200 µm or more are commonly called **giant oocytes.**

Differences between male and female gametes		
Feature	Spermatozoon	Ovum
Diameter	Small: 3 µ	Very large: 120 µ
Length	60 µ	Small
Shape	Adapted for motility	Adapted to provide ample storage of nutrition for the embryo formed after fertilization
Motility	Highly motile	Immotile
Cytoplasm	Very little	Large amount
Chromosomal types	(22 + X) or (22 + Y)	(22 + X)

2. **c. Oocyte derived Phospholipase C (PLC)-zeta mobilizes intracellular Ca^{2+} stores to induce oocyte activation**

   Ref: Yen & Jaffe's 8th/ed p 780

   ### Physiology of Sexual Reproduction Involves

   - Genetic diversity is generated through homologous recombination and random assortment of chromosomes.
   - Meiosis produces haploid (1n, 1c) gametes from diploid (2n, 4c) progenitor cells.
   - Binding of sperm to **ZP3** initiates the acrosome reaction.
   - Interaction between sperm Izumo1 and its cognate Juno receptor on the oolemma is essential for fertilization.
     - Izumo1 is the specific binding partner for Juno, a folate receptor expressed on the oolemma.
     - Binding of Izumo1 to Juno is not only essential for normal fertilization, but also conserved across mammals and is species-specific.
   - After fusion of the sperm with the oolemma, the **sperm-derived** phospholipase C (PLC)-zeta mobilizes intracellular Ca^{2+} stores to induce oocyte activation.
   - The cells of the human embryo are likely totipotent through the cleavage stage i.e. up to around the eight-cell stage. Beyond the eight-cell stage, the cells begin to undergo differentiation.
   - The first overt indication of differentiation is the morphologic distinction of inner cell mass cells from the outer cells, progenitors of the trophoectoderm.
   - Compaction ensues to form the morula stage.
   - Implantation requires adequate and timely signaling between the blastocyst and the uterine epithelium.
   - Implantation depends on three fundamental principles:
     - A developmentally competent blastocyst
     - A receptive endometrium (the "window of implantation")
     - **Synchronicity** between the blastocyst and the endometrium.

3. **c. ICSI offers better clinical pregnancy rates than IVF**

   Ref: Speroff 8th/ed p 1355

   ### Considering Each Option

   - A normally fertilized oocyte exhibits **two distinct pronuclei**, one derived from the oocyte and the other from the sperm, and **two polar bodies** in the perivitelline space.
   - Polyploidy can be observed in up to **5–10%** of embryos but is far more prevalent in immature oocytes (up to 30%) than in mature oocytes (1–2%).

- Causes of polyploidy:
  - Polyspermy
  - Digyny—fertilization of a diploid oocyte
  - Meiotic spindle errors
  - Failure to extrude a polar body (more commonly associated with immature, aging, or postmature oocytes)
- The fertilization process requires approximately **24 hours** and ends with the first mitotic division (cleavage).
- In the absence of a male factor, ICSI offers **no clinical advantage** over conventional IVF. In fact, evidence suggests that standard IVF yields higher implantation and clinical pregnancy rates.
- Conventional IVF typically achieves fertilization rates ranging between **50% and 70%**.

4. **b. Fertility preservation**
   Ref: Human Reproduction, Vol 34, No 8, pp. 1595–1607, 2019
- IVM had initially been advocated as an OHSS-free approach for patients with PCOS.
- Since GnRH agonist maturation triggering and freeze all protocols have redesigned the landscape of ART in high responders, resulting in a significant reduction of the incidence of OHSS, OHSS prevention is no longer the key incentive for IVM.
- However, urgent fertility preservation in cancer patients is now an emerging indication for IVM.

5. **b. Hypertensive disorders of pregnancy**
   Ref: Human Reproduction, Vol.34, No.8, pp. 1595–1607, 2019
- Pregnancies in the IVM patients run almost **2-fold higher** incidence of hypertensive disorders of pregnancy compared to pregnancies after COS.
- Association between IVM and HDP in the referred study could potentially be linked to:
  - Poor placentation due to unfavorable patient characteristics
  - Suboptimal hormonal preparation of the endometrium
  - Epigenetic dysregulation.

It is plausible that patients with PCOS phenotype A in the IVM group had a more unfavorable hormonal (e.g. androgen levels) and/or metabolic profile compared to their COS counterparts.

6. **c. 120 mm Hg**
   Ref: Textbook of Assisted Reproductive Techniques. D Gardner 5th/ed p 606

- High velocities of flow may strip the cumulus from the oocyte.
- Even with laminar flow, there are significant differences in velocity of the follicular fluid within the center of the needle compared to the periphery.
- This can result in "drag" on the outer layers of the cumulus, resulting in potential damage.

Oocyte Retrieval

- The longer the needle, the smaller its internal diameter, and the greater the pressure required to maintain the same velocity.
- It was found that when a 17-gauze collection needle was used, all oocytes lost their cumulus mass when the aspiration pressure reached 20 kPa (150 mm Hg). It is therefore recommended that pressures be kept **below 120 mm Hg**.
- Apart from the speed of travel, turbulent non-laminar flow can also damage the oocyte, either stripping its cumulus mass or fracturing the zona.
- It is believed that an intact cumulus may be important in preventing damage to oocytes.

7. **d. Higher risk for cancelled transfer is seen with cleavage-stage embryos**
   Ref: Speroff 8th/ed p 1359

Implantation rate for blastocysts (30–60%) is significantly higher than for cleavage-stage embryos (12–20%).

Two potential disadvantages of extended culture:
- Embryos of lesser quality that may implant if transferred on day 3 may fail to reach the blastocyst stage *in vitro*, increasing the risk there may be no embryos for transfer.
- Whereas higher blastocyst implantation rates permit transfer of fewer embryos, multiple pregnancy rates after transfer of two blastocysts are the same or higher than those observed after transfer of larger numbers of cleavage-stage embryos.

8. **c. First ART cycles**
   Ref: Textbook of Assisted Reproductive Techniques. D Gardner 5th/ed p 666; Kamini A Rao. 2nd/ed p 380

Embryos subjected to *in vitro* culture may experience zona hardening and subsequent lower rates of hatching and blastocyst expansion than occurs *in vivo*.

Thus, it was suggested that either artificially opening or thinning of the zona could facilitate the hatching process.

A variety of techniques have subsequently been developed to aid in the hatching process:
- Mechanical partial zona dissection
- Chemical drilling using acid Tyrode's solution
- Enzymatic thinning
- Laser-assisted hatching
- Piezo micromanipulation

It has been proposed that such techniques not only aid in mechanical hatching, but also could enhance transport of nutrients from incubating media by allowing for a two-way exchange of metabolites.

Assisted hatching procedures are useful in a select group of patients:
- Frozen thawed embryo as it hardens the zona
- Thickened zona pellucida
- Age > 38 years
- Elevated basal FSH levels > 10 miu/mL
- Recurrent implantation failure
- Embryos with increased fragmentation and delayed development.

Unselected patients do not seem to experience the same benefit.

9. d. Ideal volume of media for transfer 100 microlitre
Ref: Textbook of Assisted Reproductive Techniques. D Gardner 5th/ed p 723

Time interval from embryo loading to transfer
- The time interval from loading the embryos in the catheter to depositing them in the uterine cavity should be kept to a minimum in order to prevent prolonged exposure of the embryos to ambient temperature, light, or other factors.
- Time interval of more than **60 seconds** has been shown to lower the pregnancy and implantation rates.

Mock transfer
- Performing a mock ET before the IVF cycle has been shown to significantly improve the pregnancy rate.
- It is a routine procedure for some IVF specialists to place the catheter approximately **1–1.5 cm** below the fundus to avoid touching.

Avoiding the initiation of uterine contractions
- Avoid **touching** the uterine fundus.
- The use of **soft ET catheters**—The ideal catheter should be soft enough to avoid any trauma to the endometrium and malleable enough to find its way through the cervical canal into the uterine cavity.
- Removing the **cervical mucus** before ET is advisable in order to avoid embryo entrapping in cervical mucus (cobweb effect). It can be removed by repeated gentle aspiration using a 1 cm^3 syringe with its tip placed at the external cervical os.

Amount of media used
- ET catheter is filled with ET culture medium and up to 10–15 μL will be aspirated first.
- The embryos are then aspirated in another 10–15 μL of medium and moved in the catheter to stop away from the tip.
- The volume of fluid used for ET should be as small as possible to prevent flowing out of the embryos into the cervical canal or the fallopian tubes.
- A large volume (60 μL) of transfer medium and a large air bubble in the catheter result in the expulsion of the embryos. A continuous fluid column of **30 μL** without air bubbles is recommended.

The evidence based factors include:
- Soft catheters;
- Ultrasonic guidance;
- Dummy ET;
- Curving the ET catheter according to the cervico-uterine angulations;
- Not touching the fundus; and
- Small volumes of medium to deposit the embryos.

Other factors that are based on clinical experts' recommendations include:
- Gentle manipulation;
- Removing cervical mucus;
- Slow withdrawal of the catheter to avoid negative pressure; and
- Minimizing the time of the procedure.

10. b. 1, 2, 3 & 4
Ref: The Istanbul Consensus Workshop on Embryo Assessment. Human Reproduction, Vol 26, No 6 pp. 1270–1283, 2011

Consensus scoring system for cleavage-stage embryos		
Grade	Rating	Description
1	Good	• < 10% fragmentation • Stage-specific cell size • No multinucleation
2	Fair	• 10–25% fragmentation • Stage-specific cell size for majority of cells • No evidence of multinucleation
3	Poor	• Severe fragmentation (>25%) • Cell size not stage specific • Evidence of multinucleation

Consensus scoring system for day 4 embryos		
Grade	Rating	Description
1.	Good	• Entered into a fourth round of cleavage • Evidence of compaction that involves virtually all the embryo volume
2.	Fair	• Entered into a fourth round of cleavage • Compaction involves the majority of the volume of the embryo
3.	Poor	• Disproportionate compaction involving less than half of the embryo, with two or three cells remaining as discrete blastomeres

Consensus scoring system for blastocysts

	Grade	Rating	Description
Stage of development	1		• Early
	2		• Blastocyst
	3		• Expanded
	4		• Hatched/hatching
Inner cell mass ICM	1	Good	Prominent, easily discernible, with many cells that are compacted and tightly adhered together
	2	Fair	Easily discernible, with many cells that are loosely grouped together
	3	Poor	Difficult to discern, with few cells
Trophoectoderm TE	1	Good	• Many cells forming a cohesive epithelium
	2	Fair	• Few cells forming a loose epithelium
	3	Poor	• Very few cells

The scoring system for blastocysts is a combination of the stage of development, and of the grade of the ICM and of the TE.

11. a. Highly compact packaging of primary sperm DNA filament is produced by DNA-histone complexes

Ref: Textbook of Assisted Reproductive Techniques. D Gardner 5th/ed p 65

- Highly compact packaging of primary sperm DNA filament is produced by DNA- protamine complexes. (not histone)

Human Sperm Chromatin Structure

- In many mammals, spermatogenesis leads to the production of highly homogenous spermatozoa. This allows mature sperm nuclei to adopt a volume 40-times less than that of normal somatic nuclei. The final, highly compact packaging of the primary sperm DNA filament is produced by **DNA- protamine complexes**. Contrary to nucleosomal organization in somatic cells, which is provided by histones, these DNA–protamine complexes approach the physical limits of molecular compaction.
- Human sperm nuclei, on the other hand, contain considerably fewer protamines (**around 85%**) than sperm nuclei of the bull, stallion, hamster, and mouse. Human sperm chromatin is therefore less regularly compacted and frequently contains DNA strand breaks.
- The fundamental packaging unit of mammalian sperm chromatin is a **toroid** containing 50-60 kilobases of DNA. Individual toroids represent the DNA loop domains that are highly condensed by protamines and fixed at the nuclear matrix. Toroids are cross-linked by **disulfide bonds** formed by oxidation of sulfhydryl groups of cysteine present in the protamines.
- This condensed, insoluble, and highly organized nature of sperm chromatin acts to protect the genetic integrity during transport of the paternal genome through the male and female reproductive tracts.
- The retention of 15% histones, which are less basic than protamines, leads to the formation of a less compact chromatin structure.
- In contrast to the bull, cat, boar, and ram—whose spermatozoa contain only one type of protamine (P1)—human and mouse spermatozoa contain a second type of protamine called P2, which is **deficient in cysteine residues**. Consequently, the disulfide cross-linking that is responsible for more stable packaging is diminished in human sperm as compared with species containing P1 alone.
- Altered P1/P2 ratios and the absence of P2 are associated with male fertility problems. The P1/P2 ratio has been shown to correlate with sperm DNA fragmentation. The reference range reported for P1/P2 in a fertile, normozoospermic population ranges from 0.54 to 1.43.

12. b. 1, 2, 3 & 4

Ref: Yen & Jaffe's 8th/ed p 802

Oocyte Quality Assessment

- Ideally, both nuclear and cytoplasmic maturation should be assessed, because both processes are required for an oocyte to fertilize successfully and support early embryonic development.
- Typically only **70% to 80%** of retrieved oocytes have achieved nuclear maturation (i.e., have emitted the first polar body and are in metaphase II); the remaining 20% to 30% are at either prophase I or metaphase I.
- Following hyaluronidase stripping of the cumulus and corona radiata cells prior to ICSI, the nuclear maturity of an oocyte is readily apparent by the presence of a single polar body and the absence of the GV.
- For conventional IVF, nuclear maturity of the oocyte is ascertained indirectly at the fertilization check by demonstrating successful fertilization with **two pronuclei and two polar bodies** present.

- Current techniques for assessing oocyte quality fall into the two major categories:

Invasive	Noninvasive
Polar body biopsy and PGT-A	• Morphologic assessment of the surrounding cumulus oophorus with a light microscope • Polarized light microscopy to visualize the size and shape of the meiotic spindle • The thickness of the inner zona pellucida layer

Morphologic Assessment of Cumulus Oophorus with a Light Microscope

- During the periovulatory period in response to the midcycle surge of LH or exogenous hCG, the cumulus cells secrete glycosaminoglycans, resulting in expansion of the cumulus oophorus, and a radiating appearance of the inner corona radiata cells.
- Nuclear maturity and emission of the first polar body is most accurately determined by visualization of the oocyte itself.
- The imperfect prediction of oocyte maturity by morphologic assessment of the cumulus-corona radiata cells has led to the development of alternative noninvasive approaches to assess oocyte quality.

13. d. Smaller needle (19 or 20G) and a higher pressure on the aspiration pump may improve oocyte yield

Ref: Yen & Jaffe's 8th/ed p 802

In Vitro Oocyte Maturation

- In the setting of IVM, GV-stage oocytes are retrieved when the follicles reach a diameter of **6 to 12 mm**, either with or without **hCG priming**, which may improve maturation rates following culture.
- Retrieved oocytes are typically cultured for **28 to 36 hours** to allow time for progression to metaphase II, thereby simulating the timing from the LH surge in vivo.
- A specialized, **smaller needle** (19 or 20G, rather than the 16 to 17G needles generally used) is needed to remove the more adherent immature oocyte-cumulus complex from the membrana granulosa cells lining the follicle, and a **lower pressure** on the aspiration pump may improve oocyte yield.
- The efficiency of IVM varies depending upon whether the oocytes arise from polycystic ovaries, naturally cycling ovaries, or ovaries primed with low doses of gonadotropins.
- The majority of studies indicate that while more than 60% of IVM oocytes achieve nuclear maturation by progressing to metaphase II, a low percentage successfully acquire cytoplasmic maturation and exhibit the ability to support pronuclear formation and early embryonic development.
- Only 40% to 80% of fertilized IVM oocytes progress through early cleavage, and of those that do cleave and that are transferred, **implantation rates of less than 15%** are seen in the majority of studies.
- This low efficiency is further diminished for oocytes matured without their cumulus-corona cells. Therefore, attempts to salvage immature oocytes for clinical use after cumulus-corona cell removal in preparation for ICSI are not recommended with the IVM protocols currently available.

14. a. 2 pronuclei and 2 polar bodies

Ref: Yen & Jaffe's 8th/ed p 805

- Approximately 16 to 18 hours post insemination, the oocytes are examined for fertilization.
- The cumulus-corona radiata cells are gently removed from the oocyte, which is then examined under an **inverted microscope** with Hoffman illumination at around **100× magnification**.
- A zygote with **two pronuclei (PNs) and two polar bodies** is morphologic evidence of normal fertilization.
- All oocytes with either less than or more than 2PNs are discarded. The 2PN zygotes are then set up in culture either separately or in groups.

15. d. All of the above

Ref: Yen & Jaffe's 8th/ed p 805

- ICSI is primarily indicated for treatment of severe male factor infertility.

Other indications for ICSI:
- In azoospermic men where spermatozoa are microsurgically retrieved from the epididymis and the testis.
- When after sperm selection, the spermatozoa show poor progressive motility.
- Prior total fertilization failure (TFF) with conventional IVF.
- High titer of antisperm antibodies.
- Limited sperm supply from a banked specimen (e.g. in a patient who subsequently was rendered sterile by gonadotoxic treatment).
- Human immunodeficiency virus serodiscordance-ICSI avoids the interaction of oocytes with semen, thereby reducing the risk of viral exposure.
- Fertilization of cryopreserved oocytes (freezing can lead to **premature exocytosis of cortical granules** and **ZP hardening** that inhibit natural sperm penetration)
- Fertilization of oocytes following IVM

- PGT and ICSI:
  - Removal of the polar body requires the stripping of cumulus corona cells, thus supporting ICSI as the only insemination method to avoid polyspermy.
  - When embryos need to be analyzed for gene defects, the avoidance of **contaminating spermatozoa** on the ZP reduces the chance of false amplification by polymerase chain reaction.

16. **a. First medium, high in lactate and pyruvate; second medium, high in glucose**

    Ref: Yen & Jaffe's 8th/ed p 805

The "back to nature" approach	The "let the embryo choose" approach
• In contrast to the fallopian tube, the glucose concentration in the uterine fluid is relatively high, but the lactate and pyruvate concentrations are relatively low. • These observations led to the development of a pair of media, reflecting these differences in energy substrate concentration, that are used in sequence for support of human blastocyst formation: the **first medium, relatively high in lactate and pyruvate**, is used from days 1 to 3 of culture, and the **second medium, relatively high in glucose**, is used from day 3 onward. • The resultant paired media comprise the **sequential media system.**	• This approach is based on the determination of blastocyst formation rates following systematic adjustments in medium composition in numerous experiments using the simplex optimization approach. • This approach has resulted in the development of a single medium for the culture human embryos from day 1 to day 5/6. • This system is referred to as the **single-step system.**

- The weight of the evidence indicates that neither system is superior to the other.
- Limited data exist evaluating whether or not media need to be changed on day 3 for the duration of extended culture; by doing so, one might limit accumulation of toxic metabolites like ammonium, but similarly may negate any beneficial effects of autocrine, embryotrophic substances.

17. **c. 37°C, 7.2 to 7.4, 5%**

    Ref: Yen & Jaffe's 8th/ed p 806

Optimal temperature, pH, and oxygen tension for in vitro culture of human embryos		
Optimal temperature	*Optimal pH*	*Optimal oxygen tension*
• The only RCT performed to date comparing sibling embryos cultured in 37°C versus a perhaps more physiologic 36°C demonstrated that the rate of usable blastocyst formation was higher in the **37°C** group. • Therefore, this is the preferred and standard temperature in most laboratories.	• Most commercial media manufacturers recommend culture within the range of **7.2 to 7.4**, and these recommendations may vary according to the stage at which the medium is used (fertilization vs. cleavage stage vs. extended culture). • Importantly, the external pH in the media drop does not reflect the internal pH within the embryo, and varying amounts of lactate, pyruvate, and certain amino acids in culture media can lead to differences in intracellular buffering.	• A prospective randomized trial showed that culture of embryos in low **(5%)** versus atmospheric oxygen tension resulted in a significant increase in both the conversion rate of human zygotes to blastocysts, as well as the live birth rate. • As the uterine oxygen tension in the human is approximately 2%, it remains to be determined whether a further reduction in the incubator oxygen tension would prove beneficial for extended culture.

18. **c. 2, 3, 4 & 5**

    Ref: Yen & Jaffe's 8th/ed p 808

The primary goal of evaluating embryo quality is identification of an embryo marker that predicts pregnancy rate more accurately than the age of the female partner and the number of embryos transferred. Evaluation of embryo quality fall into the two broad categories of invasive and noninvasive.

Invasive	Noninvasive
• Preimplantation genetic testing-A	• Morphologic assessment conventional grading • Time-lapse imaging • Metabolomics • Noninvasive chromosomal screening

19. d. Time to 2-cell, 3-cell, and 5-cell stages

Ref: Yen & Jaffe's 8th/ed p 808

- Retrospective analysis of imaged embryos has shown that three parameters predicted development to the blastocyst stage with greater than 93% accuracy:
  - Duration of the first cytokinesis
  - Time interval between the end of the first cleavage and initiation of the second cleavage (from 1 to 2 cells embryo)
  - Synchronicity of the blastomeres in the second cleavage division, from the 2 to 4 cell stage.
- The parameters that may be associated with implantation potential:
  - Duration of the first cytokinesis
  - Time to the 2-cell, 3-cell, and 5-cell stages
  - Duration of the 2-cell and 3-cell stages
  - Abnormal cleavage (i.e. division of one cell into three daughter cells)
  - Reverse cleavage (i.e. two daughter cells fusing to form one cell).

20. a. 1. Fallopian tube, 2. Uterotubal junction, 3. Interstitial portion of fallopian tube

Ref: Yen & Jaffe's 8th/ed p 808

Stage	Days post fertilization	Location in reproductive tract
Pre-zygote	0	Fallopian tubes
2-cell embryo	1	Fallopian tubes
4-cell embryo	2	Fallopian tubes
8 cell embryo	3	Uterotubal junction
Morula	4	Interstitial portion of Fallopian tubes
Blastocyst	5-6	Intrauterine
Implanting, hatched blastocyst	6-7	Intrauterine

21. b. Inner cell mass quality may be more predictive of implantation and live birth than trophoectoderm quality

Ref: Yen & Jaffe's 8th/ed p 808-809

An important consideration at the blastocyst stage is the **quality of the trophoectoderm**.

Retrospective data indicate that TE quality may be more predictive of implantation and live birth than ICM quality.

Single vs Group Culture

- Blastocyst formation rate may be improved when embryos are cultured together within a shared drop of media.
- Embryos in group culture are significantly more likely to blastulate and to form high-quality blastocysts. Embryo density in group culture was not associated with blastulation.

Metabolomics

- Small molecules in spent culture medium can be detected using several techniques, including tandem mass spectrometry, proton nuclear magnetic resonance, and Raman and near infrared spectroscopy.
- Several studies have investigated candidate markers of viability in the culture medium, such as soluble human leukocyte antigen (sHLA-G), markers for amino acid metabolism, glucose uptake, and specific protein peaks associated either with implantation failure or success using proteomic profiling.

22. d. ICSI is performed both in MI as well as MII oocytes with almost equal pregnancy rates

Ref: Textbook of Assisted Reproductive Techniques. D Gardner 5th/ed p 143

ICSI Methodology

- Post oocyte retrieval, oocytes are examined under the inverted microscope at 100× and the cumulus–corona cell complexes are scored as mature, slightly immature, completely immature, or slightly hypermature.
- Thereafter, the oocytes are incubated for about **four hours** for stabilization of mitotic spindle and oocyte maturity.
- Immediately prior to micromanipulation, the cumulus–corona cells are removed by exposure to HTF-HEPES-buffered medium containing 40 IU/mL of **Cumulase**.
- A good and timely cumulus removal is necessary for observation of the oocyte and effective use of the **holding and/or injecting** pipette during micromanipulation.
- For final removal of the residual corona cells, the oocytes are repeatedly aspirated in and out of an EZ-Tip® 290–135 μm locked on a STRIPPER.
- Each oocyte is then examined under the microscope to assess nuclear maturity and morphology; metaphase II (MII) is assessed according to the absence of the germinal vesicle and the presence of an extruded polar body.
- ICSI is performed **only in oocytes that have reached MII level of maturity**.

Embryology

23. c. Decreased risk of monozygotic twinning
Ref: Yen & Jaffe's 8th/ed p 809

Advantages of blastocyst transfer	Disadvantages of blastocyst transfer
• Improved **temporal synchronization** between embryo and uterus at the time of transfer. • The possibility of selecting **developmentally more competent embryos**, because blastocyst stage embryos have proved their ability to progress through normal developmental milestones in vitro. • The rationale to transfer fewer embryos with higher implantation potential, thereby reducing the risk of **multiple gestations**.	• Extending culture to the blastocyst stage appears to result in attrition of some embryos, and in some cases all of the embryos undergo **developmental arrest** or degeneration, leaving no embryos for transfer. • Blastocyst transfer has been associated with an increased risk of **monozygotic twinning** in some studies, and the obstetrically more serious condition of monochorionic twinning. • Possible adverse effects of longer durations of culture on the risks of **epigenetic mutations** in offspring.

24. c. 1.5 cm
Ref: Textbook of Assisted Reproductive Techniques. D Gardner 5th/ed p 721

Depositing the embryos in the mid-fundal area of the uterus to avoid touching fundus, improves the pregnancy rates.

The majority of studies show that the optimal depth of transfer from the fundus is approximately **1.5 cm**.

25. a. 1
Ref: ASRM Practice Committee. Guidance on the limits to the number of embryos to transfer: a committee opinion. Fertil Steril. 2017;107:901-03.

As per ASRM 2017, number of euploid cleavage stage embryos that can be transferred in a woman 37 years of age undergoing her first transfer is **one**.

American society for reproductive medicine/society for assisted reproductive technologies recommendations for the limit to the number of embryos to transfer

Prognosis	Age(y)			
	<35	35–37	38–40	41–42
Cleavage-stage embryos				
Euploid	1	1	1	1
Other favorable	1	1	</=3	</=4
All others	</=2	</=3	</=4	</=5
Blastocysts				
Euploid	1	1	1	1
Other favorable	1	1	</=2	</=3
All others	</=2	</=2	</=3	</=3

Other favourable = Any ONE of these criteria: *Fresh cycle*: expectation of 1 or more high-quality embryos available for cryopreservation, or previous live birth after an IVF cycle; *FET cycle*: availability of vitrified day-5 or day-6 blastocysts, euploid embryos, first FET cycle, or previous live birth after IVF cycle.

26. c. After, 3 days
Ref: Yen & Jaffe's 8th/ed p 812

Optimal window for initiating luteal phase support begins **after** oocyte retrieval but ends by the **third day** after oocyte retrieval.

27. a. –196°c
Ref: Textbook of Assisted Reproductive Techniques. D Gardner 5th/ed p 142

Sperm Cryopreservation

- The sperm suspension (adjusted to a concentration of ~30×10^6/mL) is diluted with at least an equal amount of cryopreservation medium (**Freezing Medium**-Test Yolk Buffer with Glycerol; Irvine Scientific).
- 1 mL aliquots of the final solution are placed in 1 mL cryogenic vials (Nalgene Brand Products, Rochester, NY).
- The vials are exposed to liquid nitrogen vapor at –70°C for 15 minutes, and then plunged into liquid nitrogen at **–196°C**.
- Vials are thawed at 37°C for 15 minutes when spermatozoa are needed for injection.
- Surgically retrieved samples are cryopreserved similarly to fresh semen with an excess of cryoprotectant and, when appropriate, exposed to a **motility enhancer** (3 mmol/L pentoxifylline) to facilitate the identification of viable spermatozoa.

28. a. Slow freezing methods have been successfully used for freezing blastocysts
Ref: Textbook of Assisted Reproductive Techniques. D Gardner 5th/ed p 266

- Slow-freezing methods using cryoprotectants such as dimethyl sulfoxide (DMSO) or 1,2-propanediol have been successfully used for years for cryopreserving both 2PN zygotes and cleavage stage human embryos.
- The challenges associated with freezing blastocysts are unique due to the large fluid-filled blastocele cavity

that presents an increased risk of **intracellular ice crystal formation**.
- The high water content (75%-85%), related to the large cell size, can convert into ice crystals at low temperatures, generating significant and irreversible damage to the cellular ultrastructure.
- In addition to this, the cytoplasmic oocyte is also characterized by a high sensitivity of the cytoskeleton to low temperatures.

29. d. All of the above

Ref: Yen & Jaffe's 8th/ed p 816

Technological advancements involving three parent IVF are emerging that particularly target oocyte mitochondrial DNA (mtDNA). This focus is driven by the facts that,
1. Mutations in mtDNA can lead to devastating mitochondrial syndromes such as Leigh syndrome, Kearns-Sayre syndrome, and neurogenic weakness with ataxia and retinitis pigmentosa, for which there are currently no cures.
2. Inheritance of mtDNA is strictly through the maternal line.

Germline Nuclear Transfer (NT)

Genome of an oocyte or zygote that carries an mtDNA mutation is transferred into an enucleated donated oocyte or zygote with wild-type mtDNA.

Emerging technologies for prevention of mitochondrial diseases	
Oocyte NT	Zygote NT
Maternal spindle transfer (MST)	Pronuclear transfer (PNT)
Polar body transfer (PBT)	
Germinal vesicle transfer (GVT)	

30. d. All of the above

Ref: Yen & Jaffe's 8th/ed p 816

Risks involved with germline nuclear transfer technologies:
- **Karyoplast mtDNA carryover**—Although this may be minimal at the time of transfer (<1%), several studies with hESC lines have shown a variable increase in mutation load up to 50% to 60% in some of the lines after both PNT and MST.
- Possible **incompatibility** between the patient's nuclear genome and the mtDNA in the reconstituted donor oocyte.
- **Potential shifts in mutation copy number during development**—It is currently unknown whether the mtDNA mutation will accumulate in tissues and organs over time or not, so, prenatal screening is recommended and vigilant, long-term safety and efficacy monitoring of children born from these emerging technologies is required.

31. b. Rapid cooling

Ref: Yen & Jaffe's 8th/ed p 855

The three techniques used for cryopreservation of sperm are:
1. Slow freezing
2. Rapid cooling
3. Vitrification

The most commonly used cryoprotectant :10% glycerol supplemented with hen's egg yolk-citrate buffer.

1. **Slow freezing**
   - Programmable machine can be used.
   - In this case the specimen is prepped in the same way as in rapid cooling, but the sample is cooled in stepwise fashion.
   - A typical protocol may cool at a rate of −10°C/min to −80°C/min, after which the specimen is plunged into liquid nitrogen.
2. **Rapid cooling**
   - The **most common method** used for cryopreservation of sperm.
   - It involved initially mixing the semen sample in dropwise manner with an **equal volume** of cryoprotectant, then placing the sample in a liquid nitrogen **vapor** phase for 10 to 30 minutes. Finally, the sample is plunged into liquid nitrogen.
3. **Vitrification**
   - It is widely for embryo storage but has not been applied to routine sperm cryopreservation.
   - A potential drawback of vitrification is that only a small amount of sperm can be vitrified at one time.

32. a. Slow freezing

Ref: Yen & Jaffe's 8th/ed p 855

Ovarian Tissue Cryopreservation

- Ovarian tissue cryopreservation is much more complex in that it involves multiple cellular types.
- Only the **ovarian cortex** is preserved.
- The presence of stromal tissue may impair the permeation of the cryoprotectant into the ovarian cortex.
- Currently there is no standardized protocol for ovarian tissue cryopreservation.
- The permeable cryoprotectant of choice may be propanediol, dimethyl sulfoxide (DMSO), or ethylene glycol, with or without sucrose.
- The **slow freezing method is thought to be preferable**, as initial reports of vitrification resulted in a lower

proportion of intact oocytes, presumably because insufficient time was allowed for penetration of the cryoprotectant into the tissue.
- Slow freezing remains the **gold standard** for ovarian tissue cryopreservation.

33. c. Vitrification

Ref: Yen & Jaffe's 8th/ed p 855

Oocyte Cryopreservation

- The oocyte is a large cell, with a high water content which makes it susceptible to the formation of ice crystals, with consequent damage to the spindle and organelles.
- Due to the susceptibility of the oocyte to ice crystal formation with slow freezing, vitrification techniques have been employed.
- Clinical outcomes with cryopreserved oocytes have dramatically improved.
- To provide optimal oocyte survival, fertilization, and pregnancy outcomes, **early freezing** (within 2 hours after oocyte retrieval) should be performed.
- ICSI should be performed **2 to 3 hours** after oocyte warming to allow for optimal spindle reformation.
- Most widely used vitrification solution consists of a mixture of 7.5% EG/DMSO plus sucrose (equilibrium solution) and 15% EG/DSMO plus sucrose (vitrification solution).

34. d. Under negative pressure

Ref: Yen & Jaffe's 8th/ed p 823

In order to minimize exposures to contaminants, IVF laboratories must rigorously control air quality.
- IVF laboratories generally have their own central air handling unit (AHU) and/or mobile filter units where the outside (plus recirculating) air is forced through high efficiency particulate air (HEPA) filters, along with activated charcoal, potassium permanganate, and/or activated carbon filters.
- The HEPA filters remove particulate matter (i.e., ≥0.3 μm in size) and absorb mold spores and bacteria. The carbon or charcoal filters remove VOCs.
- To maintain the clean air environment, the laboratory should have:
  - **A high tightness factor**: walls and ceilings should have no penetrations.
  - **Multiple air exchanges per hour**: 15 to 25 air exchanges/hour.
  - **Positive pressure**: To prevent contaminants from adjacent rooms entering the laboratory.

35. d. All of the above

Ref: Textbook of Assisted Reproductive Techniques. D Gardner 5th/ed p 144

Ooplasmic Injection

- The oocyte is held in place by the suction applied to the holding pipette.
- The injection pipette is lowered and focused in accordance with the outer right border of the oolemma on the equatorial plane at three o'clock.
- The spermatozoon is then brought into proximity with the beveled opening of the injection pipette and pushed against the ZP, permitting its penetration to the inner surface of the oolemma.
- As the point of the pipette reaching the approximate center of the oocyte, a break in the membrane should occur. This is reflected by:
  - Sudden **quivering of the convexities** (at the site of invagination) of the oolemma above and below the penetration point.
  - Proximal flow of the cytoplasmic organelles.
  - Spermatozoon moving upward into the pipette.

36. b. Hyaluronic acid

Ref: Textbook of Assisted Reproductive Techniques. D Gardner 5th/ed p 108

In response to this gonadotropin, the cumulus cells produce specific glycosaminoglycans, the secretion of which results in cumulus mucification and its expansion.

The major component of the extracellular matrix secreted by the cumulus cells is **hyaluronic acid**.

The mucified cumulus mass that encapsulates the ovulated egg is penetrated by the spermatozoon that uses enzymes localized on its surface membrane to accomplish this mission.

37. c. 1 & 3

Ref: Yen & Jaffe's 8th/ed p 835

Assessment of Fertilization

- The average fertilization rates for CI are 50% to 70%.
- The fertilization rate after ICSI is usually expressed per number of injected oocytes and ranges from 70% to 80%.
- The current standard of care is to evaluate for fertilization 16 to 20 hours post insemination.
- Fertilization assessment should be performed under high magnification (at least 200×), or a suitable time-lapse microscopy device, in order to verify PN number and morphology.

2PN	• Oocytes are considered normally fertilized when two individualized or fragmented polar bodies are present together with two clearly visible pronuclei (2PN) that contain nucleoli.
0PN	• Failure of fertilization. • Failure of sperm penetration. • Premature sperm chromosome condensation • Failure of sperm head decondensation • Ejection of the sperm from the oocyte • Early syngamy—Typically syngamy occurs 20 to 24 hours after insemination. Syngamy is a time period of pronuclei nuclear breakdown before proceeding through the first mitotic division to form the two-cell embryo. • Embryos with syngamy prior to 23 to 24 hours produce higher implantation rates, while syngamy prior to 20 hours result in decreased live birth rate.
1 PN	• 1PN oocytes after CI are likely to be **parthenogenetically activated** as a result of mechanical or chemical factors. • In some cases, the zygote may be diploid and presence of 1PN may be explained by asynchronous pronuclear formation, or possibly male and female pronuclear fusion (atypical syngamy). • Evidence suggests that more than half of unipronuclear embryos after CI are diploid, which is significantly higher than what is observed after ICSI (20% to 30%)
Multipro-nuclear zygotes	• Triploidy (3PN) is the most common multipronuclear zygote. • The extra pronuclei may be of maternal (dygynic) or paternal (diandric) origin. • If CI, triploidy is most often due to insufficient protection against polyspermy (diandric). • With ICSI, the cause of triploidy is largely due to failure of meiosis II with retention of the second polar body (dygynic). • Triploid zygotes can result in pregnancies with severe congenital anomalies and should not be transferred.

Fertilization Outcomes Following CI or ICSI

Outcome	Ploidy status post CI	Transfer to be done or not	Ploidy status post ICSI	Transfer to be done or not
0PN	>50% diploid	Yes	>50% diploid	Yes
1PN	30-60% diploid	Yes	Haploid	No
2PN	Diploid	yes	Diploid	Yes
3PN	Dispermic triploidy	No	Digynic triploidy	No
>3PN	Multiploidy	No	Multiploidy	No

38. **b. 25–26 hours post-insemination/ICSI**

Ref: Textbook of Assisted Reproductive Techniques. D Gardner 5th/ed p 231

Sequential Embryo Assessment Criteria

- **18–19 hours post-insemination/ICSI**
  Identification of pronucleate oocytes
  The pronuclei are examined for:
  - Symmetry
  - The presence of even numbers of NPBs
  - The positioning of the polar bodies
- **25–26 hours post-insemination/ICSI**
  - Embryos that have already cleaved to the two-cell stage
  - Zygotes that have progressed to nuclear membrane breakdown
- **42–44 hours post-insemination/ICSI**
  - Number of blastomeres should be greater than or equal to four
  - Fragmentation of less than 20%
  - No multinucleated blastomeres
- **66–68 hours post-insemination/ICSI**
  - Number of blastomeres should be greater than or equal to eight
  - Fragmentation of less than 20%
  - No multinucleated blastomeres
- **106–108 hours post-insemination/ICSI**
  - The blastocoel cavity should be full
  - ICM should be numerous and tightly packed
  - Trophectoderm cells should be numerous and cohesive.

CHAPTER 18

Drugs in Reproductive Endocrinology

Multiple Choice Questions

1. Which of the following statement is incorrect about clomiphene citrate?
   a. Enclomiphene is more potent isomer
   b. Only FSH rises, LH remains same
   c. Miscarriage rates with clomiphene are similar to spontaneous conception cycles
   d. Reversible blurred vision by clomiphene is due to its mydriatic action

2. Most severe complication of clomiphene citrate:
   a. Renal failure
   b. Visual disturbances
   c. Hepatic enzyme derangement
   d. Syncope

3. Most common side effect of clomiphene citrate therapy:
   a. Visual floaters
   b. Nausea
   c. Hot flushes
   d. Headaches

4. Given orally in early to midfollicular phase, clomiphene causes .... percent rise in endogenous serum FSH levels:
   a. 20–30
   b. 30–40
   c. 50–60
   d. 70–80

5. For anovulatory women, ovulation and conception rate with clomiphene, respectively:
   a. 80%, 40%
   b. 60%, 20%
   c. 50%, 50%
   d. 80%, 10%

6. Which of the following is not true about recombinant gonadotropins?
   a. More purer than urinary products
   b. More batch to batch consistency
   c. Potency assessed by Steehlman and Pohley assay
   d. Recombinant FSH biosimilars have same efficacy

7. Replacing glycine by D-Amino acid at position 6 makes GnRH agonist, all *except*:
   a. More hydrophobic
   b. More resistant to enzyme degradation
   c. Easily excretable by renal system
   d. More potent

8. Incidence of severe OHSS following gonadotropin ovulation induction:
   a. 1%
   b. 5%
   c. 7%
   d. 10%

9. Multiple pregnancy rates with gonadotropins and clomiphene, respectively:
   a. 30%, 10%
   b. 15%, 5%
   c. 10%, 10%
   d. 30%, 20%

10. Which is the least practical route to administer progesterone as luteal phase support in ART?
    a. Oral
    b. Vaginal
    c. Transdermal
    d. Intramuscular

11. r-hCG 250 µg is at least as effective as .... IU of u-hCG:
    a. 2500
    b. 5000
    c. 7500
    d. 10,000

12. Minimal effective dose of GnRH antagonist to suppress a premature LH rise in most patients:
    a. 0.75 mg
    b. 0.25 mg
    c. 0.50 mg
    d. 1.0 mg

13. Maximum dose of gonadotropin beyond which any increase in live birth rates is not seen:
    a. 450 IU
    b. 300 IU
    c. 600 IU
    d. 550 IU

14. Which of the following is a contraindication to clomiphene administration?
    a. Pre-existing ovarian cysts
    b. Suspected malignancy
    c. Liver disease
    d. All

15. Which is incorrect statement regarding aromatase inhibitors?
    a. Half-life—48 hours
    b. Hepatic metabolism
    c. More teratogenic than clomiphene
    d. Ovulation rate 75%

16. Which of the following is not true regarding gonadotropins?
    a. The treatment of hypogonadotropic women with FSH alone leads to follicular development but not pregnancy
    b. Corifollitropin alpha is long-acting recombinant FSH
    c. Magnitude of FSH elevation above the threshold level is more important than the duration of elevation of FSH for single dominant follicle selection
    d. Urinary derived FSH is associated with a theoretical risk of transmission of prion proteins

17. Pulsatile GnRH administration is a novel therapy in WHO type 1 anovulatory disorders. Which of the following is incorrect about it?
    a. Intravenous route appears superior with higher bioavailability
    b. Cumulative pregnancy rates of 50% to 60% with six cycles
    c. Pulse interval of 60 to 90 minutes is used with a dose of 2.5 to 10 µg per pulse
    d. Pulsatile GnRH administration is continued throughout the luteal phase until menses or a positive pregnancy test

18. Which of the following is false about Corifollitropin-α?
    a. Produced by the fusion of recombinant FSH and the C-terminal peptide of the β-subunit of hCG
    b. Longer half life than daily recombinant FSH
    c. Increased patient friendliness during ovarian stimulation for IVF
    d. Decreased chances of OHSS

19. Which of the following does not carry substantial evidence of benefit of addition of r-LH to r-FSH in women undergoing long gonadotropin-releasing hormone agonist protocols?
    a. Prior poor responders
    b. Mid-follicular (day 6) ultrasound showing no follicle > 10 mm
    c. Age > 35 years
    d. Mid-follicular (day 6) estradiol < 200 pg/mL

20. False statement about GnRH antagonist cotreatment in COH:
    a. Cetrorelix is third generation GnRH antagonist
    b. Minimal effective dose to suppress premature LH rise is 0.25 mg
    c. No difference is seen with respect to live birth rates with antagonist protocol when compared to agonist protocol
    d. Lower pregnancy rates are seen following the fixed protocol

21. Which of the following is not an advantage of using GnRH antagonist in IVF cycles when compared to GnRH agonists?
    a. More flexibility regarding cycle programming
    b. Reduced requirement of exogenous gonadotropins
    c. Short duration of ovarian stimulation
    d. Reduced rate of OHSS

22. Once administered, within how many hours GnRH antagonist lead to blockage of gonadotropin secretion?
    a. 12 hours   b. 24 hours
    c. 72 hours   d. 120 hours

23. As shown by many RCTs, which of the following drugs when given as luteal phase support have found to be helpful in increasing pregnancy rates in fresh embryo transfer cycles?
    1. Progesterone
    2. Estrogen
    3. Aspirin
    4. Doxycycline
    5. Methylprednisone
    a. All
    b. 1 only
    c. 1 & 2
    d. 1, 2 & 3

Answer with Explanations

1. **b. Only FSH rises, LH remains same**

   Ref: Yen & Jaffe's 8th/ed p 752
   - The rise in FSH is accompanied by **a similar rise in serum LH levels.**
   - Miscarriage rates of **13% to 25%** are reported; similar to the spontaneous miscarriage rate and those observed in infertile women undergoing IVF.
   - Hot flushes occur in up to 10% of women taking CC.
   - The **mydriatic action** of CC may cause reversible blurred vision in a similar number.
   - The multiple pregnancy rate is less than **10%,** and OHSS is rare.
   - The putative increased risk of ovarian cancer reported to be associated with the use of CC for more than 12 months has led CC to be licensed for **just 6 months** of use in some countries.

2. **b. Visual disturbances**

   Ref: Textbook of Assisted Reproductive Techniques, Gardner 5th/ed p 501

   Visual symptoms include spots (floaters), flashes, or abnormal perception.
   These disappear following cessation of CC therapy.

3. **c. Hot flushes**

   Ref: Textbook of Assisted Reproductive Techniques, Gardner 5th/ed p 501

   Most common side effect of CC therapy:
   - Hot flushes—10%
   - Bloating and discomfort—5%
   - Breast discomfort—2%
   - Nausea and vomiting—2%
   - Visual symptoms and headaches—1.5%

4. **c. 50–60**

   Ref: Yen & Jaffe's 8th/ed p 752
   - Given orally in the early to midfollicular phase, clomiphene causes a **50% rise in the endogenous serum FSH level,** thus stimulating follicle growth.
   - Limitation of the duration of administration to **5 days** is aimed at allowing FSH levels to fall in the late follicular phase and the mechanisms for monofollicular development and ovulation to operate.

5. **a. 80%, 40%**

   Ref: Yen & Jaffe's 8th/ed p 753; Textbook of Assisted Reproductive Techniques. D Gardner 5th/ed p 500
   - Between 60% and 85% of anovulatory women will become ovulatory with CC, and 30% to 40% will become pregnant.
   - Why do some women who become ovulatory with CC not conceive?
   - Reasons include
     - Patient selection
     - The regimen used
     - The presence of other causes of subfertility
     - The effects of CC on the reproductive tract:
       - Antiestrogen effects on the endometrium
       - Antiestrogen effects on the cervical mucus
       - Decrease of uterine blood flow
       - Impaired placental protein 14 synthesis
       - Subclinical pregnancy loss
       - Effect on tubal transport
       - Detrimental effects on the oocytes

6. **c. Potency assessed by Steehlman and Pohley assay**

   Ref: Yen & Jaffe's 8th/ed p 746

   The recombinant products offer
   - Improved purity
   - More batch to batch consistency
   - Large-scale availability

   - The initial gonadotropin preparations were very impure with many contaminating proteins; only less than 5% of the proteins present were bioactive.
   - As purity improved, it was necessary to add human chorionic gonadotropin (hCG) to maintain this ratio of bioactivity.
   - Bioactivity of gonadotropin preparations continues to be assessed by the crude in vivo rat ovarian weight gain **Steehlman and Pohley assay.**
   - Through recombinant DNA technology and the transfection of human genes encoding for the common α subunit and hormone-specific β subunit of the glycoprotein hormone into Chinese hamster ovary cell lines, the large-scale in vitro production of human recombinant FSH (recFSH) has been realized.
   - Because of its purity, recFSH can now be administered by **protein weight** rather than bioactivity, and so-called **filled by-mass** preparations are now available for clinical use.

7. c. Easily excretable by renal system
Ref: Yen & Jaffe's 8th/ed p 747

- An increased potency could be achieved by replacing
  - Glycine for D-amino acids at **position 6**
  - Gly-NH$_2$ by ethylamide at **position 10**
- Clinically safe GnRH agonists were developed relatively easily by replacing one or two amino acids.
- Such simple structural changes render these compounds
  - More **hydrophobic** and thus less easily excretable, increasing half life.
  - More **resistant** to enzymatic degradation.
  - More **potent.**

Flare effect
The administration of GnRH agonists induces an initial stimulation of gonadotropin release for 2 to 3 weeks followed by a downregulation (or desensitization) due to the clustering and internalization of pituitary GnRH receptors.

8. a. 1%
Ref: Yen & Jaffe's 8th/ed p 748

The incidences of OHSS following gonadotropin ovulation induction:
- Mild—20%
- Moderate—6–7%
- Severe—1–2%

- Moderate to critical OHSS is very rare with CC but constitutes an important complication of gonadotropin use.
- In addition to PCOS, risk factors for the development of OHSS include young age and low body weight.
- The risk is further increased when adjuvant GnRH agonist treatment is employed.

9. a. 30%, 10%
Ref: Yen & Jaffe's 8th/ed p 750; 753

- Overall cumulative pregnancy rates with gonadotropin therapy are reported to be 33% within three cycles, but at the price of an unacceptably high multiple pregnancy rate of 20% for twins and 10% for higher-order multiple pregnancy.
- Less intense ovarian stimulation may reduce the incidence of higher-order multiple pregnancies, but probably at the expense of a reduction in overall conception rate.
- Multiple pregnancy rates with clomiphene remains less than 10%.

10. c. Transdermal
Ref: Textbook of Assisted Reproductive Techniques. D Gardner 5th/ed p 613

- Progesterone cannot be administered transdermally and probably never will be.
- Reasons:
  - The doses that need to be administered for matching corpus luteum production (25 mg/24 hours in the midluteal phase) are several orders of magnitude larger than the daily production of estradiol (from 0.05 to 0.5 mg/24 hours). This would require that skin systems be much too large for any practical application.
  - The skin is rich in **5α-reductase**, an enzyme that is capable of inactivating progesterone, thus hampering any possible efficacy.
- While transdermal administration of synthetic progestins exists (for contraception), transdermal progesterone is not available for LPS in ART.

11. b. 5000
Ref: Textbook of Assisted Reproductive Techniques. D Gardner 5th/ed p 506

- r-hCG 250 μg is at least as effective as 5000 IU of u-hCG.
- A 2016 meta-analysis compared clinical outcomes following final follicle maturation with uhCG, rhCG, or recombinant LH (rLH).
- The ongoing pregnancy/live birth rates were similar between uhCG and rhCG and also between uhCG and rLH.
- There were no differences in rates of OHSS.

12. b. 0.25 mg
Ref: Yen & Jaffe's 8th/ed p 768

- Both single high-dose and multiple low-dose GnRH antagonist regimens have been described.
- Multiple, daily dose regimens are most widely used at present.
- Initial dose finding studies suggested that a daily injection of **0.25 mg** represents the minimal effective dose to suppress a premature LH rise in most patients.
- GnRH antagonists need only be given when there is follicular development and rising E2 levels that might give rise to a premature elevation in pituitary LH release due to positive feedback mechanisms.

13. a. 450 IU
Ref: Yen & Jaffe's 8th/ed p 800

Maximum dose of gonadotropin that should be prescribed per day is 450 IU, as higher doses have not been shown to be more effective and only result in additional medication cost.

14. **d. All**

Ref: Textbook of Assisted Reproductive Techniques.
D Gardner 5th/ed p 500

Contraindications to clomiphene administration include
- Preexisting ovarian cysts
- Suspected malignancy
- Liver disease

15. **c. More teratogenic than clomiphene**

Ref: Textbook of Assisted Reproductive Techniques.
D Gardner 5th/ed p 502

Aromatase Inhibitors

The different types and generations of aromatase inhibitors		
Generation	Type I	Type II
First	None	Aminoglutethimide
Second	Formestane	• Fadrozole • Rogletimide
Third	Exemestane	• Anastrozole • Letrozole • Vorozole

- Administered **orally.**
- Half-life of approximately **48 hours**, which allows once-daily dosing.
- Metabolized mainly in the **liver.**
- Excreted through the **biliary** (85%) and the urinary (11%) systems.
- Side effects observed after long-term administration:
  - Bone pain (20%)
  - Hot flushes (18%)
  - Back pain (17%)
  - Nausea (15%)
  - Dyspnea (14%)
- Cumulative rates of teratogenicity with letrozole are <5% and comparable to rates with clomiphene.
- In patients with PCOS, ovulation rate is 75% and conception rate is 25%.
- Letrozole appears to prevent unfavourable effects on the endometrium that are frequently observed with antiestrogen use for ovulation induction.

16. **c. Magnitude of FSH elevation above the threshold level is more important than the duration of elevation of FSH for single dominant follicle selection**

Ref: Yen & Jaffe's 8th/ed p 756

The concept of the FSH "window" stresses the significance of the **duration** of FSH elevation above the threshold level rather than the magnitude of elevation of FSH for single dominant selection.
So, it is the duration for which FSH remains elevated which is more important rather than the magnitude.

17. **b. Cumulative pregnancy rates of 50% to 60% with six cycles**

Ref: Yen & Jaffe's 8th/ed p 759

Pulsatile Gonadotropin-releasing Hormone Therapy

- Effective, reliable, and safe alternative to gonadotropin therapy for treating WHO type 1 anovulation.
- Lower chances of multifollicular development and ovarian hyperstimulation.
- To mimic the normal pulsatile release of GnRH, a pulse interval of 60 to 90 minutes is used with a dose of **2.5 to 10 µg** per pulse.
- The lower dose should be used initially to minimize the likelihood of multiple pregnancies.
- Pulsatile GnRH administration may be continued throughout the luteal phase until menses or a positive pregnancy test. Alternatively, it may be discontinued after ovulation, and the corpus luteum supported by hCG.
- Cumulative pregnancy rates of **83% to 95% after six cycles** have been reported, with multiple pregnancies accounting for 3% to 8% of pregnancies.
Route?
- The intravenous route appears superior to the subcutaneous route.
- Local complications such as **phlebitis** may occasionally be encountered when intravenous administration is used. To avoid this, pulsatile GnRH can be administered subcutaneously.
- Subcutaneous route is certainly simpler than the intravenous route but plasma GnRH profiles are damped after subcutaneous administration and **bioavailability is reduced**. However, the increased convenience offered by the subcutaneous route has led to this approach being favoured.

18. **d. Decreased chances of OHSS**

Ref: Textbook of assisted reproductive techniques.
D Gardner 5th/ed p 510

Corifollitropin-α

- Produced by the **fusion** of α-subunit of r-hFSH together with a hybrid β-subunit made up of the β-subunit of hFSH and the C-terminal part of the β-subunit of hCG.
- FSH-CTP has a **longer half-life** than standard r-hFSH.
- It initiates and sustains follicular growth for **one week**, so one dose can replace the first seven daily injections of gonadotropin in COS.
- FSH-CTP is now approved for use in Europe in ART cycles in combination with a GnRH antagonist.

- Ongoing pregnancy rates per cycle initiated are not significantly different for FSH–CTP or r-hFSH.
- The reported incidence of moderate/severe **OHSS** is 4.1% with corifollitropin-α versus 2.7% with follitropin-β. (OHSS risk is higher, not lower)
- The effects of FSH–CTP cannot be adjusted to individual patient requirements; therefore, careful assessment of patient suitability is required before treatment is commenced.
- Because of some of these concerns, the recent focus of research has been in the use of corifollitropin-α in ART patients with **a known poor response** to FSH.

19. **c. Age > 35 years**

    Ref: Current opinion on use of luteinizing hormone supplementation in assisted reproduction therapy. Reproductive BioMedicine Online (2011) 23, 81–90

Consensus on recommended use of LH in Asian women undergoing long gonadotropin-releasing hormone agonist protocols	
Patient category	Indication

Substantial evidence of benefit of r-HLH in addition to r-HFSH	Prior poor responders, defined as
	• Oocyte count < 4 in previous cycle
	• Mid-follicular (day 6) suboptimal response on long agonist
	  ○ No follicles >10 mm
	  ○ Estradiol < 200 pg/mL
	  ○ Endometrial thickness < 6 mm

Some evidence of benefit of r-HLH in addition to r-HFSH	Age >35 years started on ovarian stimulation with either the long agonist or antagonist protocol
Further research is needed to determine benefit of r-HLH	• Biomarkers e.g. variant LH • Low baseline serum LH < 1.2 IU/L • Low antral follicle count • Low anti-Mullerian hormone

20. **d. Lower pregnancy rates are seen following the fixed protocol**

    Ref: Yen & Jaffe's 8th/ed p 768

- Both single high-dose and multiple low-dose GnRH antagonist regimens have been described.
- Multiple, daily dose regimens are most widely used at present.
- Initial dose finding studies suggested that a daily injection of **0.25 mg** represents the minimal effective dose to suppress a premature LH rise in most patients.
- In all phase 3 comparative trials of the daily GnRH antagonist cotreatment regimen, it was initiated on cycle day 6.
- However, in principle, GnRH antagonists need only be given when there is follicular development and rising E2 levels that might give rise to a premature elevation in pituitary LH release due to positive feedback mechanisms.
- However, a meta-analysis of four studies comparing fixed with flexible regimens showed a trend toward lower pregnancy rates following the **flexible** protocol (OR 0.7; 95% CI, 0.47 to 1.05).

21. **a. More flexibility regarding cycle programming**

    Ref: Yen & Jaffe's 8th/ed p 768

Advantages and disadvantages for the Use of GnRH Antagonists in IVF	
Advantages	Disadvantages
• Prevention of premature LH increase is easier and takes less time. • GnRH antagonists are not associated with an initial acute stimulation of gonadotropins and steroid hormones (so-called flare effect). • The initial stimulation by GnRH agonists can induce ovarian cyst formation. • No hot flushes are observed with GnRH antagonists. • Inadvertent administration of the GnRH analogue in early pregnancy can be avoided, as GnRH antagonist is administered in the follicular phase of the menstrual cycle. • Requirements for exogenous gonadotropins are reduced, rendering ovarian stimulation less costly. • Duration of ovarian stimulation protocols is shortened, improving patient discomfort. • Reduced rate of OHSS with similar efficacy.	• Still more experience with GnRH agonist cotreatment. • GnRH antagonists offer **less flexibility regarding cycle programming** as compared with the long GnRH agonist protocol. • Reduced ability to gain an orderly daily volume of oocyte retrievals compared with GnRH agonist, although this can be improved by using the oral contraceptive pill.

22. **b. 24 hours**

    Ref: Yen & Jaffe's 8th/ed p 797

- GnRH antagonists offer the possibility of acutely suppressing LH secretion without an initial increase in LH release.
- They act as competitive inhibitors of the GnRH receptor, such that they can off compete endogenous GnRH, leading to an acute decrease in gonadotropin secretion **within 24 hours**.
- GnRH antagonists are typically administered as a small daily dose (cetrorelix or ganirelix, 0.25 mg daily by subcutaneous injection), usually starting on cycle day 6 to 8 or when the lead follicle reaches 14 mm in diameter or as a single large dose (cetrorelix, 3 mg subcutaneously, which has a 4-day duration of action) on approximately cycle day 8.

23. b. 1 only

Ref: Yen & Jaffe's 8th/ed p 812

- While luteal phase support with exogenous progesterone is critical following IVF, the addition of other medications (estrogen, aspirin, doxycycline, and methylprednisone) has not been shown to be helpful.

• Progesterone	• Because oocyte retrieval is associated with the removal of a large number of granulosa cells, the adequacy of ovarian progesterone production after oocyte retrieval has been a major concern since the inception of IVF.
	• Two major methods of luteal-phase support have been used in fresh IVF cycles: progesterone supplementation (vaginal or intramuscular preparations) or hCG.
	• Both appear to be associated with an increased pregnancy rate compared with no luteal support, but hCG is associated with a higher rate of OHSS.
	• **Optimal window** for initiating luteal phase support begins after oocyte retrieval but ends by the third day after oocyte retrieval.
	• Length of time necessary for luteal phase support ?
	• A recent randomized trial in 220 women using micronized progesterone vaginally found **no difference** in miscarriage or ongoing pregnancy rates when progesterone was discontinued at 5 versus 8 weeks of gestation. However, there was substantially more bleeding in the group discontinuing treatment at 5 weeks.
	• Given the anxiety first trimester bleeding causes patients, treatment beyond 5 weeks seems reasonable.
	• A major problem with the use of progesterone for luteal phase support is the **pain and sterile abscesses** associated with daily intramuscular injections.
• Estrogens	• Role of supplemental estrogen is less clear.
	• In cycles utilizing GnRH agonists or GnRH antagonists, the profound suppression of gonadotropins in the follicular phase may carry over to the luteal phase.
	• A 2015 meta-analysis of 15 RCTs demonstrated that there was no difference in clinical pregnancy rates with luteal estradiol supplementation.
• Low-dose aspirin	• Aspirin is proposed to increase ovarian blood flow, improving folliculogenesis and promoting implantation.
	• Some practitioners begin aspirin during ovarian stimulation, while others utilize it only in the luteal phase, believing that it may contribute to excessive bleeding during oocyte retrieval.
	• A meta-analysis of seven trials included 1241 women undergoing ovarian stimulation for IVF or ICSI.
	• There was no significant improvement in IVF/ICSI outcome for women taking aspirin in terms of clinical pregnancy or live birth.
	• There were no differences between the groups with respect to miscarriage or ectopic pregnancies.
	• The authors concluded that the currently available data do not support the use of aspirin in IVF cycles.
• Doxycycline	• There are no RCTs addressing the clinical efficacy of doxycycline post oocyte retrieval; as such, its routine use is discouraged.
• Methylprednisone	• 2012 meta-analysis of 14 RCTs ($n = 1879$) showed no difference in live birth rates following glucocorticoid administration.

CHAPTER 19

Miscellaneous

Multiple Choice Questions

1. Mini hypothalamus:
   a. Hamartomas
   b. Craniopharyngiomas
   c. Ependymomas
   d. Pinealomas

2. First and second polar bodies each contain how many chromosomes?
   a. 23, 46
   b. 46, 46
   c. 23, 23
   d. 46, 23

3. An oocyte arrested in prophase of meiosis enveloped by a single layer of granulosa cells surrounded by a basement membrane:
   a. Primary follicle
   b. Primordial follicle
   c. Preantral follicle
   d. Antral follicle

4. Testes begin to differentiate at?
   a. 6–7 weeks
   b. 7–8 weeks
   c. 8–9 weeks
   d. 9–10 weeks

5. Due to fixed initial endowment of germ cells, the newborn female enters life having lost .... percent of her oocytes:
   a. 30
   b. 50
   c. 10
   d. 80

6. Which of the following statement is false?
   a. In female fetus, loss of Wolffian system is due to lack of circulating testosterone
   b. Primitive germ cells are unable to survive in locations other than genital ridge
   c. Girls with Turner syndrome experience normal migration and mitosis of germ cells, but oogonia do not undergo meiosis
   d. Hypothalamic-pituitary portal circulation is functional by 12th week

7. False about AMH in male fetus:
   a. Secreted at 7 weeks
   b. Comes from leydig cells
   c. After involution of Müllerian ducts, AMH continues to be secreted, but there is no known function
   d. Causes Müllerian duct regression by 8th week

8. A 20-year-old girl presents with cramping pain which starts along with menses and stays for first two days. She is otherwise fine. What is this condition?
   a. Secondary dysmenorrhea
   b. Mittelschmerz
   c. Congestive dysmenorrhea
   d. Primary dysmenorrhea

9. Which of the following is by-product of female gametogenesis?
   a. Polar body
   b. Mature oocyte
   c. Oogonia
   d. Primary oocyte

10. How much it takes for a single sperm to form in total?
    a. 64 hours
    b. 12 days
    c. 64 days
    d. 12 hours

11. Which of following male cell contain 23 chromosomes and is followed by spermiogenesis?
    a. Spermatid
    b. Primary spermatocyte
    c. Secondary spermatocyte
    d. Spermatogonia

12. Which hormone promotes proliferation of glandular and stromal elements of endometrium?
    a. Progestrone
    b. FSH
    c. Estradiol
    d. Activin

13. Most suitable dynamic test for evaluation of growth hormone secretion:
    a. Growth hormone releasing hormone and arginine test
    b. Oral glucose tolerance test
    c. Insulin tolerance test
    d. Clonidine stimulation test

14. Line of separation during menstruation runs from:
    a. Stratus spongiosum
    b. Stratum basalis
    c. Stratus functionalis
    d. Any layer

15. All of the following will lead to increased endogenous estrogen levels, *except*:
    a. Decreased SHBG
    b. Obesity
    c. Decreased aromatization
    d. Liver diseases

16. Mid cycle LH surge induces all *except*:
    a. Resumption of meiosis
    b. Formation of corpus luteum
    c. Luteinization of theca and granulosa cells
    d. Early production of estrogen

17. FSH and LH ratio in Human menopausal gonadotropin:
    a. 1:1
    b. 2:1
    c. 3:1
    d. 1:2

18. Local side effects such as pain and allergic reactions in urinary products are attributed to:
    a. FSH
    b. LH
    c. Both FSH and LH
    d. Nongonadotropin proteins

19. Which of the following is incorrect for Danazol?
    a. Danazol is orally administered isoxazol derivative of 17α-ethinyltestosterone
    b. Acts primarily by inhibiting the midcycle urinary LH surge
    c. Creates low androgen, high estrogen environment
    d. Inhibits steroidogenic enzymes and increases free testosterone levels

20. Most common cause of recurrent pregnancy loss in 1st trimester:
    a. Genetic factors
    b. Uterine factors
    c. Medical problems
    d. Immunologic factors

21. Most common chromosomal abnormalities observed among abortuses:
    a. Monosomy X
    b. Autosomal trisomies
    c. Polyploidies
    d. Structural abnormalities

22. Timely appearance of embryonic heart activity in normal woman decreases risk of pregnancy loss from global risk of 15% to:
    a. <5%
    b. 5-10%
    c. 10-15%
    d. Remains same

23. In woman <35 years of age with recurrent pregnancy loss, miscarriage rate after timely appearance of embryonic heart activity:
    a. 25-35%
    b. 35-55%
    c. 60%
    d. 15-25%

24. Most common congenital uterine anomaly associated with recurrent pregnancy loss:
    a. Bicornuate uterus
    b. Unicornuate uterus
    c. Septate uterus
    d. Uterus didelphys

25. Which of the following is incorrect regarding infertility?
    a. Fecundability is the probability that cycle will result in live birth
    b. Rate of conception within one year of regular unprotected sexual act is 80%
    c. Infertility affects 10-15% of couples
    d. Rate of infertility increases as couple ages

26. Incorrect regarding luteal phase defect:
    a. Lag of more than 2 days in histological development of endometrium compared to day of cycle
    b. Very rare phenomenon in normal woman
    c. Inadequate progesterone secretion or action
    d. Higher incidence seen in women with recurrent pregnancy loss

27. Average monthly fecundability in normal couple:
    a. 25%
    b. 10%
    c. 50%
    d. 75%

28. Unexplained infertility will be labelled with evidence of all of the following, *except*:
    a. Normal postcoital test
    b. Normal semen analysis
    c. Normal documented ovulation
    d. Bilateral patent tubes

29. Which of the following is not correct regarding drug most commonly used for ovulation induction?
    a. Weak estrogenic actions are clinically apparent only when endogenous estrogen levels are very low
    b. Steroidal triphenylethylene derivative that acts as a selective estrogen receptor modulator (SERM)
    c. Clomiphene is cleared through the liver and excreted in the stool
    d. Enclomiphene is the more potent isomer and the one responsible for its ovulation-inducing actions

30. Which of the following is not true regarding post-coital test?
    a. Shaking movement of sperm in post-coital test is suggestive of immunologic infertility
    b. Intrauterine insemination can be an appropriate treatment for poor post-coital test
    c. Has a good validity
    d. Clinically useful in patient who is going to have superovulation combined with IUI

31. Which of the following statement incorrect?
    a. Menstrual period for 10 years before menopause show progressive prolong follicular phase followed by short follicular phase
    b. A progesterone concentration more than 3 ng/mL implies ovulation
    c. In cycles monitored with BBT, the interval of highest fertility spans the 7-day interval immediately before the midcycle rise in BBT.
    d. A low AFC has high specificity for predicting poor response to ovarian stimulation

32. Measurement of which of the following antibodies does not form part of criteria for diagnosis of antiphospholipid antibody syndrome?
    a. Lupus anticoagulant
    b. Anticardiolipin antibody
    c. Anti-β2-glycoprotein 1 antibody
    d. Antiphosphatidylserine antibody

33. Which of the following is not correct regarding antiphospholipid antibody syndrome?
    a. Prevalence of antiphospholipid syndrome among women with recurrent pregnancy loss is very high (>15%)
    b. Abnormal laboratory test results must be observed on at least two separate occasions at least 12 weeks apart
    c. Antiphospholipid antibodies are directed against platelets and the vascular endothelium
    d. Live birth rates for women with antiphospholipid syndrome who receive combined treatment with aspirin and unfractionated heparin during pregnancy are 70–80%

34. Which of the following is incorrect regarding thromobophilias as cause of recurrent pregnancy loss?
    a. Tests to detect antinuclear and antithyroid antibodies have no clinical utility in euthyroid women with recurrent pregnancy loss
    b. Factor V Leiden mutation and prothrombin gene mutation are the most common causes of thrombophilia
    c. Have strong association for first trimester pregnancy loss
    d. Hyperhomocystinemia is a known risk factor for thrombosis

35. Maximum fertilizable life span for sperm and egg, respectively:
    a. 5 days, 24 hours
    b. 3 days, 12 hours
    c. 3 days, 24 hours
    d. 5 days, 12 hours

36. Which of the following statements is incorrect?
    a. If anovulation is the only factor, most couples will become pregnant within 3 months of ovulation induction
    b. Age related decline in fecundity is primarily due to uterine factor
    c. Majority of early abortions after age 35 are due to autosomal trisomies
    d. Risk of ectopic pregnancy is increased 7 fold after pelvic infection

37. All of the following are at risk of luteal phase defect, except:
    a. Taking gonadotropin for ovulation induction
    b. History of recurrent pregnancy loss
    c. Showing short luteal phases on basal body temperature charts
    d. Taking clomiphene citrate for ovulation induction

38. Which of the following statements is incorrect regarding primary dysmenorrhea?
    a. Prostaglandin E2 is primary mediator of dysmenorrhea
    b. Caused by myometrial ischemia due to frequent and prolonged uterine contractions
    c. Pain coincident with onset of menses
    d. Intrauterine pressures can reach as high as 400 mm Hg

39. Amount of menstrual bleeding to label as menorrhagia and hypomenorrhea, respectively:
    a. 50 mL, 10 mL
    b. 80 mL, 10 mL
    c. 80 mL, 5 mL
    d. 50 mL, 5 mL

40. Examples of estrogen withdrawal bleeding include all *except*:
    a. Following bilateral oophorectomy during the follicular phase
    b. Following cyclic estrogen-only hormone therapy in castrate or postmenopausal women
    c. Midcycle bleeding that can accompany the transient but abrupt fall in estrogen levels immediately preceding ovulation
    d. Following estrogen progestin cyclic hormone therapy

41. All of the following are features of adenomyosis, *except*:
    a. Myometrial cysts on transvaginal ultrasound is the most specific diagnostic criterion
    b. Adenomyosis is a disorder characterized by the extension of endometrial glands into the myometrium
    c. Thickening of the junctional zone on MRI T2 weighted imaging is characteristic
    d. Patient presents as multiparous woman with dysmenorrhea and menorrhagia

42. Which of the following is incorrect regarding Mirena?
    a. Not useful if ovulatory woman presents with menorrhagia
    b. Consist of 52 mg levonorgestrel
    c. Approved for 5 years
    d. Menstrual blood loss in women with heavy menstrual bleeding can be reduced by 75–95%

43. All of the following are role of prolactin in amniotic fluid, *except*:
    a. Protecting the human fetus from dehydration
    b. To allow labour to proceed in a timely manner
    c. Promote surfactant production
    d. All are true

44. Which of the following is not true regarding lactation?
    a. Human placental lactogen has very strong lactogenic effect
    b. The increase in prolactin parallels the increase in estrogen beginning at 7–8 weeks' gestation
    c. Increase in prolactin secretion is due to estrogen suppression of dopamine
    d. Full lactation is inhibited by progesterone

45. Galactorrhea is least likley associated with:
    a. Antipsychotic drugs
    b. Hypothyroidism
    c. Low dose estrogen progesterone oral contraceptive pills
    d. Severe renal diseases

46. Which is not true for AMH?
    a. Participant in feedback relationship between ovary and pituitary gonadotropins
    b. Can be measured in any phase of menstrual cycle
    c. Marker of ovarian reserves of follicles
    d. Product of granulosa cells

47. Which of the following conditions are not associated with early menopause?
    a. Irregular menses in 40's
    b. Frequent consumption of alcohol
    c. History of hysterectomy
    d. Smokers

48. Which of the following statements is not true regarding menopause?
    a. Age of menopause has changed very little since early Greek times
    b. Overweight women have more hot flushes
    c. Hot flushes coincides with surge of FSH
    d. Vaginal pH >4.5 suggests estrogen deficiency

49. Which of the following statements is not true regarding endocrinology of menopause?
    a. Both FSH and LH rises to 10 fold postmenopause
    b. Androstenedione is principal steroid secreted by postmenopausal ovary
    c. The circulating estradiol level after menopause is approximately 10-20 pg/mL
    d. Most of the circulating estradiol derived from peripheral conversion of estrone

50. Which of the following medication is not associated with osteoporosis?
    a. Thyroxine
    b. SSRI
    c. Proton pump inhibitors
    d. Teriparatide

51. Most important hormone responsible for spermatogenesis:
    a. Testosterone   b. DHEA
    c. Dihydrotestosterone   d. Androsterone

52. **Most common cause of non-obstructive azoospermia:**
    a. Kallmann syndrome
    b. 47, XXY
    c. 47, XYY
    d. 46, XX male syndrome

53. **Cardinal feature of men with 47, XXY, irrespective of clinical spectrum of syndrome:**
    a. Gynecomastia
    b. Eunuchoid habitus
    c. Learning difficulties
    d. Small testes

54. **Which gene is most likely involved in cryptorchidism?**
    a. INSL-3
    b. GREAT
    c. SPATA-16
    d. AKT

55. **Primary cells involved in testosterone production in males:**
    a. Sertoli cells
    b. Leydig cells
    c. Germ cells
    d. Peritubular myoid cells

Answer with Explanations

1. **a. Hamartomas**

   Ref: Yen & Jaffe's 8th/ed p 393; Endotext. Aug 2015. Normal and abnormal puberty

   - Hypothalamic hamartomas are congenital malformations composed of a heterotropic gray matter, neurons, and glial cells usually located on the floor of the third ventricle or attached to the tuber cinereum, are a common etiology of precocious gonadarche.
   - The tumors can be classified as parahypothalamic, attached or suspended from the floor of the third ventricle, or as intrahypothalamic, in which the mass is enveloped by the hypothalamus and distorts the third ventricle.
   - The lesions do not grow over time and do not metastasize.
   - Extreme precocity or the absence of circulating tumor markers such as β-hCG and α-fetoprotein suggests a hamartoma.

   Points to be remembered regarding hamartomas:
   - Heterotopic neuronal masses containing GnRH neurons that attach to tuber cinereum or floor of third ventricle.
   - Function as **ectopic hypothalamic pulse generators** divorced from central inhibitory mechanisms.
   - Most common tumors associated with **central** precocious puberty.
   - Can be associated with **gelastic seizures.**

2. **c. 23, 23**

   Ref: Oogenesis. Giovanni Coticchio et al. p 220

   - Both polar bodies contain 23 chromosomes each.
   - In response to LH surge, the oocyte resumes meiosis; chromosomes condense and during anaphase, at the end of first meiosis (MI), the separations of the bivalents, which move to the opposite poles of the meiotic spindle, occur.
   - 23 chromosomes (each composed by two chromatids) enter the polar body (PB), while the remaining 23 are maintained within the oocyte.
   - After MI, a second meiotic spindle forms immediately, the remaining chromosomes align at the spindle equator, and the cell cycle stops again until fertilization, when fusion of the sperm and egg plasma membranes triggers the resumption and completion of MII.
   - Sister chromatids, which have been held together until this step, are separated passing one into the second PB and the other remaining in the oocyte.
   - Thus, female meiosis takes a very long period to be completed, since this process starts during fetal life and reaches the conclusion until years later with the fertilization of an ovulated mature oocyte.

3. **b. Primordial follicle**

   Ref: Oogenesis. Giovanni Coticchio et al. p 40

   - The female germline is stored within the ovary in the form of primordial follicles, which are comprised of non-growing, meiotically arrested oocytes surrounded by a **single layer** of **flattened pre-granulosa cells.**
   - Although recently challenged, it remains widely accepted that the population of primordial follicles established during fetal life is finite.
   - Throughout life, the number of primordial follicles progressively declines, and eventually, the supply becomes so low that the menopause or reproductive senescence begins.
   - Primordial follicles have one of two fates:
     - Recruitment into the growth phase, with the possibility of ovulation
     - Death.
   - An oocyte arrested in prophase of meiosis enveloped by a single layer of granulosa cells surrounded by a basement membrane is primordial follicle
   - As oocyte enlarges and gets surrounded by a membrane, the zona pellucida, it becomes preantral follicle

4. **a. 6-7 weeks**

   Ref: Cambridge. Infertility in the male. 4th/ed p 8

   - By the sixth week of development, if the embryo is chromosomally XY, cells in the sex cords in the medulla will grow and become Sertoli cells, under the influence of SRY (sex-determining region of the Y sex chromosome), and the cortex will disappear.
   - The Sertoli cells will start to produce AMH, which will halt the development of the paramesonephric ducts and eventually cause rapid regression during the eighth to tenth week of development.
   - The pimordial germ cells are embedded in testicular cords.

- Mature sertoli cells are site of production of ABP (Androgen binding protein) and inhibin.

5. d. 80

Ref: Speroff 8th/ed p 115

The cortical content of germ cells falls to **2 million** by birth as a result of prenatal oocyte depletion. This occurs over a short time period of 20 weeks.

Due to fixed initial endowment of germ cells, the newborn female enters life having lost **80 percent** of her oocytes.

6. a. In female fetus, loss of Wolffian system is due to lack of circulating testosterone

Ref: Speroff 8th/ed p 339

- Testosterone can reach the developing Wolffian duct system via the systemic fetal circulation, but the paracrine actions of testosterone produced in nearby Leydig cells are more important for the stabilization and differentiation of the wolffian duct.
- High local concentrations of testosterone stimulate the ipsilateral Wolffian duct to differentiate into the epididymis, vas deferens, and seminal vesicle.
- Duct system differentiation proceeds, therefore, according to the nature of the adjacent gonad. High concentrations of testosterone are required because the duct does not have the ability to convert testosterone to dihydrotestosterone (DHT).
- For the same reason, the Wolffian ducts do not develop in female fetuses exposed to excess endogenous adrenal androgens or to excess maternally-derived androgens, as occurs in women with pregnancy luteoma.
- Testosterone acts via binding to androgen receptors in the Wolffian duct, which are detectable in both males and females, but androgen production in females does not approach the levels required to promote wolffian duct differentiation.
- Thus, in female fetus, loss of Wolffian system is due to lack of **locally** produced testosterone.

7. b. Comes from leydig cells

Ref: Yen & Jaffe's 8th/ed p 833

- AMH is produced by the **granulosa cells** of pre-antral and small antral follicles and its values are virtually undetectable at the birth but increase gradually until puberty and then remain relatively stable during the early reproductive period.
- In the third decade (30s), AMH levels start declining and become very low during perimenopausal period.
- The measurement of AMH in blood is mainly used to assess ovarian reserve but may be useful also to diagnose alterations of follicle recruitment and initial growth.
- In fact, measurement of AMH has been used in evaluation of sexual ambiguity (male neonates have much higher levels than female neonates) and to distinguish between hypogonadism and delayed puberty.
- Low levels of AMH are found in Turner syndrome and hypogonadotropic hypogonadism.
- In fetus, AMH is secreted at the time of Sertoli cell differentiation at 7 weeks leading to regression of Müllerian duct by 8 weeks with no known function after involution of Müllerian ducts.

8. d. Primary dysmenorrhea

Ref: Speroff 8th/ed p 579

- Dysmenorrhea is cyclical cramping pains occurring before or during menstruation.
- Primary dysmenorrhea is a benign condition mostly associated with **ovulatory cycles** often dating since menarche.

Dysmenorrhea

- Primary dysmenorrhea is caused by myometrial ischemia due to frequent and prolonged uterine contractions. Studies of uterine blood flow using Doppler ultrasonography have revealed that uterine and arcuate artery resistance on the first day of menses is significantly higher in women with primary dysmenorrhea than in women without dysmenorrhea, suggesting that constriction of uterine vessels is the proximate cause for pain.
- The secretory endometrium contains substantial stores of arachidonic acid, which is converted to prostaglandin F_{2a} (PGF_{2a}), prostaglandin E_2 (PGE_2), and leukotrienes during menses. PGF_{2a} always stimulates uterine contractions and is the primary mediator of dysmenorrhea. Endometrial concentrations of PGF_{2a} and PGE_2 correlate with the severity of dysmenorrhea.
- Classically, primary dysmenorrhea begins just before or coincident with the onset of menses and declines gradually over the subsequent 72 hours. The menstrual cramps are intermittent, vary in intensity, and usually are centered in the suprapubic region. Typically, the pattern is consistent across cycles.
- In contrast, women with secondary dysmenorrhea related to pelvic pathology, such as endometriosis, frequently report increasingly severe pain that often occurs at midcycle and during the week preceding menses, in addition to symptoms of deep dyspareunia and dyschezia (painful bowel movements).

- In those with secondary dysmenorrhea related to uterine myomas, pain results primarily from menorrhagia, with an intensity that correlates with the volume of menstrual flow.

9. **a. Polar body**

   Ref: Oogenesis. Giovanni Coticchio et al. p 13

The polar body is merely a **useless by-product** of gametogenesis which subsequently degenerates.

10. **c. 64 days**

    Ref: Cambridge. Infertility in the male. 4th/ed p 74

- Spermatogenesis refers to the production and development of spermatozoa, the mature male gametes of most sexually reproducing species.
- In mammals, spermatogenesis begins with diploid stem cells that resemble other somatic cells; it ends with highly specialized motile haploid cells that are remarkably unique in appearance and function.
- While somewhat lengthy, taking about **64 days** in humans, spermatogenesis is a highly efficient procedure leading to the production of an estimated 70 million spermatozoa daily.

11. **a. Spermatid**

    Ref: Cambridge. Infertility in the male. 4th/ed p 75

Starting cell type	Ploidy
A spermatogonium	Diploid
B spermatogonium	Diploid
Primary spermatocyte	Diploid
Secondary spermatocyte	Haploid
Spermatid	Haploid
Spermatozoon	Haploid

Spermatid contains 23 chromosomes and it is followed by spermiogenesis.

12. **c. Estradiol**

    Ref: Speroff 8th/ed p 61

Estrogen is major proliferating and progesterone is major differentiating hormone in body.

13. **b. Oral glucose tolerance test**

    Ref: Yen & Jaffe's 8th/ed p 843

Growth Hormone Deficiency

- It leads to **short stature** associated with **delayed bone age**.
- There is history of a **normal growth rate until 6–12 months** of age, then growth velocity tails off.
- GH deficiency is associated with **neonatal hypoglycemia** and, jaundice and doll like face.
- It should be differentiated from hypothyroidism as hypothyroidism is often associated with short stature but there will be weight gain and other signs of thyroid disease like dry skin, constipation and bradycardia.

Oral Glucose Tolerance Test

- The OGTT is the **primary test** used for the diagnosis of GH hypersecretion.
- After an overnight fast, 75 to 100 g of oral glucose will cause a suppression of serum GH.
- Blood samples are taken every 30 minutes for 2 hours.
- With usual polyclonal RIAs, a GH decrease to below 2 ng/mL is found in normal subjects while 80% of acromegalic subjects will not suppress to this level.
- The monoclonal assays are much more sensitive for testing, and failure of GH to suppress to below 1 ng/mL is diagnostic of acromegaly.

14. **a. Stratus spongiosum**

    Ref: Speroff 8th/ed p 129

Line of separations runs from **stratum spongiosum** leaving behind stratum basale from which new endometrial lining is formed.

15. **c. Decreased aromatization**

    Ref: Speroff 8th/ed p 204

There are 4 mechanisms that could result in increased endogenous estrogen levels:
i. Increased precursor androgen
ii. Increased aromatization
iii. Increased direct secretion of estrogen
iv. Decreased SHBG leading to increased levels of free estrogen.

16. **d. Early production of estrogen**

    Ref: Kamini A Rao 2nd/ed p 25; Speroff 8th/ed p 229

Mid cycle LH surge leads to:
- Resumption of meiosis
- Formation of corpus luteum
- Luteinization of theca and granulosa cells
- Expansion of the cumulus
- Synthesis of prostaglandins and other eicosanoids essential for follicle rupture.

17. **a. 1:1**

    Ref: Textbook of Assisted reproductive technique. D Gardner. 5th/ed p 507

One 75 IU ampule of hMG contains an equivalent amount of 75 IU FSH and 75 IU LH in vivo bioactivity.

18. **d. Nongonadotropin protein**

    Ref: Textbook of Assisted reproductive technique. D Gardner. 5th/ed p 507

hMG preparations contain up to five different FSH isohormones and up to nine LH species. These differences may cause discrepancies in patients' responses, which are occasionally observed when using various lots of the same preparation.

FSH, which is the major active agent, accounts for <5% of the local protein content in extracted urinary gonadotropin products. The specific activity of these products does not usually exceed 150 IU/mg protein.

The different proteins found in various hMG preparations include tumor necrosis factor binding protein I, transferrin, urokinase, Tamm–Horsfall glycoprotein, epidermal growth factor, and immunoglobulin-related proteins. Local side effects, such as pain and allergic reactions, have been reported and attributed to immune reactions related to nongonadotropin proteins.

19. **c. Creates low androgen, high estrogen environment**

Ref: Speroff 8th/ed p 1242

Danazol

- First drug ever approved for the treatment of endometriosis in the US.
- It is an orally administered **isoxazol derivative** of 17α-ethinyltestosterone.
- Acts primarily by **inhibiting the midcycle urinary LH surge** and inducing a chronic anovulatory state.
- Inhibits steroidogenic enzymes and increases free testosterone levels.
- The many different effects of danazol combine to yield a **high androgen, low estrogen** environment that inhibits growth of endometriosis.

20. **a. Genetic factors**

Ref: Speroff 8th/ed p 1194

- Genetic factor accounts for the **most common cause** of 1st trimester abortion.

Analyses using newer techniques not dependent on cell culture (fluorescence in situ hybridization, FISH; comparative genomic hybridization, CGH), and more recent careful cytogenetic studies of early missed abortions suggest that the true incidence of chromosomal abnormalities in miscarried early pregnancies is closer to **75%**.

21. **b. Autosomal trisomies**

Ref: Speroff 8th/ed p 1194

- Among women with history of recurrent pregnancy loss, chromosomally normal (euploid) abortuses are more common, particularly in those age 35 and under.

Over 90% of the chromosomal abnormalities observed among abortuses are numerical (aneuploidy, polyploidy); the remainder are split between structural abnormalities (translocations, inversions) and mosaicism.

Overall, **autosomal trisomies** are the most common abnormality (usually involving chromosomes 13-16, 21, or 22), followed by monosomy X (45, X) and polyploidies.

22. **a. <5%**

Ref: Speroff 8th/ed p 1194

- In both normal and infertile asymptomatic young women, the timely appearance of embryonic heart activity decreases the risk of pregnancy loss from the global risk of 12–15% to between 3% and 5%.
- The prognostic value of embryonic heart activity declines with increasing maternal age.
  - 35 years or below: <5%
  - 36–39 years: 10%
  - 40 years or above: 29%

The risk for miscarriage decreases as the duration of pregnancy increases.

The risk of pregnancy loss as per the following milestones are achieved:
- Gestational sac: 12%
- Yolk sac: 8%
- Embryonic crown-rump length
  - >5 mm: 7%
  - 6–10 mm: 3%
  - >10 mm: <1%

23. **d. 15–25%**

Ref: Speroff 8th/ed p 1194

In women with past histories of recurrent pregnancy loss, the miscarriage rate after detection of embryonic heart activity is still three to five times higher: 15–25%.

24. **c. Septate uterus**

Ref: Speroff 8th/ed p 1203

- The septate uterus is by far the most common uterine developmental anomaly, accounting for 80–90% of all major malformations in both women with recurrent pregnancy loss (3.5% prevalence) and in the general population. It is also the malformation most highly associated with poor pregnancy outcomes.
- Data from numerous case series indicate that the miscarriage rate associated with septate uteri is approximately 65%.

A septate uterus results from incomplete resorption of the medial septum separating the two otherwise normally fused hemiuteri.

Septum resorption normally occurs only after urologic development is completed; the prevalence of urinary tract anomalies, therefore, is not increased in women with septate uteri.

25. **a. Fecundability is the probability that cycle will result in live birth**

    Ref: Yen & Jaffe's 8th/ed p 556

- Approximately 85-90% of healthy young couples conceive within 1 year, most within 6 months.
- Infertility therefore affects approximately 10-15% of couples and is an important part of the practice of many clinicians.
- Fecundability is the probability of achieving a pregnancy in one menstrual cycle (approximately 0.25 in healthy couples).
- Fecundity is the ability to achieve a pregnancy that results in a live birth in one menstrual cycle.

26. **b. Very rare phenomenon in normal woman**

    Ref: Speroff 8th/ed 1165

Luteal Phase Defect

- Histologic and sampling dates that agreed, within a 2-day interval are considered normal, whereas a date more than 2 days are considered "out of phase".
- Traditionally, diagnosis of LPD required abnormal results in two (preferably consecutive) cycles, reasoning that reproductive failure could only be attributed to LPD if it was consistent or recurring, and acknowledging that LPD also could occur in normal fertile women, at least occasionally.
- Endometrial dating cannot guide the clinical management of women with reproductive failure and has no place in the diagnostic evaluation of infertility.

27. **a. 25%**

    Ref: Yen & Jaffe's 8th/ed p 556

    Average monthly fecundability in normal couple is 25%

28. **a. Normal postcoital test**

    Ref: Speroff 8th/ed p 1185; Kamini A Rao 2nd/ed p 250

Unexplained Infertility

- It is a diagnosis of exclusion, after systematic evaluation fails to identify a cause.
- The incidence of unexplained infertility ranges from 10% to as high as 30% among infertile populations.
- At a minimum, the diagnosis of unexplained infertility implies evidence of normal semen quality, ovulatory function, a normal uterine cavity, and tubal patency.

- In the past, the diagnosis also required a "positive" postcoital test (excluding cervical factor infertility) and "in phase" endometrial dating (excluding luteal phase deficiency), but no longer, because the tests have proven invalid.
- In the past, the diagnosis also required laparoscopy (excluding pelvic adhesions and endometriosis), but **laparoscopy is no longer performed routinely**, because evidence indicates it has very limited impact on overall outcomes among women with unexplained infertility.
- Instead, transvaginal ultrasonography is performed to detect unsuspected ovarian pathology, such as endometriomas.
- Consequently, much of infertility previously attributed to cervical factors, luteal phase deficiency, and mild endometriosis or adhesions is now "unexplained."

29. **b. Steroidal triphenylethylene derivative that acts as a selective estrogen receptor modulator (SERM)**

    Ref: Textbook of Assisted Reproductive Technique. D Gardner. 5th/ed p 499; Speroff 8th/ed p 1296

Clomiphene

- Non-steroidal triphenylethylene derivative
- Acts as a selective estrogen receptor modulator (SERM), having both estrogen agonist and antagonist properties. However, in almost all circumstances, clomiphene acts purely as an antagonist or antiestrogen; its weak estrogenic actions are clinically apparent only when endogenous estrogen levels are very low.
- Clomiphene is cleared through the **liver** and excreted in the stool; approximately 85% is eliminated within a week, but traces can remain in the circulation for longer.
- Clomiphene is a racemic mixture of two different stereoisomers, enclomiphene (62%; originally known as cis-clomiphene) and zuclomiphene (38%; originally known as trans-clomiphene).
- **Enclomiphene is the more potent** isomer and the one responsible for its ovulation-inducing actions.
- The half-life of enclomiphene is relatively short, so serum concentrations rise and fall quickly during and after treatment.
- Zuclomiphene is cleared much more slowly; serum levels remain detectable for weeks after a single dose and may even accumulate gradually over a series of cycles, but there is no evidence that residual zuclomiphene has any important clinical effects or consequences.

30. d. Clinically useful in patient who is going to have superovulation combined with IUI

Ref: Speroff 8th/ed p 1169

The Postcoital Test

- No longer recommended.
- Abnormalities of cervical mucus production or sperm/mucus interaction are rarely, if ever, the sole or principal cause of infertility.
- Chronic cervicitis or cervical stenosis resulting from conization or other treatment for cervical disease that might impair sperm-mucus interaction can be identified by speculum examination, and in the absence of such findings, the likelihood that cervical mucus represents an important obstacle is remote.
- Semen analysis identifies couples with significant male factor infertility.
- The only randomized trial comparing outcomes in women with normal and abnormal post-coital tests found the test invalid because neither test results nor treatment for abnormal tests affected outcome.

31. a. Menstrual period for 10 years before menopause show progressive prolong follicular phase followed by short follicular phase

Ref: Speroff 8th/ed p 1185

Perimenopausal Transition

- Menstrual period for 10–15 years before menopause show progressive shorter follicular phase due to rising levels of FSH and early recruitment of follicles. This is followed by progressive lengthening of follicular phase.
- When women are in their 40s, anovulation becomes more prevalent, and prior to anovulation, menstrual cycle length increases, beginning 2 to 8 years before menopause.
- Cycles greater than 40 days in length are prevalent in the year before menopause.
- In an Australian longitudinal study, when cycle length exceeded 42 days, menopause predictably followed within 1 or 2 years.
- The duration of the follicular phase is the major determinant of cycle length.
- This menstrual cycle change prior to menopause is marked by elevated FSH levels and decreased levels of inhibin, but normal levels of LH and slightly elevated levels of estradiol.

Progesterone levels generally remain **below 1 ng/mL** during the follicular phase, rise slightly on the day of the LH surge (1–2 ng/mL) and steadily thereafter, peak 7–8 days after ovulation, and decline again over the days preceding menses.

A progesterone concentration less than 3 ng/mL implies anovulation, except:
- When drawn immediately after ovulation
- Just before the onset of menses, when lower levels naturally might be expected.

In cycles monitored with BBT, the interval of highest fertility spans the 7-day interval immediately before the midcycle rise in BBT.

32. d. Antiphosphatidyl serine antibody

Ref: Recurrent pregnancy loss. Howard J. A. Carp. 2nd/ed p 168

International consensus definition for the diagnosis of antiphospholipid syndrome

Diagnosis requires one of the clinical criteria and one of the laboratory findings

Clinical criteria:
- Vascular thrombosis
- Pregnancy morbidity
  A. One or more losses after the 10th week of a morphologically normal fetus.
  B. One or more premature births of a normal neonate before the 34th week because of preeclampsia or eclampsia or placental insufficiency.
  C. Three or more unexplained consecutive early miscarriages.

Laboratory tests:
1. Lupus anticoagulant present on two or more occasions at least 12 weeks apart.
2. Anticardiolipin antibody of IgG or IgM isotype in medium to high titer on two or more occasions at least 12 weeks apart.
3. Anti-β2-glycoprotein 1 antibody of IgG or IgM isotype in 99th percentile titer on two or more occasions at least 12 weeks apart.

33. a. Prevalence of antiphospholipid syndrome among women with recurrent pregnancy loss is very high (>15%)

Ref: Speroff 8th/ed 1206

Although the prevalence of antiphospholipid syndrome among all women with recurrent pregnancy loss is quite low **(3–5%)**, the disorder is nonetheless a potentially treatable cause of recurrent pregnancy loss.

Tests for the detection of a lupus anticoagulant and antiphospholipid antibodies are minimally invasive, relatively inexpensive, and, therefore, justified in the evaluation of most if not all women with recurrent pregnancy loss.

34. c. Have strong association for first trimester pregnancy loss

Ref: Recurrent pregnancy loss. Howard J. a. Carp. 2nd/ed p 188

The association between thrombophilias and pregnancy loss varies with the type of pregnancy loss (early, late) and the thrombophilia.

A meta-analysis including data from 31 studies found that although thrombophilias are associated with both early and late pregnancy loss, the association is stronger for **second trimester and later losses** than for early miscarriage.

The observation is not surprising when one considers that **maternal intervillous blood flow does not develop to any appreciable degree** before approximately 8 weeks' gestation (at the earliest); thrombosis related to a thrombophilia, therefore, is less likely to explain earlier pregnancy losses.

35. a. 5 days, 24 hours

Ref: Speroff 8th/ed p 1156

Normal sperm can survive in the female reproductive tract and retain the ability to fertilize an egg for at least 3 and up to 5 days, but an oocyte can be fertilized successfully for only approximately 12-24 hours after ovulation.

Consequently, virtually all pregnancies result from intercourse occurring sometime within the 6-day interval ending on the day of ovulation.

36. b. Age related decline in fecundity is primarily due to uterine factor

Ref: The Boston IVF Handbook of infertility. 3rd/ed p 11

Age related decline in fecundity is primarily due to aging oocytes. A pregnancy rate in older women of approximately 30% can be achieved in a donor oocyte program.

37. a. Taking gonadotropin for ovulation induction

Ref: Kamini A Rao 2nd/ed p 165

Diagnosis of luteal phase defect should be considered in:
- Women with normal cycles and unexplained infertility
- Short luteal phase demonstrated by basal body temperature chart
- Recurrent pregnancy loss
- Clomiphene citrate for ovulation induction

38. a. Prostaglandin E2 is primary mediator of dysmenorrhea

Ref: Speroff 8th/ed p 580

- The secretory endometrium contains substantial stores of arachidonic acid, which is converted to prostaglandin F_{2a} (PGF_{2a}), prostaglandin E_2 (PGE_2), and leukotrienes during menses.
- PGF_{2a} always stimulates uterine contractions and is the **primary mediator** of dysmenorrhea.
- Endometrial concentrations of PGF_{2a} and PGE_2 correlate with the severity of dysmenorrhea.
- Treatment with cyclooxygenase (COX) inhibitors decreases prostaglandin levels in menstrual fluid and uterine contractile activity; response curves correlate closely with serum drug levels.

39. c. 80 mL, 5 mL

Ref: Speroff 8th/ed p 592

Menorrhagia is abnormally long or heavy menses, lasting > 7 days or involving blood loss > 80 mL.

Hypomenorrhea is blood loss less than 5 mL.

40. d. Following estrogen progestin cyclic hormone therapy

Ref: Speroff 8th/ed p 598

Estrogen Withdrawal Bleeding

- Following bilateral oophorectomy during the follicular phase of the cycle.
- Cyclic estrogen-only hormone therapy in castrate or postmenopausal women.
- Midcycle bleeding that can accompany the transient but abrupt fall in estrogen levels immediately preceding ovulation.
- In women receiving cyclic hormone therapy with exogenous estrogen and progestin, bleeding follows withdrawal of progestin even if estrogen treatment continues and this is known as progestin withdrawal bleeding.

41. b. Adenomyosis is a disorder characterized by the extension of endometrial glands into the myometrium

Ref: Kamini A Rao 2nd/ed p 386

Adenomyosis

- Disorder characterized by the extension of both **endometrial glands and stroma** into the myometrium
- It is a relatively common finding in hysterectomy specimens from women with menorrhagia unrelated to uterine myomas or endometrial pathology.
- Hypertrophy and hyperplasia in the surrounding myometrium generally results in diffuse uterine enlargement. However, some women develop focal nodular lesions called adenomyomas (exaggerated myometrial proliferation around foci of ectopic endometrium), which resemble leiomyomas clinically.
- **Myometrial cysts** on transvaginal ultrasound is the most specific diagnostic criterion
- MRI is a more sensitive diagnostic technique, particularly in the presence of uterine myomas; thickening of the junctional zone on T2 weighted imaging is characteristic.

42. **a. Not useful if ovulatory woman presents with menorrhagia**

Ref: Speroff 8th/ed p 614

LNG-IUS

- Consist of **52 mg** levonorgestrel mixed with poly-dimethylsiloxane, which controls the rate of hormone release.
- Levonorgesterel released at the rate of **20 mcg/day**.
- For contraceptive purposes, the device is approved for **5 years**, but lasts for 7 years, and perhaps up to 10 years.
- Menstrual blood loss in women with heavy menstrual bleeding can be reduced by 75-95%, due to progestin-induced decidualization of the endometrium.
- The LNG-IUS is an attractive option for ovulatory women with heavy menstrual bleeding and for women with intractable bleeding associated with chronic illnesses (renal failure).

43. **d. All are true**

Ref: Speroff 8th/ed p 628

Amniotic fluid prolactin plays a role in:
- Modulating **electrolyte economy**, protecting the human fetus from dehydration by control of salt and water transport across the amnion.
- Modulate **prostaglandin synthesis** within the chorion and amnion to allow labor to proceed in a timely manner.
- Amniotic fluid PRL may pass into the fetal tracheobronchial system to promote **surfactant production**.

44. **a. Human placental lactogen has very strong lactogenic effect**

Ref: Yen & Jaffe's 8th/ed p 262

Human Placental Lactogen

- The increase in prolactin parallels the increase in estrogen beginning at **7-8 weeks** gestation, and the mechanism for increasing prolactin secretion is believed to be estrogen suppression of the hypothalamic prolactin-inhibiting factor, dopamine.
- Human placental lactogen is a **single-chain polypeptide** of 191 amino acids with two disulphide bridges having 96% homology with growth hormone.
- Made by the placenta and actively secreted into the maternal circulation from the sixth week of pregnancy, human placental lactogen (hPL) rises progressively, reaching a level of approximately 6,000 ng/mL during third trimester. hPL, though displaying less activity than prolactin, is produced in such large amounts that it may exert a lactogenic effect. But, although HPL is produced in very large quantities, it appears to be a **redundant hormone**.

- It is detectable in serum and urine in both normal and molar pregnancies, and it disappears rapidly from serum and urine after delivery of placenta-it cannot be detected after first postpartum day.

45. **c. Low dose estrogen progesterone oral contraceptive pills**

Ref: Speroff 8th/ed p 634

- Excessive estrogen can lead to milk secretion via hypothalamic suppression, causing reduction of dopamine and release of pituitary prolactin, and direct stimulation of the pituitary lactotrophs.
- Galactorrhea developing during oral contraceptive administration may be most noticeable in the traditional dosing regimen during the 7 days free of medication (when the steroids are cleared from the body and the prolactin interfering action of the estrogen and progestin on the breast wanes).
- Galactorrhea caused by excessive estrogen disappears within 3-6 months after discontinuing medication. This is now a rare occurrence with the lower-dose pills.

46. **a. Participant in feedback relationship between ovary and pituitary gonadotropins**

Ref: Yen & Jaffe's 8th/ed p 853; Speroff 8th/ed p 684

Unlike inhibin B, AMH is not a participant in the feedback relationship between the ovary and the pituitary gonadotropins, rather AMH, a product of granulosa cells, reflects the number of follicles present in the ovaries awaiting FSH stimulation.

47. **b. Frequent consumption of alcohol**

Ref: Speroff 8th/ed p 686

Diet and Menopause

- Undernourished women and vegetarians experience an earlier menopause.
- Because of the contribution of body fat to estrogen production, thinner women experience a slightly earlier menopause.
- Frequent consumption of alcohol is associated with a later menopause. This is consistent with the reports that women who consume alcohol have higher blood and urinary levels of estrogen, and greater bone density.

48. **c. Hot flushes coincides with surge of FSH**

Ref: Speroff 8th/ed p 696

Hot Flush

- It is the most common problem of the postmenopause.
- It presents no inherent health hazard.
- It coincides with a surge of LH (not FSH).

- It is preceded by a subjective prodromal awareness.
- This aura is followed by measurable increased heat over the entire body surface.
- A flush is triggered by a small elevation in core body temperature.

Unlike the decline in age of menarche that occurred with an improvement in health and living conditions, most historical investigation indicates that the age of menopause has changed little since early Greek times.

49. a. Both FSH and LH rises to 10 fold postmenopause
Ref: Speroff 8th/ed p 689

Endocrinology of Menopause

- FSH increases by 10-20 fold
- LH increases by 3 fold
- Gonadotropins reach maximal level 1-3 years after menopause, after which there is a gradual, but slight, decline in both gonadotropins.
- **FSH levels are higher than LH** because
  - LH is cleared from the blood faster (half-live 20 min for LH and 3-4 h for FSH)
  - There is no specific negative feedback peptide for LH like inhibin for FSH.
- The age-related decline in gonadotropin levels in the later years of postmenopausal life is believed to reflect aging of the pituitary gonadotropin-secreting cells, specifically a decrease in the ability to respond to GnRH.
- The circulating estradiol level after menopause is approximately 10-20 pg/mL, most of which is derived from peripheral conversion of estrone, which in turn is mainly derived from the peripheral conversion of androstenedione.

50. d. Teriparatide
Ref: Speroff 8th/ed p 742; Yen & Jaffe's 8th/ed p 323

- Teriparatide (Forteo) is the recombinant human 1-34 amino acid fragment of parathyroid hormone. This is the only treatment, besides fluoride, that directly stimulates osteoblasts to form new bone.

Being expensive, its use is reserved for women who are difficult to treat and have a history of fractures.

Bone losing medications:
- Thyroxine
- Glucocorticoids
- SSRIs
- Proton pump inhibitors
- Aromatase inhibitors
- Heparin
- Anticonvulsants
- GnRH agonists

51. a. Testosterone
Ref: Infertility in the male. Cambridge. 4th/ed p 19

FSH increases spermatogonial number and maturation of spermatocytes but it is unable to complete spermatogenesis.

LH participates in regulating spermatogenesis by stimulating synthesis of testosterone, which plays an essential role in spermatid maturation.

It is the intratesticular testosterone which is most important for spermatogenesis.

52. b. 47, XXY
Ref: Infertility in the male. Cambridge. 4th/ed p 251

Most common cause in non-obstructive azoospermia patients is 47, XXY Klinefelter syndrome, which occurs in 1/500 to 1/1000 live births.

It is underlying genetic anomaly in 10% of NOA men.

53. d. Small testes
Ref: Infertility in the male. Cambridge. 4th/ed p 252

Small testes are common to all 47, XXY men, no matter where on the clinical spectrum they may fall. They typically measure about 8–10 cm^3 in volume.

Gynecomastia and eunuchoid body habitus is seen only at the severe end of phenotypic spectrum.

54. a. INSL-3
Ref: Infertility in the male. Cambridge. 4th/ed p 262

The insulin-like 3 hormone (INSL-3), also known as Ley I-L (Leydig insulin-like) and Rlf (relaxin-like factor), is the main testicular hormone that induces gubernacular development.

Animal studies showed that deficiency of INSL-3 resulted in the testis and genital tract being freely mobile within the abdomen because there were no cranial or caudal attachments of the testis to the inguinal region.

The protein is similar to relaxin, a hormone produced by the ovaries and prostate.

55. b. Leydig cells
Ref: Infertility in the male. Cambridge. 4th/ed p 252

Leydig cells are involved in testosterone production.

EU GSPR Authorised Reprsentative
Logos Europe, 9 rue Nicolas Poussin
1700, La Rochelle, France
Phone: +33 (0) 6 67 93 73 78
E-mail: contact@logoseurope.eu

www.ingramcontent.com/pod-product-compliance
Ingram Content Group UK Ltd.
Pitfield, Milton Keynes, MK11 3LW, UK
UKHW050431150426
5217IPUK00019B/1333